A cognitive theory of consciousness

A cognitive theory of consciousness

BERNARD J. BAARS

The Wright Institute
Berkeley, California

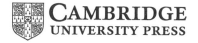

CAMBRIDGE
UNIVERSITY PRESS

Published by the Press Syndicate of the University of Cambridge
The Pitt Building, Trumpington Street, Cambridge CB2 1RP
40 West 20th Street, New York, NY 10011-4211, USA
10 Stamford Road, Oakleigh, Melbourne 3166, Australia

First published 1988
Reprinted 1990
First paperback edition 1993
Reprinted 1995

Printed in the United States of America

Library of Congress Cataloging-in-Publication Data is available
A catalogue record for this book is available from the British Library

ISBN 0-521-30133-5 hardback
ISBN 0-521-42743-6 paperback

This book is gratefully
dedicated to the pioneers in cognitive science
who made it possible

We shall not cease from exploration
and the end of all our exploring
will be to come back
to the place from which we came
and know it for the first time.

T. S. Eliot

Contents

Figures and tables

Figures

xi

Tables

Preface

Conscious experience is notoriously the great, confusing, and contentious nub of psychological science. We are all conscious beings, but consciousness is not something we can observe directly other than in ourselves, and then only in retrospect. Yet as scientists we aim to gather objective knowledge even about subjectivity itself. Can that be done? This book will sketch one approach, and no doubt the reader will come to his or her own judgment about its inadequacies. Of one thing, however, we can be very sure – that we cannot pursue scientific psychology and hope to avoid the problem for very long.

Indeed, historically, psychologists have neither addressed nor evaded consciousness successfully, and two major psychological metatheories, introspectionism and behaviorism, have come to grief on the horns of this dilemma. Having perhaps gained some wisdom from these failures, most scientific psychologists now subscribe to a third metatheory for psychology, the cognitive approach (Baars, 1986a). Whether cognitive psychology will succeed where others have not depends in part on its success in understanding conscious experience – not just because "it is there," but because consciousness, if it is of any scientific interest at all, must play a major *functional* role in the human nervous system.

The first obstacle in dealing with consciousness as a serious scientific issue comes in trying to make sense of the tangled thicket of conflicting ideas, opinions, facts, prejudices, insights, misunderstandings, fundamental truths, and fundamental falsehoods that surrounds the topic. Natsoulas (1978a) counts at least seven major definitions of the word "consciousness" in English. One topic alone, the mind–body issue, has a relevant literature extending from the Upanishads to the latest philosophical journals – perhaps three thousand years of serious thought. We can only nod respectfully to the vast philosophical literature and go our own way; in doing so we do not discount the importance of philosophical questions. But one time-honored strategy in science is to side-step philosophical issues for a time by focusing on empirically decidable ones in the hope that, eventually, new scientific insights may cast some light on the perennial philosophical concerns.

How are we to discover empirical evidence about consciousness? What is a theory of consciousness a theory of? Nineteenth-century psychologists like Wilhelm Wundt and William James believed that consciousness was the fundamental constitutive problem for psychology, but they had remarkably little to say about it *as such*. Freud and the psychodynamic tradition have much to say about *un*conscious motivation, but take conscious experience largely for granted. Behaviorists tended to discourage any serious consideration of consciousness in the first half of this century; and even cognitive psychologists have studiously avoided it until the last few years.

In truth, the facts of consciousness are all around us, ready to be studied. Practically all psychological findings involve conscious experience. Modern psychologists find themselves in much the position of Molière's Bourgeois Gentleman, who hires a scholar to make him as sophisticated as he is wealthy. Among other absurdities, the scholar tries to teach the bourgeois the difference between *prose* and *poetry*, pointing out that the gentleman has been speaking *prose* all his life. This unsuspected talent fills the bourgeois gentleman with astonished pride – speaking *prose*, and without even knowing it! In just this way, some psychologists will be surprised to realize that they have been studying consciousness all of their professional lives. The physicalistic philosophy of most psychologists has tended to disguise this fundamental fact, and our usual emphasis on sober empirical detail makes us feel more secure with less glamorous questions. But a psychologist can no more evade consciousness than a physicist can side-step gravity.

Even if the reader is willing to grant this much, it may still be unclear how to approach and define the issue empirically. Here, as elsewhere, we borrow a leaf from one of William James's books. In *The Principles of Psychology* (1890/1983), James suggests a way of focusing on the issue of consciousness by *contrasting* comparable conscious and unconscious events. James himself was hindered in carrying out this program because he believed that psychology should not deal with *un*conscious processes; unconscious events, he thought, were physiological. In contrast, our current cognitive metatheory suggests that we can indeed talk psychologically about both conscious *and* unconscious processes *if* we can infer the properties of both on the basis of public evidence. In cognitive psychology, conscious and unconscious events have the same status as any other scientific constructs. A wealth of information has now accumulated based on this reasoning.

Now, we can compare a reliably reported conscious image of this morning's breakfast to the memory of breakfast *before* it became conscious; a conscious stream of speech may be compared to the same stream when it is not attended (there is considerable evidence that unattended speech is nevertheless processed up to a point); we can also compare a conscious interpretation of an ambiguous word to the same word when the interpretation is not conscious, because the alternative meaning is being accessed (again there is evidence that unconscious word meanings are still briefly processed); or a barely subliminal stimulus may be compared to one presented above threshold; or a habitual unconscious action may be compared to the same act before it fades from consciousness. The "Contrastive Analysis" tables throughout this book list many such pairs of conscious and unconscious phenomena, which are widely accepted in the experimental literature. In all these examples we know that *both* the conscious *and* the unconscious cases involve a mental representation of a very similar stimulus that is apparently processed in a comparable way. Thus, each pair of cases creates a controlled experiment with consciousness as the dependent variable. Now we can ask, given that these paired events are so similar, why is *one* member of each pair conscious but *not* the other? This question requires a theoretical answer. Indeed, the set of such contrastive pairs imposes empirical constraints on any theory of conscious experience; and a complete theory must explain all the contrastive pairs, in the simplest and most plausible way (Baars, 1986b).

Contrastive analysis makes it possible, for example, to take Pavlov's findings about the Orienting Response (OR), the massive wave of activity that affects all parts of the nervous system when we encounter a novel situation. We can contrast our conscious experience of a stimulus that elicits an OR to our unconscious representation of the same stimulus after the OR has become habituated due to repetition of the stimulus (Sokolov, 1963; see Chapters 1 and 5, this volume). Now we can ask: What *is* the difference between the conscious and the unconscious representation of this stimulus? After all, the physical stimulus is the same, the inferred stimulus representation is the same, and the organism itself is still much the same; but in the first case the stimulus is conscious, in the second it is not. In this way, we focus on the *differential implications* of conscious experience in otherwise very similar circumstances. It makes not a bit of difference that Pavlov was a devout physicalist who felt that a scientific treatment of conscious experience was impossible. In time-honored scientific fashion, good data outlast the orientation of the investigators who collected them.

Although a number of investigators have discussed contrasts like this, there has been a very unfortunate tendency to focus on the most difficult and problematic cases, rather than on the simplest and most revealing ones. For instance, there has been extensive debate about subliminal perception and "blind sight" – the kind of brain damage in which people can identify visual stimuli without a sense of being conscious of them. These are important phenomena, but they are methodologically and conceptually very difficult and controversial. They are very poor sources of evidence at this stage in our understanding. Trying to tackle the most difficult phenomena first is simply destructive of the normal process of science. It leads to confusion and controversy, rather than clarity. When Newton began the modern study of light, he did not begin with the complicated question of wave–particle duality, but with a simple prism and a ray of sunlight. Only by studying simple, clear cases first can we begin to build the solid framework within which more complex and debatable questions can be understood. We will adopt this standard scientific strategy here. First, we consider the clear contrasts between comparable conscious and unconscious events. Only then will we use the resulting framework to generate ideas about the very difficult boundary questions.

One could easily generate dozens of tables of contrasts, listing hundreds of facts about comparable conscious and unconscious phenomena (Baars, 1986b). In Chapter 1, some of the contrastive pairs of facts that invite such an analysis are surveyed. However, in the theoretical development, starting in Chapter 2, we prefer to present only a few simplified tables, summarizing many observations in a few statements. Others might like to arrange the data differently, to suggest different theoretical consequences. The reader may find it interesting to build a model as we go along, based on the contrastive facts laid out throughout the book.

The use of cumulative empirical constraints

Although a great deal of research must still be done to resolve numerous specific issues, many useful things can already be said about the picture as a whole. Integrative theory can be based on "cumulative constraints." This is rather different from the usual method of inquiry in psychology, which involves a careful investigation of precise *local* evidence. Let me illustrate the difference.

Suppose we are given four hints about an unknown word:

    1 It is something to eat,
    2 one a day keeps the doctor away,
    3 it is as American as Mom's unspecified pie, and
    4 it grows in an orchard.

One way to proceed is to take each hint in isolation, and investigate it carefully. For "growing in an orchard," we may survey orchards to define the probability of peaches, pears, plums, cherries, and apples. That is a *local, increasingly precise* approach. Another approach is to accept that by itself each hint may only partly constrain the answer, and to use the set of hints as a whole to support the best guess. After all, there are many things to eat. The doctor could be kept away by a daily aspirin, or by bubonic plague, or by regular exercise. Mom *could* bake blueberry pie. And many fruits grow in an orchard. But "growing in an orchard" *plus* "one a day keeps the doctor a way" eliminates bubonic plague and regular exercise. Each hint is locally incomplete. But, taken together, the combination of locally incomplete facts help to support a single, highly probable answer for the whole puzzle.

Scientific psychologists are trained to perform local, increasingly precise investigations. This has the advantage of producing more and more accurate information, though sometimes about smaller and smaller pieces of the puzzle. Alternatively, we could use all the local sources of evidence *together* to constrain global hypotheses. Of course, global models should make novel local predictions. But sometimes we can develop a compelling global picture, even if some of the local evidence is still missing.

The two methods are complementary. In this book we will largely pursue the second, global method.

A suggestion to the reader

This book is in the nature of a scouting expedition, exploring a territory that is not exactly unknown, but at least uncharted by modern psychologists. After a self-imposed absence of many decades, the psychological community seems poised to explore this territory once again. In that process it will no doubt probe both the evidence and the theoretical issues in great detail. This work aims to produce a preliminary map to the territory. We try here to cover as much ground as possible, in reasonable detail, to make explicit our current knowledge, and to define gaps therein.

There are two ways to read this book. First, it can be taken at face value, as a theory of conscious experience. This entails some work. Though I have tried very hard to make the theory as clear and understandable as possible, the job of understanding each hypothesis, the evidence *pro* and *con*, and its relation to the rest of the theory will take some effort. An easier way is to take the theory as one way of organizing what we know today about conscious experience – a vast amount of evidence. I believe this book considers nearly all the major cognitive and neuroscientific findings about conscious and unconscious processes. Rather than testing each hypothesis, the theory can be taken as a convenient "as if" framework for understanding this great literature.

The second approach is easier than the first, and may be better for students and the general reader. Graduate students, professional psychologists, and others with a deeper commitment to the issues will no doubt wish to scrutinize the theory with greater care. The Glossary and guide to theoretical claims at the end of the book defines each major concept formally and relates it to the theory as a whole; this may be helpful to those wishing to examine the theory in more detail.

A brief guide to the book

This book sketches the outlines of a theory of conscious experience. Although it may seem complicated in detail, the basic ideas are very simple and can be stated in a paragraph or two. In essence, we develop only a single theoretical metaphor: a *publicity metaphor* of consciousness, suggesting that there is a "global workspace" system underlying conscious experience. The global workspace is the publicity organ of the nervous system; its contents, which correspond roughly to conscious experience, are distributed widely throughout the system. This makes sense if we think of the brain as a vast collection of specialized automatic processors, some nested and organized within other processors. Processors can compete or cooperate to gain access to the global workspace underlying consciousness, enabling them to send global messages to any other interested systems. Any conscious experience emerges from cooperation and competition between many different input processors. One consequence of this is that a global message must be *internally consistent*, or else it would degrade very rapidly due to internal competition between its components (see Chapter 2). Further, conscious experience requires that the *receiving systems* be adapting to, matching, or acting to achieve whatever is conveyed in the conscious global message (see Chapter 5). Another way of stating this is to say that any conscious message must be globally *informative*. But any adaptation to an informative message takes place within a stable but unconscious *context*.

Contexts are relatively enduring structures that are unconscious, but that can evoke and be evoked by conscious events (Chapter 4). Conscious contents and unconscious contexts interweave to create a "stream of consciousness" (Chapter 6). The interplay between them is useful in solving a great variety of problems, in which the conscious component is used to access novel sources of information while unconscious contexts and processors deal with routine details. Voluntary control of action can be treated as a special kind of problem solving, with both conscious and unconscious components (Chapter 7). And if we take one plausible meaning of "self" as the dominant, enduring context of many conscious experiences, we may also say that conscious experience provides information to the self-as-context (Chapter 9). This framework seems to unify the great bulk of empirical evidence in a reasonable way.

There are other ways to think about conscious experience, but these can be seen to follow from the extended publicity metaphor. Properties like selectivity, limited capacity, self-consciousness, the ability to report conscious contents, knowledge of the world, reflective consciousness; consciousness as the domain of rationality; consciousness as the "glue" for combining different perceptual features, as the domain of error-correction and trouble-shooting, as a tool for learning; the relationship between consciousness and novelty, voluntary control, and self – all these points are consistent with and appear to follow from the present framework.

The theory is developed as a cumulative set of models, from Model 1 – which is a bare-bones first approximation – to Model 7, which aims to place the entire system in a single coherent framework. Each model is captured graphically in a global workspace diagram, and all the diagrams are cumulative; each is intended to include all the previous diagrams. Thus, we present a graphic notation as an explicit formalism, which may be translated into other theoretical languages at will. For a quick preview of the entire theory, the reader may wish to peruse all the theoretical figures and captions (see the list of figures and tables).

The global workspace metaphor results in a remarkable simplification of the evidence presented in the conscious–unconscious contrasts. This great simplification provides one cause for confidence in the theory. Further, a number of specific, testable predictions are generated throughout the book. The ultimate fate of the theory depends of course on the success or failure of those predictions.

Where we cannot suggest plausible answers, we will try at least to ask the right questions. This is done throughout by marking *theoretical choice-points* whenever we are forced to choose between equally plausible hypotheses. At these points reasonable people may well disagree. In each case we state arguments for and against the course ultimately taken, with some ideas for testing the alternatives. For example, in Chapter 2 we suggest that perception and imagery – so-called qualitative conscious contents – play a special role as global input that is broadcast very widely. Although there is evidence consistent with this proposal, it is not conclusive; therefore, it is marked as a "theoretical choice-point" to indicate a special need for further evidence. It is still useful to explore the implications of this idea with the proviso that further facts may force a retreat to a previous decision-point.

No theory at this stage can expect to be definitive. But we do not treat theory here as a once-and-for-all description of reality. Theories are tools for thinking and, like other tools, they tend sooner or later to be surpassed.

The need to understand conscious experience

Imagine the enterprise of scientific psychology as a great effort to solve a jig-saw puzzle as big as a football field. Several communities of research-ers have been working for decades on the job of finding the missing pieces in the puzzle, and in recent years many gaps have been filled. However, one central missing piece – the issue of conscious experience – has been thought to be so difficult that many researchers have sensibly avoided that part of the puzzle. Yet the gap left by this great central piece has not gone away, and surrounding it are numerous issues that cannot be solved until it is addressed. If that is a reasonable analogy, it follows that the more pieces of the jig-saw puzzle we discover, the more the remaining uncertainties will tend to cluster about the great central gap where the missing piece must fit. The more we learn while continuing to circumvent conscious experience, the more it will be true that the remaining unanswered questions require an understanding of consciousness for their solution.

Certainly not everyone will agree with our method, conclusions, theoretical metaphor, or ways of stating the evidence. Good theory thrives on reasoned dissent, and the ideas developed in this book will no doubt change in the face of new evidence and further thought. We can hope to focus and define the issues in a way that is empirically responsi-ble, and to help scotch the notion that conscious experience is something psychology can safely avoid or disregard. No scientific effort comes with a guarantee of success. But if, as the history suggests, we must choose in psychology between trying to understand conscious experience and trying to avoid it, we can in our view but try to understand.

Acknowledgments

Explicit development of this theory began in 1978. Since then, a number of psychologists and neuroscientists have provided valuable input, both encouraging and critical. Among these are Donald A. Norman, David Galin, George Mandler, Lester Luborsky, Michael Wapner, Benjamin Libet, Anthony Marcel, James Reason, Donald G. MacKay, Michael J. Apter, Donald E. Broadbent, Paul Rozin, Richard Davidson, Ray Jacken-doff, Wallace Chafe, Thomas Natsoulas, Peter S. White, Matthew

Erdelyi, Arthur Reber, Jerome L. Singer, Theodore Melnechuk, Stephen Grossberg, Mardi J. Horowitz, David Spiegel, James Greeno, Jonathan Cohen, Albert I. Rabin, James Newman, George Stone, and Diane Kramer. I am especially grateful to Donald Norman, David Galin, and Mardi J. Horowitz for their open-minded and encouraging attitude, which was at times sorely needed.

I am grateful for support received as a Cognitive Science Fellow at the University of California, San Diego, funded by the Alfred P. Sloan Foundation, in 1979–80; and for a Visiting Scientist appointment in 1985–6 at the Program for Conscious and Unconscious Mental Processes, Langley Porter Neuropsychiatric Institute, University of California, San Francisco, supported by the John D. and Catherine T. MacArthur Foundation, and directed by Mardi J. Horowitz. The MacArthur Foundation is to be commended for its thoughtful and historically significant decision to support research on conscious and unconscious functions. Finally, the Wright Institute and its president, Peter Dybwad, were extremely helpful in the final stages of this work.

The editorial board of Cambridge University Press showed rare intellectual courage in accepting this book for its distinguished list at a time when the theory was largely unknown. I think that is admirable, and I trust that the result justifies their confidence.

Bernard J. Baars
Berkeley, California

Part I

Introduction

After a brief historical survey, Chapter 1 suggests a workable (though by no means perfect) operational definition of consciousness, one that is already widely used, and which will apply throughout the book. We can focus on the issue of consciousness *as such* by comparing pairs of events that seem to differ only in that one event is conscious while the other is not. There are many such minimally contrastive pairs of well-established facts. This method of "contrastive analysis" will provide the empirical basis of theoretical development.

Chapter 1 continues with contrastive analyses for perception and imagery. We review current ideas about consciousness, culminating with the introduction of the Global Workspace theory, which combines the most viable hypotheses into a single, simple framework. Finally, we describe some recurrent questions to be addressed in the coming chapters.

1   What is to be explained?
Some preliminaries

> The study . . . of the *distribution* of consciousness shows it to be exactly
> such as we might expect in an organ added for the sake of steering a
> nervous system grown too complex to regulate itself.
>
> *William James*, 1890 (p. 141)

1.0   Introduction

Chances are that not many hours ago, you, the reader, woke up from what
we trust was a good night's sleep. Almost certainly you experienced the
act of waking up as a discrete beginning of something new, something
richly detailed, recallable and reportable, something that was not happening even a few minutes before. In the same way we remember going to
sleep as an *end* to our ability to experience and describe the world. The
world this morning seemed different from last night – the sun was out, the
weather had changed, one's body felt more rested. Hours must have
passed, things must have happened without our knowledge. "We were
not conscious," we say, as if that explains it.

At this moment you can probably bring to mind an image of this
morning's breakfast. It is a conscious image – we can experience again,
though fleetingly: the color of the orange juice, the smell of hot coffee, the
taste and texture of corn flakes. Where were those images just before we
made them conscious? "They were unconscious," we say, or "in
memory," as if that explains it.

At this instant you, the reader, are surely conscious of some aspects of
the act of reading – the color and texture of this page, and perhaps the
inner sound of *these words*. Further, you can become conscious of certain
beliefs – a belief in the existence of mathematics, for example – although
beliefs do not consist of sensory qualities in the same way that orange
juice has taste, or the way a mental image of corn flakes recreates the
experience of a certain crunchy texture. In contrast to your conscious
experiences, you are probably *not* conscious of the feel of your chair at
this instant; nor of a certain background taste in your mouth, of that
monotonous background noise, of the sound of music or talking in the
background, of the complex syntactic processes needed to understand

3

this phrase, of your intentions regarding a friend, of the multiple meanings of ambiguous words, as in *this case*, of your eye movements, of the complex vestibular processes that are keeping you oriented to gravity, of your ability to drive a car. Even though you are not currently conscious of them, there is a great deal of evidence to support the idea that all of these unconscious events are being represented and actively processed in your nervous system.

The fact that we can predict all these things with considerable confidence indicates that conscious experience is something knowable, at least in its boundaries. But what does it mean that at this moment *this* event is likely to be conscious, and *that* one unconscious? What role does the distinction between conscious and unconscious events play in the running of the nervous system? That is the central question explored in this book. Asking the question this way allows us to use the very large empirical literature on these matters, to constrain theory with numerous reliable facts. A small set of ideas can explain many of these facts. These ideas are consistent both with modern cognitive theory and with many traditional notions about consciousness. We will now briefly review some of these traditional ideas.

1.1   Some history and a look ahead

Consciousness seems so obvious in its daily manifestations, yet so puzzling on closer examination. In several millenia of recorded human thought it has been viewed, variously,

> as a fact that poses fundamental questions about the nature of reality;
> as the natural focus for scientific psychology;
> as a topic psychology must *avoid* at any cost;
> as a nonexistent or "epiphenomenal" by-product of brain functioning; and finally
> as an important unsolved problem for psychology and neuroscience.

Consciousness has had its ups and downs with a vengeance, especially in the last hundred years. Even today, more sense and more nonsense is spoken of consciousness, probably, than of any other aspect of human functioning. The great problem we face here is how to tip the balance in favor of sense and against nonsense.

In thinking about conscious experience we are entering a stream of ideas that goes back to the earliest known writings. Any complete account of human thought about human experience must include the great technical literatures of Vedanta Hinduism, Buddhism, and Taoism; but it must also include European philosophy from Plato to Sartre, as well as the various strands of mystical thought in the West. Indeed, the history of ideas in all developed cultures is closely intertwined with ideas about perception, knowledge, memory, imagination, and the like, all involving conscious experience in different ways. We cannot trace this fascinating story here in detail. Our main purpose is not to interpret the great historical literature, but to develop a *theory* that will simplify our understanding of conscious experience, just as any good theory simplifies its subject matter. But we will very briefly set the historical context.

When scientific psychology began in the nineteenth century it was intensely preoccupied with consciousness. By contrast, the twentieth century so far has been remarkable for its rejection of the whole topic as "unscientific." Some psychologists in this century have even argued that conscious experience does not exist, a view that has never been seriously held before. Nevertheless, many of these same radical skeptics have uncovered evidence that is directly relevant to the understanding of conscious experience. Though their findings are often described in ways that avoid the word "consciousness," their evidence stands, no matter what we call it. We shall find this evidence very useful.

Usually when we wish to study something – a rock, a chemical reaction, or the actions of a friend – we begin with simple observation. But conscious experience is difficult to observe in a straightforward way. We cannot observe someone else's experience directly, nor can we study our own experience in the way we might study a rock or a plant. One great problem seems to be this: Conscious experience is hard to study because we cannot easily stand *outside* of it to observe the effects of its presence and absence. But generally in science, we gain knowledge about any event by comparing its presence and absence; that is after all what the experimental method is about. If we try to vary the degree of our own consciousness – between waking, drowsiness, and sleep, for example – we immediately lose our ability to observe. How do you observe the coming and going of your own consciousness? It seems futile, like a dog chasing its own tail. There is a vicious circle in attempting to observe conscious experience, one that hobbles the whole history of scientific attempts to understand consciousness.

The difficulty in studying *unconscious* processes is even more obvious – by definition we cannot directly observe them at all. Unconscious processes can only be inferred, based on our own experience and on observation of others. Throughout recorded history, individual thinkers have held that much more goes on unconsciously than common sense would have us believe, but this realization did not catch on very widely until the middle of the nineteenth century, and then only in the face of much resistance (Ellenberger, 1970; Whyte, 1962). Acknowledging the power of unconscious processes means giving up some of our sense of control over ourselves, a difficult thing to do for many people.

In sum, throughout recorded history it has been remarkably difficult for philosophers and scientists to study and talk sensibly about *either* conscious or unconscious events. Even as scientific psychology was being founded in the nineteenth century, psychologists became caught up in these difficulties. Such early luminaries as Wilhelm Wundt and William James *defined* psychology as the quest for the understanding of conscious experience. William James, the preeminent American psychologist of the nineteenth century, is still an extraordinary source of insight into conscious functioning, and we will quote him throughout this book. But James must be treated with great caution because of his strong philosophical preconceptions. He insisted, for example, that all psychological facts must ultimately be *reduced* to conscious experiences. For James, conscious experience, one of the most puzzling phenomena in psychology, was to be the foundation for a scientific psychology. But building on a foundation that is itself puzzling and badly understood is a recipe for futility – it undermines the scientific enterprise from the start (Baars, 1986a).

James raised a further problem by getting hopelessly entangled in the great foundation problem of psychology, the mind/body problem, which Schopenhauer called "die Weltknoten" – the "world-knot." At various points in his classic *Principles of Psychology* (1890) James tried to reduce all phenomena to conscious experiences (mentalism), whereas at others he tried to relate them to brain processes (physicalism); this dual reduction led him to mind/body dualism, much against his will. Conflicting commitments created endless paradoxes for James. In some of his last writings (1904/1977) he even suggests that "consciousness" should be dispensed with altogether, though momentary conscious *experiences* must be retained. And he insistently denied the psychological reality of *un*conscious processes. These different claims are so incompatible with each other as to rule out a clear and simple foundation for psychological science. Thus many psychologists found James to be a great source of confusion, for all his undoubted greatness, and James himself felt confused. By 1892 he was writing in despair, "The real in psychics seems to 'correspond' to the unreal in physics, and *vice versa*; and we are sorely perplexed" (p. 460).

Toward the end of the nineteenth century other scientific thinkers – notably Pierre Janet and Sigmund Freud – began to infer unconscious processes quite freely, based on observable events such as posthypnotic suggestion, conversion hysteria, multiple personality, slips of the tongue, motivated forgetting, and the like. Freud's insights have achieved extraordinary cultural influence (Ellenberger, 1970; Erdelyi, 1985). Indeed the art, literature, and philosophy of our time are utterly incomprehensi-

ble without his ideas and those of his opponents like Jung and Adler. But
Freud had curiously little impact on scientific psychology, in part because
his demonstrations of unconscious influences could not be brought easily
into the laboratory – his evidence was too complex, too rich, too
idiosyncratic and evanescent for the infant science of psychology to
digest.

1.1.1 The rejection of conscious experience: Behaviorism and the positivist philosophy of science

The controversy and confusion surrounding consciousness helped lead to
the behavioristic revolution, starting about 1913. Behaviorism utterly
denied that conscious experience was a legitimate scientific subject, but it
promised at least a consistent physicalistic basis on which psychology
could build. For some radical behaviorists the existence of consciousness
was a paradox, an epiphenomenon, or even a threat to a scientific
psychology: "Consciousness," wrote John Watson, "is nothing but the
soul of theology" (Watson, 1925; see p. 3; Baars, 1986a). Watson's
behaviorism quickly achieved remarkable popularity. In various forms
this philosophy of science held a dominant position in American universities until very recently.

But physicalistic psychology was not limited to America. Similar
philosophies became dominant in other countries under different labels.
In Russia, Pavlov and Bekhterev espoused a physicalistic psychophysiology, and in England and parts of the European continent, the positivist
philosophy of science had much the same impact. Thus at the beginning
of the twentieth century many psychologists rejected consciousness as a
viable topic for psychology. Naturally they rejected *un*conscious processes as well – if one cannot speak of conscious phenomena, one cannot
recognize unconscious ones either.

The conventional view is that nineteenth-century psychology was
rejected by behaviorists and others because it was unreliable and subjec-
tivist, because it was mired in fruitless controversy, and because it was
unscientific. However, modern historical research has cast doubt on this
view in all respects (Baars, 1986a; Blumenthal, 1979; Danziger, 1979). It
now appears that psychologists like Wilhelm Wundt used objective
measures most of the time, and employed introspection only rarely. Even
a cursory reading of James's great text (1890/1983) indicates how many
"modern" empirical phenomena he knew. Numerous important and
reliable effects were discovered in the nineteenth century, and many of
these have been rediscovered since the passing of behaviorism: basic
phenomena like selective attention, the capacity limits of short-term

memory, mental imagery, context effects in comprehension, and the like. Major controversies occurred, as they do today, but primarily about two topics we must also address in this book: (1) the evidence for imageless thought, indicating that much "intelligent" processing goes on unconsciously (e.g., Woodworth, 1915), and (2) the question whether there is such a thing as a conscious command in the control of action (Baars, 1986b, esp. Ch. 7; James, 1890/1983). But these were important, substantive controversies, not mere metaphysical argumentation. They were perhaps unsolvable at the time because of conceptual difficulties faced in the late nineteenth century, some of which have been resolved today. These include the difficulties encountered by William James with unconscious processes and mentalistic reductionism.

As for introspection itself – reports of conscious experience, sometimes by trained observers – it is used almost universally in contemporary psychology, in studies of perception, imagery, attention, memory, explicit problem solving, and the like (e.g., Ericsson & Simon, 1984; Kosslyn, 1980; Stevens, 1966). No doubt methodological improvements have been made, but the basic technique of asking subjects, "What did you just perceive, think, or remember?" is extremely widespread. We do not call it "introspection," and we often avoid thinking that subjects in experiments answer our questions by consulting their own experience. But surely our subjects themselves think of their task in that way, as we can learn simply by asking them. They may be closer to the truth in that respect than many experimenters who are asking the questions.

In rejecting consciousness as well as the whole psychology of common sense, behaviorists were supported by many philosophers of science. Indeed, philosophers often tried to dictate what was to be genuine psychology and what was not. Ludwig Wittgenstein, in his various phases of development, inveighed against "mentalistic language" – the language of psychological common sense – as "a general disease of thinking" (Malcolm, 1967). In his later work he argued against the possibility of a "private language" – that is, that people can really know themselves in any way. His fellow philosopher Gilbert Ryle presented very influential arguments against inferred mental entities, which he ridiculed as "ghosts in the machine" and "homunculi." Ryle believed that all mentalistic inferences involved a mixing of incompatible categories, and that their use led to an infinite regress (1949).

From a modern psychological point of view, the problem is that these philosophers made strong empirical claims that are more properly left to science. Whether people can reliably report their own mental processes is an empirical question. Whether inferred mental entities like "consciousness," "thinking," and "feeling" are scientifically useful is a decision that should be left to psychological theory. In fact, there is now extensive evidence that mental images can be reported in very reliable and revealing ways (Cooper & Shepard, 1973; Kosslyn, 1980). Other mental events, like intentions, may be more difficult to report, as we shall see (Chapters 6, 7, and 8). Similarly, a vast amount of research and theory over the past twenty years indicates that inferred mental entities can be scientifically very useful, as long as they are anchored in specific operational definitions and expressed in explicit theory (e.g., Anderson, 1983; Miller & Johnson-Laird, 1976; Neisser, 1967). Sometimes mentalistic inferences are indeed flawed and circular, as Ryle argued so strongly, but not always. The job is to make scientific inferences properly. If we were to avoid all inference we would lose the power of theory, an indispensable tool in the development of science.

In one way, however, philosophies of science like behaviorism may have advanced the issue – namely by insisting that all psychological entities could be viewed "from the outside," as objects in a single physical universe of discourse. For some psychologists consciousness could now be treated as a natural phenomenon (to be sure, with a subjective aspect), basically like any other event in the world. In this light the most significant observations about consciousness may be found in remarks by two well-known psychologists of the time: Clark Hull, a neobehaviorist, and Edwin G. Boring, an operationist and the preeminent historian of the period. In 1937 Hull wrote that

to recognize the existence of a phenomenon [i.e., consciousness] is not the same as insisting upon its basic, i.e., logical, priority. Instead of furnishing a means for the solution of problems, consciousness appears to be itself a problem needing solution. (p. 855)

And Boring some years later (1953) summarized his own thinking about introspection by saying that

operational logic, in my opinion . . . shows that human consciousness is an inferred construct, a capacity as inferential as any of the other psychological realities, and that literally immediate observation, the introspection that cannot lie, does not exist. All observation is a process that takes time and is subject to error in the course of its occurrence.

This is how we view conscious experience in this book: as a theoretical construct that can often be inferred from reliable evidence; and as a basic problem needing solution. Within the behavioristic framework it was difficult to build theory, because of resistance to inferred, unobservable constructs. Today, the new cognitive metatheory has overcome this reluctance. The cognitive metatheory encourages psychologists to go beyond raw observations, to infer explanatory entities if the evidence for them is compelling (Baars, 1986a). This is not such a mysterious process – it is what human beings are always doing in trying to understand their world. No one has ever publicly observed a wish, a feeling of love or hate, or even a pain in the belly. These are all inferred constructs, which we find useful to understand other people's actions, and sometimes even our own.

It cannot be overemphasized that such inferences are not unique to psychology. All sciences make inferences that go beyond the observables. The atom was a highly inferential entity in the first century of its existence; so was the gene; so was the vastness of geological time, a necessary assumption for Darwinian theory; and other scientific constructs too numerous to list here. Cognitive psychology applies this commonsensical epistemology in a way that is more explicit and testable than it is in everyday life. In this way, scientific psychologists have once again begun to speak of meaning, thought, imagery, attention, memory, and, recently, conscious and unconscious processes – all inferred concepts that have been tested in careful experiments and stated in increasingly adequate theories. Our view here is that *both* conscious and unconscious processes involve inferences from publicly observable data. Thus conscious and unconscious events reside in the same domain of discourse: the domain of inferred psychological events. From this perspective William James was wrong to insist that all psychological events must be reduced to conscious experiences, and behaviorists were equally wrong to insist that we cannot talk about consciousness at all. Once we accept a framework in which we simply try to understand the factors underlying the observations in exactly the way geologists try to understand rocks – that is to say, by making plausible and testable inferences about the underlying causes – the way becomes much clearer.

Today we may be ready to think about conscious experience without the presuppositional obstacles that have hobbled our predecessors (e.g., Mandler, 1975a,b; Posner, 1978; Shallice, 1972). If that is true, we are living at a unique moment in the history of human thought. We may have a better chance to understand human conscious experience now than ever before. Note again – this is not because we are wiser or harder-working than our predecessors, or even because we have more evidence at our disposal. We may simply be less encumbered by restrictive assumptions that stand in the way of understanding. Many scientific advances occur simply when obstructive assumptions are cleared away (see Chapter 5). Such "release from fixedness" is noteworthy in the work of Copernicus and Galileo, Darwin, Freud, and Einstein. While I cannot compare my work with theirs, the fact remains that progress can often be made simply by giving up certain presupposed blind spots.

1.1.2 Empirical evidence about conscious experience:
Clear cases and fuzzy cases

There are many clear cases of conscious experience (see Figure 1.1). The
reader may be conscious of this page, of images of breakfast, and the like.
These clear cases are used universally in psychological research. When
we ask a subject in a perception experiment to discriminate between two
sounds, or to report on a perceptual illusion, we are asking about his or
her conscious experience. Commonsensically this is obvious, and it is
clearly what experimental subjects believe. But scientific psychologists
rarely acknowledge this universal belief. For example, there is remarkably little discussion of the conscious aspect of perception in the research
literature. The twenty-volume *Handbook of Perception* has only one
index reference to consciousness, and that one is purely historical
(Carterette & Friedman, 1973–78). Nevertheless, reports about the subjects' experiences are used with great reliability and accuracy in psychological research.

    In addition to so many clear cases, there are many fuzzy cases where
it may be quite difficult to decide whether some psychological event is
conscious or not. There may be fleeting "flashes" of conscious experience that are difficult to report, as William James believed. There are
peripheral "fringe" experiences that may occur while we focus on
something else. Early psychologists reported that abstract concepts have
fleeting conscious images associated with them (Woodworth, 1915), and
indeed the writings of highly creative people like Mozart and Einstein
express this idea. Such examples are much more difficult to verify as
conscious than the clear cases discussed above.

The zero-point problem

This kind of uncertainty sometimes leads to seemingly endless controversy. For example, there is much debate about whether subliminal
perceptual input is conscious or not (Cheesman & Merikle, 1984; Holender, 1986; Marcel, 1983a,b). Likewise there is great argument about
the evidence for "blind sight," where patients with occipital damage can
name objects they claim not to experience (Holender, 1986; Natsoulas,
1982b; Weisskrantz, 1980). It is regrettable that so much current thinking
about consciousness revolves around this "zero-point problem," which
may be methodologically quite beyond us today. Progress in most
scientific research comes from first looking at the easy, obvious cases.
Only later, using knowledge gained from the clear cases, can one resolve
the truly difficult questions. Newton first used prisms to analyze light;
only later was his analysis extended to difficult cases like color filters and

Clearly conscious phenomena

↑
Attended percepts
Clear mental images
Deliberate inner speech
Material deliberately retrieved from memory
Fleeting mental images
Peripheral or "background" perceptual events
Abstract but accessible concepts

Fuzzy, difficult-to-determine events

Active but unrehearsed items in immediate memory
Presuppositions of conscious concepts
Fully habituated stimuli
Subliminal events that prime later conscious processes
"Blind sight" in occipital brain damage
Contextual information, set
Automatic skill components
Unretrieved material in long-term memory
Perceptual context
↓
Abstract rules, as in syntax

Clearly unconscious events

Figure 1.1. The continuum of clear and fuzzy events. Some things, such as clear percepts, are indisputably conscious; others, such as active but unrehearsed items in immediate memory, are debatable; and still others, such as unretrieved material in Long Term Memory, are clearly unconscious. We proceed here by contrasting the clearly conscious and unconscious cases, using those contrasts to constrain theory, and finally making some plausible theoretical inferences about the disputable, "fuzzy" cases. One problem in the scientific literature has been a tendency to focus first on the disputable cases, such as subliminal perception and "blind sight" in certain kinds of brain damage. However, scientific progress is generally made by moving from clear cases to fuzzy cases, not vice versa.

the wave–particle issue. If Newton had begun with these difficult cases, he would never have made his discoveries about light. In science, as in law, hard cases make bad law.

In this book we will make an effort to build on clear cases of conscious and unconscious processes. We will try to circumvent the "zero-point problem" as much as possible (e.g., 5.7). We use a "high criterion" for consciousness. We want people to report a conscious experience that is independently verifiable. Ordinary conscious perception obviously fits this definition, but it also includes such things as the conscious aspects of mental images, when these can be verified independently. On the unconscious side, we also set a high criterion: Unconscious processes must be inferrable on the basis of strong, reliable evidence, and they must *not* be voluntarily reportable even under the optimum conditions (Ericsson & Simon, 1984). Syntactic processing provides a strong example of such a clearly unconscious event. Even professional linguists who study syntax every working day do not claim to have conscious access to their own syntactic processes.

Between these clear cases of conscious and unconscious events there is a vast range of intermediate cases (Figure 1.1). In this book we start with clear cases of conscious and unconscious events, seek a plausible theory to explain them, and then use this theoretical scaffolding to decide some of the fuzzier cases. But we will start simply.

We began this chapter with some claims about the reader's own experience. The reader is momentarily conscious of most words in the act of reading, but at the same time competing streams of potentially conscious information are likely to be unconscious (or barely conscious); syntactic processes are unconscious; most conceptual presuppositions are unconscious (Chapter 4); habituated stimuli are unconscious; image-able memories, as of this book's cover, can be momentarily conscious but are currently unconscious; and so on. These inferences are supported by a great deal of solid, reliable evidence. Such clear cases suggest that we can indeed speak truthfully about some conscious and unconscious events.

1.1.3 Modern theoretical languages are neutral with respect to conscious experience

Current theories speak of information processing, representation, adaptation, transformation, storage, retrieval, activation, and the like, without assuming that these are necessarily conscious events. This may seem obvious today, but is is actually a painfully achieved historic insight into the right way to do psychological theory (Baars, 1986a; Jackendoff, 1987). William James, as noted above, felt strongly that all psychological events must be reducible to conscious experiences, while the behaviorists denied the relevance of either consciousness or unconsciousness. Either position makes it impossible to compare similar conscious and unconscious events, and to ask the question, "Precisely what is the difference between them?" Because it is neutral with respect to conscious experience, the language of information processing gives us the freedom to talk about inferred mental processes as either conscious or unconscious. This is a giant step toward clarity on the issues.

1.2 What is to be explained? A first definition of the topic

What is a theory of consciousness a theory of? In the first instance, as far as we are concerned, it is a theory of the nature of experience. The reader's private experience of *this* word, his or her mental image of yesterday's breakfast, or the feeling of a toothache – these are all contents of consciousness. These experiences are all *perceptual* and *imaginal*. (In this book we will use the word "imaginal" to mean internally generated quasi-perceptual experiences, including visual and auditory images, inner speech, bodily feelings, and the like.)

For present purposes we will also speak of *abstract but immediately expressible concepts* as conscious – including our currently expressible beliefs, intentions, meanings, knowledge, and expectations. Notice that these abstract concepts are experienced differently from perceptual and imaginal events (Baars, 1986b; Natsoulas, 1978a; and throughout this volume). Abstract concepts do not have the same rich, clear, consistent qualities that we find in the visual experience of this book: no color, texture, warmth, size, location, clear beginning and ending, and so forth. Perceptual and imaginal experiences are characterized by such qualities. Conceptual events are not. In contrast to qualitative *conscious experiences* we will sometimes refer to abstract conceptual events in terms of conscious *access*. This issue is closely related to the question of *focal* versus *peripheral* consciousness. The reader right now is conscious of *these words*. But much ancillary information is immediately available, as if it exists vaguely in some periphery of awareness. Some of it is in short-term memory and can be immediately brought to mind (1.3.4); some of it is in the sensory periphery, like a kind of background noise; and some of it may consist of ideas and skills that are always readily available, such as one's ability to stand up and walk to the next room. Again, it is probably better to think about peripheral events in terms of rapid conscious *access*, rather than prototypical conscious *experience*.

Common sense calls both qualitative experiences and immediately expressible, nonqualitative concepts "conscious." For the time being we will follow this usage *if* the events in question meet our operational criteria, discussed below. A complete theory must explain both the similarities *and* differences between these reports. Later in this book we will also explore the notion of *conscious control*, as a plausible way of thinking about volition (Chapter 7).

In reality, of course, every task people engage in involves all three elements: conscious experience, access, and control. Ultimately we cannot understand the role of consciousness if we do not explore all three. However, one can make the case that conscious qualitative experience is fundamental to the understanding of the other aspects and uses of consciousness. Thus we first address the puzzle of conscious experience (Chapters 2 and 3), then explore conscious access (Chapters 4 and 5), proceed to conscious control (Chapters 6 and 7), and finally consider the integrated functioning of all three elements (Chapters 8, 9, and 10).

The first order of business, then, is to find a usable objective criterion for the existence of a conscious event. When would any reasonable person agree that someone just had some experience? What is reliable objective evidence that a person just saw a banana, felt a sharp toothache, remembered the beauty of a flower, or experienced a new insight into the nature of conscious experience?

1.2.1 Objective criteria: Gaining access to the phenomena

In the course of this book we will often appeal to the reader's personal experience, but only for the sake of illustration. From a scientific point of view, all evidence can be stated in entirely objective terms. We can define a useful (though not perfect) objective criterion for conscious events. There may be arguments against this first operational definition, but it marks out a clear domain almost everyone would consider conscious. Within this domain we can proceed with theory construction, and then consider more difficult cases.

For now, we will consider people to be conscious of an event if (1) they can say immediately afterwards that they were conscious of it *and* (2) we can independently verify the accuracy of their report. If people tell us that they experience a banana when we present them with a banana but not with an apple, we are satisfied to suppose that they are indeed conscious of the banana. *Verifiable, immediate consciousness report* is in fact the most commonly used criterion today. It is exactly what we obtain already in so many psychological experiments.

It is important not to confuse a useful operational definition with the reality of conscious experience. Surely many conscious events are not conveniently verifiable – dreams, idiosyncratic images, subtle feelings, etc. But this is not necessary for our purpose, since we can rely upon the many thousands of experiences that can indeed be verified. In the usual scientific fashion, we are deliberately setting a high criterion for our observations. We prefer to risk the error of doubting the existence of a conscious experience when it is actually there, rather than the opposite error of assuming its existence when it is not there.

For example, in the well-known experiment by Sperling (1960), subjects are shown a 3×3 grid of letters or numbers for a fraction of a second (Figure. 1.2). Observers typically claim that they can see all the letters, but they can only recall three or four of them. Thus they pass the "consciousness report" criterion suggested above, but they fail by the criterion of verifiability. However, it is troubling that subjects – and experimenters serving as subjects – continue to insist that they are momentarily conscious of *all* the elements in the array. Sperling brilliantly found a way for observers to reveal their knowledge objectively, by

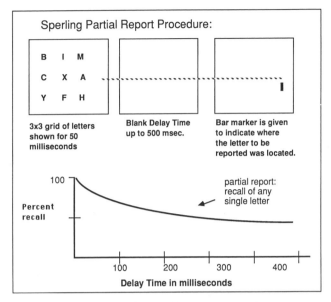

Figure 1.2. The Sperling Experiment: Momentary conscious events may be difficult to recall. People briefly exposed to the letter grid claim they are conscious of all letters briefly, though they cannot report them; reporting takes too long, and the very act of reporting may interfere with conscious access. Sperling (1959) found however that several hundred msec after the letters are turned off, a bar marker just below the location of any letter can serve as a signal to retrieve that particular, arbitrarily chosen letter. This implies that the observer has access to all the letters momentarily, even though he or she cannot report them all. Conscious access is thus very real, but it fades quickly and may be subject to interference from recall efforts.

asking them *after* the exposure to report *any* randomly cued letter. Under these circumstances people can accurately report any arbitrary letter, suggesting that they do indeed have fleeting access to all of them. Since the response cue is only given after the physical information has disappeared, it is clear that the correct information must have come from memory, and not from the physical display. Now we can be quite confident that subjects in the Sperling experiment do have momentary conscious access to all the elements in the visual display. Both the criteria of "consciousness report" and verifiability are satisfied.

The Sperling experiment serves as a reminder that conscious events may decay in a few hundred milliseconds, so that immediate report is often essential (Ericsson & Simon, 1984). Sometimes even very recent events can be hard to recall – very fleeting ones for example, or novel stimuli that cannot be "chunked" into a single experience, or stimuli that are followed by distraction or surprise. Indeed, the very act of retrieving and reporting recent material may interfere with accurate recall. But in general, recent events make for the best consciousness reports.

There are many ways to verify the accuracy of report. In perception, psychophysics, and memory experiments, we can check the stimulus directly. Studies of mental imagery typically look for internal consistency. For example, the well-known experiments by Cooper and Shepard (1973) show that in rotating mental images, the time of rotation is a highly predictable linear function of the degree of rotation. This very precise result helps validate the subjects' claim that they are indeed representing the rotating image mentally. Studies of explicit problem solving typically look for accuracy of results, subgoals, timing, and characteristic errors (Ericsson & Simon, 1984), and so on. Notice, by the way, that verifiable accuracy does not guarantee consciousness by itself. Aspects of mental rotation may not be conscious, for instance, although the Cooper and Shepard experiments suggest that unconscious rotation is quite precise even when it is unconscious. Likewise, reports of a conscious experience do not guarantee that it has actually occurred. There is much evidence that people sometimes manufacture memories, images, perceptual experiences, and intentions that are demonstrably false (e.g., Nisbett and Wilson, 1977). This is why we set the criterion of *both* the report of a conscious experience *and* verifiability.

Notice that saying "I just experienced a banana" is a metacognitive act – it is a report *about* a previous mental event. Consciousness no doubt exists even without this kind of metacognition – it surely continues if we do not report it afterwards, even to ourselves. In states of deep absorption in a novel or a film, or in hypnosis, people may not be able to report on their experiences without disrupting the absorbed state, but they are quite conscious all the same (7.7.1). This suggests that there may be more direct ways of assessing conscious experience than the operational definition that is used here. In fact, as we discover more evidence that correlates with this definition, better operational criteria will no doubt emerge. If we find that people who are conscious by the two criteria used above also have excellent recognition memory for the experience, we may "bootstrap" upward, and "accurate recognition memory" may then supersede verifiable consciousness report. Or someone might discover a neural event that correlates infallibly with conscious experience, defined by verifiable consciousness report; the neural event may also work when people cannot report their experience. Over time, as confidence grows in this measure, it may begin to supersede the current definition. But for now, "verifiable, immediate consciousness report" is still the most obviously valid criterion.

Our first operational definition extends beyond perceptual events to purely mental images, bodily feelings, inner speech, and the like, when people can give verifiable reports of having been conscious of such events. These kinds of conscious events are often called "qualitative conscious contents," because they have qualities like color, weight, taste, location in space and time, etc. In addition to qualitative conscious events, people talk about other mental contents as "conscious" if they are immediately available and expressible. Thus people can give verifiable reports about their current beliefs, ideas, intentions, and expectations: But these things do not have qualities like taste or texture or color. Ideas like democracy or mathematics, a belief in another person's good intentions, and the like – these events are nonqualitative or abstract. Nevertheless, they can in principle satisfy our operational definition, and certainly in the common meaning of "consciousness" we speak often of our conscious beliefs, ideas, and intentions. The relationship between qualitative and nonqualitative conscious contents will be a running theme in this book. Chapter 7 suggests a resolution of this problem.

Note that verifiable, immediate consciousness report takes for granted a whole cognitive apparatus that any complete theory must explain. For example, it presupposes the ability to act voluntarily; this is closely related to conscious experience (see Chapter 7). Further, any theory must eventually give a principled account of the operational definitions that led to it in the first place. In the beginning we can choose measures simply because they seem plausible and useful. But eventually, in the spiraling interplay of measure and theory, we must also explain them.

1.2.2 Contrastive analysis to focus on conscious experience as such

We will focus on the notion of consciousness *as such* by contrasting pairs of similar events, where one is conscious but the other is not. The reader's conscious image of this morning's breakfast can be contrasted with the same information when it was still in memory, and unconscious. What is the difference between conscious and unconscious representations of the same thing? Similarly, what is the difference between the reader's experience of his or her chair immediately after sitting down, and the current habituated representation of the feeling of the chair? What is the difference between the meaning conveyed by this sentence, and the same meaning in memory, and therefore not currently available? Or between currently accessible ideas and the presupposed knowledge that is necessary to understand those ideas, but which is not currently available? All these cases involve contrasts between closely comparable conscious and unconscious events.

These contrasts are like experiments, in the sense that we vary one thing while holding everything else constant, and assess the effect on conscious access and experience. Indeed, many experiments of this type have been published. In studies on selective attention, on subliminal perception, and on automaticity, similar conscious and unconscious events are routinely compared (e.g., Libet, 1978; MacKay, 1973; Marcel, 1983a; Shiffrin & Schneider, 1977; Sokolov, 1963). If contrastive analysis is just like doing an experiment, what is the difference between it and any perceptual experiment? It lies only in what is being compared. In perceptual experiments we might compare a 20-decibel sound to a 30-decibel sound, both conscious events. But in contrastive analysis, we compare two mental representations, one of a 30-decibel sound before habituation (which is conscious) to the mental representation of the same sound after habituation, when it is unconscious (1.4.1, Sokolov, 1963). Contrastive analysis allows us to observe the difference between the presence and absence of conscious experiences "from the outside." We can do this through reliable inferences from observed behavior to some inferred mental event, which may be inferrable even when the subject's experience of it is lost.

1.2.3 Using multiple contrasts to constrain theory

This book is concerned with "cumulative constraints" on conscious experience (Posner, 1982). As we noted in the Preface, we can look to multiple domains of evidence, so that strengths in one domain may compensate for weaknesses in another. A great deal of empirical work is required before the hypotheses advanced in this book can be considered solid. But the power of theory is precisely to make inferences about the unknown, based on what is known. As Broadbent (1958) has noted,

> The proper road for progress . . . is to set up theories which are not at first detailed, although they are capable of disproof. As research advances the theory will become continually more detailed, until one reaches the stage at which further advance is made by giving exact values . . . previously left unspecified in equations whose general form was known. (Quoted by Posner, 1982, p. 168)

Our approach in this book is integrative and global rather than local. We will also find a strong convergence between the "system architecture" suggested in this book and other current cognitive theories, even though the evidence we consider is quite different (e.g., Anderson, 1983; Norman & Shallice, 1980; Reason, 1983). This is encouraging.

1.2.4 Some examples of the method: Perception and imagery

Perception as conscious stimulus representation

Perception is surely the most richly detailed domain of conscious experience. In perceptual research we are always asking people what they

Table 1.1. *Contrastive evidence in perception*

Conscious events	Comparable unconscious events
1 Perceived stimuli	1 Processing of stimuli lacking in intensity or duration and centrally masked stimuli
	2 Pre-perceptual processing
	3 Habituated or automatic stimulus processing
	4 Unaccessed meanings of ambiguous stimuli
	5 Contextual constraints on the interpretation of percepts
	6 Unattended streams of perceptual input

experience, or how one experience compares to another. And we always check the accuracy of those reports. Thus research in perception and psychophysics almost always fits the criterion of "accurate report of consciousness." Someone might argue that perceptual illusions are by definition inaccurate, so that the study of illusions seems to be an exception to the rule (viz., Gregory, 1966). But in fact, even perceptual illusions fit our operational definition of conscious experience: That definition is concerned after all with *verifiable report with respect to the subject's experience*, not with whether the experience itself matches the external world. We cannot check the accuracy of reported illusions by reference to the external world, but other validity checks are routinely used in the laboratory. Perceptual illusions are highly predictable and stable across subjects. If someone were to claim an utterly bizarre illusory experience that was not shared by any other observer, that fact would be instantly recognized. For such an idiosyncratic illusory experience we would indeed be in trouble with our operational definition. Fortunately, there are so many examples of highly reliable perceptual reports that we can simply ignore the fuzzy borderline issues and focus on the clear cases.

Now we can apply a contrastive analysis to perceptual events. We can treat perception as input representation (e.g., Lindsay & Norman, 1977; Marr, 1982; Rock, 1983), and contrast perceptual representations to stimulus representations that are not conscious. Table 1.1 shows these contrasts. There is evidence suggesting that "unattended" streams of information are processed and represented even though they are not conscious (e.g., MacKay, 1973; but see Holender, 1986). Further, habituated perceptual events – those to which we have become accustomed – apparently continue to be represented in the nervous system (Sokolov, 1963; see section 1.4.1). There is evidence that perceptual events are processed for some time before they become conscious, so that there are apparently unconscious input representations (Libet, 1978; Neisser, 1967). Then there are numerous ambiguities in perception, which involve two ways of structuring the same stimulus. Of these two interpretations, only one is conscious at a time, though there is evidence that the other is also represented (e.g., Swinney, 1979; Tanenhaus, Carlson, & Seidenberg, 1985). There is evidence, though somewhat controversial, that visual information that is centrally masked so that it cannot be experienced directly continues to be represented and processed (Cheesman & Merikle, 1984; Holender, 1986; Marcel, 1983a). And finally, there are many contextual representations and processes that shape a perceptual interpretation, but which are not themselves conscious (see 4.0).

Any theory of the conscious component of perception must somehow explain all of these contrasts. The problem is therefore very strongly bounded. One cannot simply make up a theory to explain one of the contrasts and expect it to explain the others.

Several psychologists have suggested that perception has a special relationship to consciousness (Freud, 1895/1966; Merleau-Ponty, 1964; Skinner, 1974; Wundt, 1912/1973). This is a theme we will encounter throughout this book. A rough comparison of major input, output, and intermediate systems suggests that consciousness is closely allied with the *input* side of the nervous system. While perceptual processes are obviously not conscious in detail, the outcome of perception is a very rich domain of information to which we seem to have exquisitely detailed conscious access. By comparison, imagery seems less richly conscious, as are inner speech, bodily feelings, and the like. Action control seems even less conscious – indeed, many observers have argued that the most obviously conscious components of action consist of feedback from actions performed, and anticipatory images of actions planned. But of course, action feedback is itself perceptual, and imagery is quasi-perceptual (see 1.2.5 and Chapter 7). The conscious components of action and imagery resemble conscious perception.

Likewise, thought and memory seem to involve fewer conscious details than perception. Even in short-term memory we are only conscious of the item that is currently being rehearsed, not of the others; and the conscious rehearsed item in Short Term Memory often has a quasi-perceptual quality. We are clearly not conscious of information in long-term memory or in the semantic, abstract component of memory. In thinking and problem solving we encounter phenomena like incubation to remind us that the details of problem solving are often carried out unconsciously (Chapter 6). Again, the most obviously conscious components in thinking and memory involve imagery or inner speech – and these resemble perceptual events. The thoughts that come to mind after incubation often have a perceptual or imaginal quality (John-Steiner, 1985). In sum, when we compare input events

Table 1.2. *Contrastive evidence in imagery**

Conscious events	Comparable unconscious events
1 Images retrieved and generated in all modalities	1 Unretrieved images in memory
2 New visual images	2 Automatized visual images
3 Automatic images that encounter some unexpected difficulty	——
4 Inner speech: currently rehearsed words in Short-Term Memory	4 Currently unrehearsed words in Short Term Memory
	5 Automatized inner speech?

* "Images" are broadly defined here to include all quasiperceptual events occurring in the absence of external stimulation, including inner speech and emotional feelings.

(perception and imagery) with output (action) and mediating events (thought and memory), it is the input that seems most clearly conscious in its details. This kind of comparison is very rough indeed, but it does suggest that perception has a special relationship to consciousness (viz., 1.5.4).

Imagery: Conscious experience of internal events

We can be conscious of images in all sensory modalities, especially vision; of inner speech; and of feelings associated with emotion, anticipatory pleasure, and anticipatory pain. These experiences differ from perception in that they are internally generated. There are now a number of techniques for assessing imagined events that can meet our operational definition of conscious experience, though the imagery literature has been more concerned with verifiability of the imagery reports than with asking whether or not the image was conscious. For example, a famous series of experiments by Cooper and Shepard (1973) shows that people can rotate mental images, and that the time needed for rotation is a linear function of the number of degrees of rotation. This very precise result has been taken as evidence for the accuracy and reliability of mental images. But it is not obvious that subjects in this task are continuously conscious of the image. It is possible that in mentally rotating a chair, we are conscious of the chair at 0, 90, and 180 degrees, and less conscious at other points along the circle (Table 1.2).

Assessing the consciousness of mental images

Fortunately researchers in imagery have begun to address the issue of consciousness more directly. Pani (1982) solicited consciousness reports

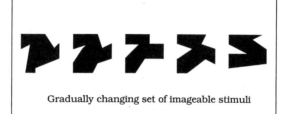

Gradually changing set of imageable stimuli

Figure 1.3. The Pani Experiment: Predictable mental images become unconscious with practice. Pani (1982) showed that mental images used in a matching task fade from consciousness with practice and return to consciousness with increased difficulty of the task. Even when the image faded, however, its contents were still available to perform the task, showing that consciousness is not needed in highly skilled and routine actions. The range of stimuli shown above differ only gradually, so that two neighboring figures differ very little, while those that are far apart are easy to distinguish. Pani asked subjects to memorize one figure, and then presented pairs of stimuli selected from the above. The subject was to choose which of the pair was most similar to the mental image. Difficulty was controlled by showing a pair of very similar, hard-to-distinguish stimuli. As subjects practiced the task, the image faded from consciousness even as the responses became faster and more accurate. (After Pani, 1982, Figure 2.)

in a verifiable mental imagery task. His results are very systematic, and consistent with historical views of imagery. Pani's subjects were asked to memorize several visual shapes, which were arbitrary so that previous learning would not be a factor. As shown in Figure 1.3, the test shapes were designed along a similarity dimension, so that any two adjacent shapes would be relatively similar, while more distant shapes were correspondingly different. Now Pani asked his subjects to perform a discrimination task: They were to keep one shape in mind and select which of two stimulus figures came closer to the one they had in mind. By making the two visual figures more or less similar to each other, he was also able to vary the difficulty of the task. The more similar the two stimuli were, the more difficult the discrimination.

Imagery reports were collected as a function of practice and difficulty, and the results were quite clear-cut: The *more* practice, the *less* subjects were conscious of the mental figure. Indeed, consciousness of the imaged figure drops very predictably with practice, even over 18 trials, with a correlation of −90 percent. When the discrimination was made more difficult, the mental image tended to come back to consciousness.

Pani's is in many ways a prototype experiment, one we will return to several times. It shows several important things. First, it suggests that even though the mental representation of the figure becomes less consciously available with practice, it continues to be used in the task.

Discrimination accuracy did not drop off with practice, even though conscious access did. This result invites a contrastive analysis: After all, some sort of mental representation of the target image continues to exist, whether conscious or not; what is the difference between the conscious image and the unconscious representation? Note also the rapid recovery of the conscious image when difficulty increased. In Chapter 5 we will argue that both fading and recovery of the conscious image can be explained in terms of novelty, informativeness, and predictability. The more predictable the mental representation, the more likely it is to fade; the more novel, informative, and difficult it is, the more likely it is to be conscious.

The importance of inner speech

Inner speech is one of the most important modes of experience. Most of us go around the world talking to ourselves, though we may be reluctant to do so out loud. We may be so accustomed to the inner voice that we are no longer aware of its existence "metacognitively," leading to the paradox of people asking themselves, "*What* inner voice?" But experiments on inner speech show its existence quite objectively and reliably (e.g., Klapp, Greim, & Marshburn, 1981). For several decades Singer and his colleagues have studied inner speech simply by asking people to talk out loud, which they are surprisingly willing to do (e.g., Pope and Singer, 1978). There is good evidence from this work that the inner voice maintains a running commentary about our experiences, feelings, and relationships with others; it comments on past events and helps to make plans for the future (Klinger, 1971). Clinical researchers have trained children to talk to themselves in order to control impulsive behavior (Meichenbaum & Goodman, 1971), and there are many hundreds of experiments in the cognitive literature on verbal Short Term Memory, which is roughly the domain in which we rehearse telephone numbers, consider different ideas, and talk to ourselves generally (e.g., Baddeley, 1976). Thus we actually know a great deal about inner speech, even though much of the evidence is listed under other headings.

Short Term Memory is the domain of rehearsable, usually verbal memory. It has been known since Wundt that people can keep in immediate memory only 7 or so unrelated words, numbers, and even short phrases. If rehearsal is blocked, this number drops to three or four (Peterson & Peterson, 1959). It is quite clear that we are not conscious of everything in conventional Short Term Memory. In rehearsing a telephone number we are qualitatively conscious only of the currently rehearsed item, not of all seven numbers, although all seven are readily available. STM raises not just the issue of conscious experience, but also that of voluntary control. We can ask people to rehearse numbers voluntarily, or we can interfere with rehearsal by asking them to do some competing, voluntary task, like counting backward by threes from 100 (Peterson & Peterson, 1959). A complete account of Short Term Memory must also include this voluntary control component (see Chapter 8).

There is considerable speculation that inner speech may become automatic with practice. Some clinical researchers suggest that people who are depressed may have rehearsed depressive ideation to the point of automaticity, so that they have lost the ability to control the self-denigrating thoughts (e.g., Beck, 1976). While this idea is plausible, I know of no studies that support it directly. This is a significant gap in the scientific literature. An experiment analogous to Pani's work on visual imagery may be able to provide the missing evidence.

1.2.5 Are abstract concepts conscious?

Philosophers have noted for many centuries that we are conscious of the perceptual world in ways that differ from our awareness of concepts. Perception has qualities like color, taste, and texture. Concepts like "democracy" or "mathematics" do not. And yet, ordinary language is full of expressions like "I am conscious of his dilemma," "I consciously decided to commit murder" and the like. Abstract beliefs, knowledge, intentions, decisions, and the like, are said to be conscious at times. And certainly our operational definition would allow this: If someone claims to be conscious of a belief in mathematics, and we can verify the accuracy of this claim somehow, it would indeed fit the definition of an "accurate report of being conscious of something." But can we really say that people are conscious of a belief that has no experienced qualities such as size, shape, color, or location in time and space?

We will suppose that it is meaningful to be conscious of some abstract concept, although the nature of the relationship between qualitative and nonqualitative experiences will be a theme throughout the book. We can point to a number of contrastive facts about our consciousness of abstract concepts. For example, the reader is probably not conscious right now of the existence of democracy, but if we were to ask whether democracy exists, this abstract fact will probably become consciously available. That is, we can contrast occasions when a concept is in memory but not "conscious" to the times when it is available "consciously." Further, there are reasons to believe that conscious access to concepts becomes less conscious with practice and predictability, just as images become less conscious with practice (5.1.3). Thus consciousness of abstract concepts seems to behave much like the conscious experience of percepts and images. We will speak of conscious *experience* of percepts and images, and *conscious access* to abstract concepts, intentions, beliefs, and the like. Chapter 7 suggests a solution to the problem of the relationship between qualitative experiences and nonqualitative conscious access.

In sum, we can find several contrasts between matched conscious and unconscious events in the realms of perception, imagery, and even abstract concepts. These are only two examples of the contrastive analysis method (see Baars, 1986b, for more examples). In the remainder of the book, we perform several others, as follows:

> In Chapter 2 we contrast the *capabilities* of comparable conscious and unconscious processes;
>
> in Chapter 3 neural mechanisms involved in *sleep and coma* are contrasted with those involved in wakefulness and arousal;
>
> in Chapter 4 we contrast *unconscious contextual factors* with the conscious experiences they influence. Contextual constraint seems to explain the difference between attended and unattended streams of information as well;
>
> in Chapter 5 *habituated or automatic* events are contrasted with similar events that are clearly conscious;
>
> in Chapter 6 we contrast *conscious access to problems and their solutions* with "incubation" and many other unconscious problem-solving phenomena;
>
> in Chapter 7 we extend contrastive analysis to the issue of voluntary control by comparing *voluntary* actions to very similar ones that are involuntary;
>
> in Chapter 8 we compare the *conscious control of attention* to automatic, unconscious control of attention; and, finally,
>
> in Chapter 9 *self-attributed* experiences to comparable *self-alien* experiences.

Thus we gain a great deal of mileage from contrastive analysis in this book.

1.2.6 Some possible difficulties with this approach

The logic of contrastive analysis is much like the experimental method, and some of the same arguments can be raised against it. In an experiment, if A seems to be a necessary condition for B, we can always question whether A does not disguise some other factor C. This question can be raised about all of the contrasts: What if the contrasts are not minimal; what if something else is involved? What if automatic skills are unconscious because they are coded in a different, procedural format that cannot be read consciously (Anderson, 1983)? What if subliminal stimulation is unconscious not because the stimulus has low energy, but because the duration of the resulting neural activity is too short? These are all possibilities. In the best of all possible worlds we would run experiments to test all the alternative hypotheses. For the time being, we will rely mainly on the extensive evidence that is already known, and try to account for it with the smallest set of principles that work. But any explanation is open to revision.

1.2.7 . . . but is it really consciousness?

A skeptical reader may well agree with much of what we have said so far, but still wonder whether we are truly describing conscious experience, or whether, instead, we can only deal with incidental phenomena associated with it. Of course, in a scientific framework one cannot expect to produce some ultimate, incorrigible understanding of "the thing itself." Rather, one can aim for an incremental advance in knowledge. No matter how much we learn about conscious experience, there may always be some irreducible core of "residual subjectivity" (Natsoulas, 1978b). In this connection it is worth reminding ourselves that physicists are still working toward a deeper understanding of gravity, a centerpiece of physical science for almost 400 years. Yet early developments in the theory of gravity were fundamental, and provided the first necessary steps on the road to current theory. We can work toward a reasonable theory, but not an ultimate one.

These considerations temper the quest for better understanding. And yet, scientific theories in general claim to *approach* the "thing itself," at least more so than competing theories. Physics does claim to understand and explain the planetary system, and biology really does seem to be gaining a genuine understanding of the mechanism of inheritance. These topics, too, were considered shocking and controversial in their time. Generally in science, if it looks like a rabbit, acts like a rabbit, and tastes like a rabbit, we are invited to presume that it is indeed a rabbit. Similarly, if something fits all the empirical constraints one can find on conscious experience, it is likely to be as close to it as we can get at this time. Of course, any claim that the current theory deals with conscious experience *as such* depends on the reliability, validity, and completeness of the evidence.

It is customary in cognitive psychology to avoid this debate through the use of scientific euphemisms like "attention," "perception," "exposure to the stimulus," "verbal report," "strategic control," and the like. These terms have their uses, but they also tend to disguise the real questions. "Strategic control" is a good way to refer to the loss of voluntary control over automatic skills (Schneider & Shiffrin, 1977; Shiffrin & Schneider, 1977). But using this term skirts the question of the connection between conscious experience and voluntary, "conscious" control. Once we label things in terms of conscious experience, this question can no longer be evaded (see Chapter 7). In this book we will find it helpful to call things by their usual names, because that tends to bring up the major issues more directly. None of the current crop of euphemisms for conscious experience conveys precisely what we mean by "conscious experience," either in life, or in this book.

1.3 Some attempts to understand conscious experience

There is now once more a rising tide of scientific interest in conscious experience. G. A. Miller (1986) has called consciousness one of the three major "constitutive" problems of psychology – the problems that define psychology as a discipline. It therefore makes sense to take another look at existing efforts to understand the topic. We will briefly review some common explanatory metaphors, explore some current models, and finally sketch the themes that will be developed further in this book. Again, the reader should not become discouraged by the apparent complexity and divergence of the evidence – the rest of this book aims to capture it all in terms of a few basic ideas.

1.3.1 Four common hypotheses

The Activation Hypothesis
One common suggestion is that consciousness involves *activation* of elements in memory that reach consciousness once they cross some activation threshold. We will call this the Activation Hypothesis; it is a current favorite, because many of today's cognitive theories use the concept of activation for reasons of their own. The Activation Hypothesis was stated as early as 1824 by Johann Herbart. In a very modern vein, he wrote:

> As it is customary to speak of an entry of the ideas into consciousness, so I call *threshold of consciousness* that boundary which an idea appears to cross as it passes from the totally inhibited state into some . . . degree of actual [conscious] ideation. . . . As we may speak of the intensification and weakening of ideas, so I refer to an idea as *below the threshold* if it lacks the strength to satisfy those conditions. . . . it may be *more* or *less far below the threshold*, according as it lacks more or less of the strength which would have to be added to it in order for it to reach the threshold. Likewise, an idea is *above the threshold* insofar as it has reached a certain degree of actual [conscious] ideation. (Herbart, 1824/1961, p. 40. Italics in original.)

Studies of perception, imagery, and memory all provide some evidence for this idea. Low-intensity stimuli in a normal surround do not become conscious. When two stimuli both evoke the same association, it is more likely to become conscious than when only one stimulus evokes the association (Anderson, 1983). And so on. Numerous phenomena involving consciousness can be explained naturally with the idea of an activation threshold. In recent years a number of models have been proposed involving "spreading activation," which are in spirit not far removed from Herbart's thoughts. These models view knowledge as a network of related elements, whether they be phonemes, words, or abstract concepts. Information can spread from node to node; the degree of involvement of any element is indicated by an activation number that is assigned to each node. These models are very effective, providing a flexible and powerful theoretical language for psychology. They have been applied to modeling language, visual perception, word perception, imagery, memory retrieval, speech production, and the like (see Rumelhart, McClelland & the PDP Group, 1986). However, in these models the strength of activation is not interpreted as the likelihood of the activated material becoming conscious.

Several theorists have made tentative suggestions that consciousness may in fact involve high-level activation. This is attractive in some ways, and indeed the model we propose in Chapter 2 may be stated in terms of activation (2.3.3). But we will sound the following note of caution about the use of activation alone to represent access to consciousness.

The trouble with unaided activation

Activation by itself is not sufficient to produce a conscious experience. This is shown especially by phenomena like habituation and automatization of conscious experience when an event is presented over and over again. We will call these phenomena *Redundancy Effects*. They are quite important in this book (Chapter 5). Redundancy Effects show that we generally *lose* consciousness of repeated and predictable events. This applies to perceived stimuli, but also to repeated mental images, to any practiced, predictable skill, and even to predictable components of meaning (see Chapter 5). Later in this chapter we will give arguments to the effect that Redundancy Effects involve not merely decay of activation, but an active learning process (1.41; 5.0).

In general, if we are to accept that conscious experience corresponds to activation above some threshold, as Herbart's Activation Hypothesis suggests, we must also accept the paradoxical idea that too much activation, lasting too long, can lead to a *loss* of conscious experience. Perhaps activation first rises and then declines? But then one would have to explain how a well-learned automatic skill can have low activation and still be readily available and very efficient! In learning to ride a bicycle, we lose consciousness of the details of riding even as we gain efficiency and availability of the skill. Hence activation cannot be used to explain both consciousness *and* efficiency and availability. If activation is used to explain consciousness, then something else is needed to account for availability and efficiency.

One is caught on the horns of a dilemma: Either consciousness and activation are the same, in which case activation cannot be used to explain the efficiency and availability of unconscious automatic skills, or activation and consciousness are different, in which case activation cannot be the only necessary condition for conscious experience. Later in this book we interpret Redundancy Effects as evidence that conscious experience always must be *informative* as well as highly activated; that is, it involves a process that works to reduce uncertainty about the input (Chapter 5). We are conscious of some event only as long as its uncertainty is not completely resolved. This view breaks the circularity of the unaided Activation Hypothesis by adding another necessary condition.

We will use activation in this book as one way to model the chances of an event becoming conscious. But activation is only a necessary, not a sufficient condition of consciousness (2.3.3).

The Novelty Hypothesis

The role suggested above for informative stimulation is not entirely new. It follows from another stream of thought about conscious experience. This trend, which we can call the Novelty Hypothesis, claims that consciousness is focused on mismatch, novelty, or "anti-habit." (Berlyne, 1960; Sokolov, 1963; Straight, 1977). Of course novelty is closely connected with the concept of information, and in Chapter 5 we suggest that the mathematical definition of information may be adapted to create a modern version of the Novelty Hypothesis (Shannon & Weaver, 1949).

The Tip-of-the-Iceberg Hypothesis

Another long tradition looks at consciousness as the tip of the psychological iceberg. The "Tip-of-the-Iceberg" Hypothesis emphasizes that conscious experience emerges from a great mass of unconscious events (Ellenberger, 1970). In modern cognitive work conscious experience is closely associated with *limited capacity mechanisms* (see 1.3.4), which represent the tip of a very large and complex iceberg of unconscious memories and mechanisms. In a different tradition, Freud's censorship metaphor attempts to explain the fact that conscious experience is only the tip of a great motivational iceberg (Erdelyi, 1985).

Curiously enough, few researchers seem to ask *why* our conscious capacity is so limited. The limitations are quite surprising, compared to the extraordinary size, capacity, and evolutionary sophistication of the nervous system. Some psychologists suppose that there must be a physiological reason for conscious limited capacity, but of course this begs the question of its functional role. Even physiological mechanisms evolve for functional reasons. We suggest an answer to this puzzle in Chapter 2.

The Theater Hypothesis

A fourth popular metaphor may be called the "searchlight" or Theater Hypothesis. This idea is sometimes called "the screen of consciousness." An early version may be found in Plato's classic Allegory of the Cave. Plato compared ordinary perception to the plight of bound prisoners in a cave, who can see only the cave wall with the shadows projected on it of people moving about in front of a fire. The people projecting the shadows are themselves invisible; they cannot be seen directly. We humans, according to Plato, are like those prisoners – we only see the shadows of reality. Modern versions of the Theater Hypothesis may be found in Lindsay and Norman (1977); Crick (1984) – and throughout this book. It has been beautifully articulated by the French historian and philosopher Hyppolite Taine (1828–93):

One can therefore compare the mind of a man to a theater of indefinite depth whose apron is very narrow but whose stage becomes larger away from the apron. On this lighted apron there is room for one actor only. He enters, gestures for a moment, and leaves; another arrives, then another, and so on. . . . Among the scenery and on the far-off stage or even before the lights of the apron, unknown evolutions take place incessantly among this crowd of actors of every kind, to furnish the stars who pass before our eyes one by one, as in a magic lantern. (Quoted in Ellenberger, 1970, p. 270)

Taine managed to combine several significant features in his theater image. First, he includes the observation that we are conscious of only one "thing" at a time, as if different mental contents drive each other from consciousness. Second, he incorporates the Tip-of-the-Iceberg Hypothesis, the idea that at any moment much more is going on than we can know. And third, his metaphor includes the rather ominous feeling that unknown events going on behind the scenes are *in control of* whatever happens on our subjective stage (cf. Chapters 4 and 5).

The Theater Hypothesis can easily incorporate an Activation Hypothesis: We can simply require that "actors" must have a certain amount of activation in order to appear in the limelight. Indeed, the theory developed in this book is a modern version of the Theater Hypothesis, attempting to include all of the partial metaphors into a single coherent model.

Some psychologists speak of consciousness in terms of a "searchlight" metaphor, a variant of the Theater Hypothesis. It compares conscious experience to a spotlight playing over elements in the nervous system (Crick, 1984; Lindsay & Norman, 1977). One can make a spotlight go wherever wanted, but a theater director can also control whatever will appear on stage. The two metaphors seem very similar, though the searchlight emphasizes control processes (see Chapter 8).

The common sense

One version of the Theater Hypothesis has had great influence in Western and Eastern thought; that is the notion of a "common sense," a domain in which all the special senses meet and share information. The original meaning of "common sense" is not the horse sense we are all born with to keep us from the clutches of used-car salesmen and politicians. Rather, "common sense," according to Aristotle (who introduced the term in Western philosophy) is a general sense modality that mediates between the five special senses. His arguments in favor of the common sense have a distinctly modern, cognitive flavor. They are as follows:

1 The five senses of popular psychology are each of them a special sense – visual only, or auditory only or tactual only, and so on. As the organs for each of them are distinct and separate it seems remarkable that the visible, auditory, tactual, and other sense qualities of an object should be localized in one and the same object. Hence the postulation of a "common" sense in addition to the "special" senses in order to account for the synthesis in question.

2 Again, there are some things apprehended in sense perception which are not peculiar to any one of the special senses but are common to two or more of them – such are, for instance, motion, rest, number, size, shape. It seemed therefore reasonable to Aristotle to assume a common sense for the apprehension of "common sensibles."

3 Once more, the different special sense-impressions are frequently compared and commonly differentiated. This likewise seemed to be the function of a common sense capable of comparing the reports of the several special senses.

And finally, Aristotle

4 also credited the common sense *with the function of memory, imagination, and even awareness of the fact that we are having sense-experiences. (Encyclopedia Britannica,* 1957, p. 128; italics added)

Thus the common sense is somehow associated with consciousness, and with introspective capabilities that tell us something about what we are conscious of. There is a remarkable resemblance between Aristotle's conclusions and the arguments found in Chapters 2 and 3 of this book. Interestingly, the notion of a common sense also appears in classical Eastern psychology about the time of Aristotle.

Each of the four hypotheses can be developed into a modern model. All four have some truth, and in a way, our job in this book is to find a viable and testable mix of these metaphors.

1.3.2 Contemporary ideas

There are currently a few psychological models with implications for attention and consciousness, but most current thinking is stated as single hypotheses, with no specified relationship to other hypotheses. For example, Mandler (1984) suggests that conscious experience often involves "trouble shooting" and interruption of ongoing processes (see Chapters 7 and 10). Posner and his co-workers have provided evidence for a number of specific properties of conscious experience, without working out an overarching theoretical position (e.g., Posner, 1982). The single-hypothesis approach has pros and cons. Single hypotheses can remain viable when models fall apart. On the other hand, model-building incorporates more information, and comes closer to the ultimate goal of understanding many properties of consciousness at the same time in a coherent way. We need both. In this book I focus on theory construction, referring to single hypotheses wherever appropriate.

1.3.3 Limited capacity: Selective attention, competing tasks, and immediate memory

The brain is such an enormous, complex, and sophisticated organ that the narrow limits on conscious and voluntary capacity should come as a great surprise. Cognitive psychologists rely on three sources of evidence about this "central limited capacity."

First, in *selective-attention* experiments subjects are asked to monitor a demanding stream of information, such as a stream of reasonably difficult speech or a visual display of a fast-moving basketball game. Under these conditions people are largely unconscious of alternative streams of information presented at the same time, even to the same sensory organ. Similarly, in absorbed states of mind, when one is deeply involved with a single train of information, alternative events are excluded from consciousness (Chapter 8).

Second, in *dual-task paradigms* people are made to do two things at the same time, such as reacting as quickly as possible to a momentary visual signal while beginning to say a sentence. In general, performance in each of the two tasks degrades as a result of competition. The more predictable, automatic, and unconscious a task becomes, the less it will degrade, and the less it will interfere with the other task as well.

Third, *immediate memory* is quite limited and fleeting. It includes sensory memories (notably the visual and auditory sensory stores), which can be consciously experienced. Sensory memories decay rapidly and are limited to relatively few separate stimuli (e.g., Sperling, 1960). Immediate memory also includes Short Term Memory, which is essentially the capacity to retain unrelated, rehearsable items of information longer than the immediate sensory stores allow.

Let us explore these facts in more detail.

Selective attention: People can be conscious of only one densely coherent stream of events at a time

The first return to consciousness in modern times can be credited to Donald E. Broadbent, who adapted a simple and instructive experimental technique for the purpose, and suggested a basic theoretical metaphor to explain it (Broadbent, 1958; Cherry, 1953). Broadbent and his colleagues asked subjects to "shadow" a stream of speech – to repeat immediately what they heard, even while continuing to listen for the next word – something that people can learn to do quite well (Moray, 1959). Rapid shadowing is a demanding task, and if one stream of speech is fed into one ear, it is not possible to experience much more than a vague vocal quality in the other ear. At the time, this seemed to indicate that human beings can fully process only one channel of information at a time. The role of attention, therefore, seemed to be to select and simplify the multiplicity of messages coming through the senses (Broadbent, 1958; James, 1890/1983). Attention was a *filter*; it saved processing capacity for the important things. In spite of empirical difficulties, the concept of "attention as a selective filter" has been the dominant theoretical metaphor for the past thirty years.

However, it quickly became clear that information in the unattended "channel" was indeed processed enough to be identified. Thus Moray (1959) showed that the subject's name in the unattended channel would break through to the conscious channel. Obviously this could not happen if the name were not first identified and distinguished from other alternatives, indicating that stimulus identification could happen unconsciously. MacKay (1973) and others showed that ambiguous words in the conscious channel were influenced by disambiguating information on the unconscious side. In a conscious sentence like, "They were standing near the bank," the word "river" in the unconscious ear would lead subjects to interpret the word "bank" as "river bank," while the unconscious word "money" would shift the interpretation to "financial bank." Finally, it became clear that the ears were really not channels at all: If one switched two streams of speech back and forth rapidly between the two ears, people were perfectly able to shadow one stream of speech, in spite of the fact that it was heard in two different locations. The important thing was apparently the *internal coherence* of the conscious stream of speech, not the ear in which it was heard (4.3.4).

Attempts were made to cope with these problems by suggesting that filtering took place rather late in the processing of input (Treisman, 1964, 1969). Speech was filtered not at the level of sound, but of meaning. However, even this interpretation encountered problems when the meaning of the unconscious speech was found to influence the interpretation of the conscious message, suggesting that even meaning penetrates *beyond* the unconscious channel under some circumstances (MacKay, 1973). Norman (1968) has emphasized the importance of semantic selectivity in determining what is to become conscious, and Kahneman (1973) has pointed out that selective attention is also influenced by long-term habits of mind or Enduring Dispositions, and by Momentary Intentions as well. Thus the filter model became enormously enriched with semantic, intentional, and dispositional factors. All these factors are indeed relevant to the issues of consciousness and attention, and yet it is not clear that they helped to resolve fundamental difficulties in the filter metaphor.

The purpose of filtering is to save processing capacity (Broadbent, 1958). If information is processed in the unattended channel as much as in the attended channel, filtering no longer has any purpose, and we are left in a quandary. We can call this the "filter paradox" (Wapner, 1986). But what is the function then of something becoming conscious? In this book we argue that consciousness involves the *internal distribution of information* (see 2.2, 2.5). Apparently both conscious and unconscious stimuli are analyzed quite completely by automatic systems. But once unattended inputs are analyzed, they are not broadcast throughout the nervous system. Conscious stimuli, on the other hand, are made available throughout, so that many different knowledge sources can be brought to bear upon the input. This creates an opportunity for *novel* contextual influences, which can help shape and interpret the incoming information in new ways. In this way the nervous system can learn to cope with truly novel information and develop innovative adaptations and responses (5.1).

Thus consciousness involves a kind of a filter – not an input filter, but a distribution filter. The nervous system seems to work like a society equipped with a television broadcasting station. The station takes in information from all the wire services, from foreign newspapers, radio, and from its own correspondents. It will analyze all this information quite completely, but does not broadcast it to the society as a whole. Therefore all the various resources of the society are not focused on all the incoming information, but just on whatever is broadcast by the television station.

From inside the society it seems as if external information is totally filtered out, although in fact it was analyzed quite thoroughly by automatic systems. Consciousness thus gives access to *internal unconscious resources* (Navon & Gopher, 1979).

> *Dual-task paradigms: Any conscious or voluntary event competes with any other*

There is a large experimental literature on interference between two tasks (e.g., Posner, 1982). In general, the findings from this literature may be summarized by three statements:

1. *Specific interference*: Similar tasks tend to interfere with each other, presumably because they use the same specific processing resources (Norman, 1976). We encounter limits in some specialized capacity when we do two tasks that both involve speech production, visual processes, and the like, or perhaps when the two tasks make use of closely connected cortical centers (Kinsbourne & Hicks, 1978).

2. *Nonspecific interference*: Even tasks that are very different interfere with each other when they are conscious or under voluntary control. When these tasks become automatic and unconscious with practice, they cease to interfere with each other (Shiffrin, Dumais, & Schneider, 1981). Similarly, two simultaneous stimuli in two different senses will degrade each other, they will fuse, or they will be experienced one after the other (Blumenthal, 1977).

3. *Competing tasks that take up limited capacity tend to become automatic and unconscious with practice. As they do so, they stop competing.*

Because there is such a close relationship between consciousness and limited capacity, we can sometimes use the dual-task situation to test hypotheses about conscious experience. Later in this book I will offer a theoretical interpretation of this kind of interference, and suggest some experiments to help decide cases where "accurate consciousness reports" may prove to be a less than reliable guide. The existence of nonspecific interference does not argue for consciousness as such, of course. It provides evidence for a central limited capacity that underlies consciousness. In general we can say that conscious experiences take up central limited capacity, but that there are capacity-limiting events that are not reported as conscious (e.g., Chapters 6 and 7).

> *Immediate memory is fleeting, and limited to a small number of unrelated items*

Another important source of evidence for a relationship between consciousness and a narrow-capacity bottle-neck is the study of immediate memory. We have already discussed the work of Sperling (1960), who showed that we can have momentary access to a visual matrix of numbers or letters. This has been interpreted as evidence for a momentary sensory memory, and evidence for similar sensory memories has been found in hearing and touch. Sensory memories can be conscious, though they need not be. For instance, we can have the experience of being very preoccupied with reading, and having someone say something we did not hear. For a few seconds afterwards, we can go back in memory and recall what was said, even though we were not conscious of it in detail at the time (Norman, 1976). It seems that even the vocal quality of the speech can be recalled, indicating that we have access to auditory sensory memory, not merely to the higher-level components.

The best-known component of immediate memory is called Short Term Memory (STM). This is the rehearsable, usually verbal component of immediate memory – the domain in which we rehearse new words and telephone numbers. There is a remarkably small limit to the number of unrelated words, numbers, objects, or rating categories that can be kept in Short Term Memory (Miller, 1956; Newell & Simon, 1972). With rehearsal, we can recall about 7 plus or minus 2 items, and without rehearsal, between 3 and 4. This is a fantastically small number for a system as large and sophisticated as the human brain; an inexpensive calculator can store several times as many numbers. Further, STM is limited in duration as well, to perhaps ten seconds without rehearsal (Simon, 1969).

Short Term Memory is a most peculiar memory, because while it is limited in size, the "size" of each item can be indefinitely large. For example, one can keep the following unrelated items in STM: consciousness, quantum physics, mother, Europe, modern art, love, self. Each of these items stands for a world of information – but it is highly organized information. That is, the relationship between two properties of "mother" is likely to be closer than the relationship between "mother" and "modern art." This is one aspect of *chunking*, the fact that information that can be organized can be treated as a single item in Short Term Memory. For another example, consider the series: 6771249100 91660129418891. It far exceeds our Short Term Memory capacity, being 24 units long. But we need only read it backwards to discover that the series is really only six chunks long, since it contains the well-known years 1776, 1492, 1900, 1066, and 1988. Chunking greatly expands the utility of Short Term Memory. It serves to emphasize that STM is always measured using a *novel, unintegrated* series of items. As soon as the items become permanently memorized, or when we discover a single principle that can generate the whole string, all seven items begin to behave like a single one.

All this suggests that STM depends fundamentally on Long Term

Memory (LTM) – the great storehouse of information that can be recalled or recognized. The fact that 1066 was the year of the Norman invasion of England is stored in LTM, and part of this existing memory must somehow become available to tell us that 1066 can be treated as a single, integrated chunk. Not surprisingly, several authors have argued that Short Term Memory may be nothing but the currently activated, separate components of Long Term Memory (Atkinson & Juola, 1974).

Short Term Memory is not the same as consciousness. We are only conscious of currently rehearsed STM items, not of the ones that are currently "in the background." Indeed, the unrehearsed items in current STM are comparable to peripheral events in the sensory field. They are readily available to focal consciousness, but they are not experienced as focal. Nevertheless, conscious experience and STM are somehow closely related. It is useful to treat consciousness as a kind of momentary working memory in some respects (Chapter 2). STM then becomes a slightly larger current memory store, one that holds information a bit longer than consciousness does, with more separate items.

Note also that STM involves *voluntary* rehearsal, inner speech, and some knowledge of our own cognitive capacities (metacognition). That is to say, STM is not something primitive, but a highly sophisticated function that develops throughout childhood. We argue later in this book that voluntary control itself requires an understanding of conscious experience, so that voluntary rehearsal in STM first requires an understanding of conscious experience. Thus STM cannot be used to explain conscious experience; perhaps it must be the other way around. In a later chapter (8.0) we will suggest that all of these functions can be understood in terms of systems that interact with conscious experience.

In conclusion, Short Term Memory is not the same as consciousness, although the two co-occur. It involves conscious experience, voluntary control over rehearsal and retrieval, the ability to exercise some metacognitive knowledge and control, and, in the case of chunking, a rather sophisticated long-term storage and retrieval system. STM is by no means simple. We will find it useful to build on a conception of conscious experience, develop from it some notions of voluntary control (see 7.0) and metacognition (see 8.0), and ultimately make an attempt to deal with some aspects of Short Term Memory (see pp. 310-3).

We have briefly reviewed the three major sources of evidence for limited capacity associated with conscious experience: the evidence for narrow limitations in selective attention, competing tasks, and immediate memory. It consistently shows an intimate connection between conscious experience, limited capacity processes, and voluntary control. There can be little doubt that the mechanisms associated with conscious experience are remarkably small in capacity, especially compared to the enormous size and sophsitication of the unconscious parts of the nervous system.

1.3.4 The Mind's Eye and conscious experience

In recent years our knowledge of mental imagery has grown by leaps and bounds. Not so long ago, "mental imagery" was widely thought to be unscientific, relatively unimportant, or at least beyond the reach of current scientific method (Baars, 1986a). But in little more than a decade we have gained a great amount of solid and reliable information about mental imagery (Cooper & Shepard, 1973; Kosslyn, 1980; Paivio, 1971).

In general there is a remarkable resemblance between the domain of mental imagery and ordinary visual perception – between the Mind's Eye and the Body's Eye (Finke, 1980; Kosslyn & Schwartz, 1981). The visual field is a horizontal oval, as anyone can verify by simply fixating at one point in space, and moving one's hands inward from the sides to the fixation point. Coming from the right and left sides, the hands become visible at approximately 65 degrees from the fixation point, long before the hands can be seen when they are moving inward vertically, from above and below. The same kind of experiment can be done mentally with the eyes closed, and yields similar results (Finke, 1980). Likewise, in the Mind's Eye we lose resolution with distance. We can see an elephant from thirty paces, but to see a fly crawling along the elephant's ear, we must "zoom in" mentally to get a better mental look. As we do so, we can no longer see the elephant as a whole, but only part of its ear. There are many other clever experiments that suggest other similarities between vision and visual imagery (see Kosslyn & Schwartz, 1981).

The best current theory of mental imagery suggests that the Mind's Eye is a domain of representation much like a working memory, with specifiable format, organization, and content (Kosslyn & Schwartz, 1981). Notice also that we can exercise some voluntary control over mental images – we can learn to rotate them, zoom in and out of a scene, change colors, and so forth. Mental imagery cannot be the same as conscious experience, but it is certainly a major mode of consciousness.

1.3.5 Perceptual feature integration and attentional access to information-processing resources

Two more current ideas deserve discussion before we can go on. They are, first, the idea that the function of consciousness is to "glue" together separable perceptual features (Treisman & Gelade, 1980) and, second, that consciousness or attention creates access to information-processing resources in the nervous system (Navon & Gopher, 1979). If we combine these ideas with the previous conceptions of attention and immediate memory, we come very close to the theoretical approach advanced in this book.

In an elegant series of experiments Treisman and her co-workers have provided evidence for the existence of separable features in vision. Treisman & Gelade (1980) showed that separable components of large, colored letters add linearly to search times. That is, to detect that something is red takes a short time; to detect that it is a red letter S takes a bit longer. Similarly, Sagi and Julesz (1985) found that people can detect the location of a few stray vertical lines in an array of horizontal lines very quickly; however, to tell whether these lines were vertical or horizontal, more time was needed. The more features were added, the more time was needed. They interpreted this to mean that integration of separable visual features takes up limited capacity. One problem with this idea is that a rich visual scene may have many thousands of separable visual features, and it is quite unlikely that all of them are processed serially. Watching a football team playing in a stadium full of cheering fans must involve large numbers of features, which surely cannot all be scanned serially, one after another. Focusing on a single, conspicuous feature, such as deciding which team is wearing the red uniforms, does seem to be a serial process.

Nevertheless there is something fundamentally important about the findings of Treisman and her co-workers. In almost any rich visual scene we may be doing a partial search. In a grocery store we search for a particular package, in a crowd we may look for a friendly face, or in a dictionary for a word. Eye movements are highly functional, scanning the parts of a scene that are most informative and personally relevant (Yarbus, 1967). This searching component may generally be serial, while the automatic, predictable components of a scene may be integrated either very quickly or in parallel; both serial and parallel processes work together to create our visual experience.

Mandler (1983, 1984) and Marcel (1983a) have argued along similar lines that consciousness has a *constructive* function, one that unifies disparate components into a coherent whole. There are many sources of evidence for such a constructivist view (e.g., Bransford, 1979), and it should be made clear at this point that the integration of perceptual features, as suggested by Treisman and Gelade and others, does not imply a passive "glueing" process; it is entirely compatible with an active, integrative construction of a set of components into a coherent whole, one that goes beyond the sum of its parts.

A very different approach is advocated by Navon & Gopher (1979), who treat limited capacity as a resource-allocation problem, much like a problem in economics. The idea that attention or consciousness involves *access to processing resources* is very powerful, and is a major aspect of the theory advanced in this book. Notice that most of the processing resources in the nervous system are unconscious, so that we have the remarkable situation of conscious events being used to gain access to unconscious processing resources. To put it slightly differently: a narrow, limited-capacity system seems to be involved in communicating with a simply enormous marketplace of processing resources.

How can these apparently different views be accomodated in a single coherent theory? After all, Treisman and her colleagues find evidence for conscious perception as an *integrative capacity* while Navon & Gopher (1979) argue for this same system as a *widely diverging* access system. We resolve this tension by speaking of a "global-workspace architecture," in which conscious events are very limited, but are broadcast system-wide, so that we have both a narrow, convergent bottle-neck and a widely diverging processing capacity (2.4, 2.5). The specialized processors in this view mobilize around centrally broadcast messages, so that the processing resources "select themselves." The situation is much like a television broadcasting station that may call for volunteers in an emergency; the volunteers are self-selected, though one may be able to recruit more of them by broadcasting more messages in the limited-capacity medium.

Models of all these phenomena have much in common. Selective attention, feature integration, immediate memory, and access to resources all suggest the existence of some sort of domain of integration related to consciousness, perhaps a "working memory" that can be worked on by both voluntary and involuntary operators. All the models involve limited capacity, and in recent years, there has been increasing emphasis on the fact that access to the limited-capacity system also gives one access to a great number of mental resources that are otherwise inaccessible (Baars, 1983). In Chapter 2, I propose a model that combines the most useful features of all these proposals.

The most recent models propose an overall *architecture* for the nervous system that incorporates these properties, as we see next.

1.3.6 Cognitive architectures: Distributed systems with limited-capacity channels

A recent class of psychological models treats the cognitive system as a society of modules, each with its own special capabilities (Minsky, 1986; Rumelhart, McClelland, and the PDP Group, 1986). These distributed systems suppose that much of the problem-solving ability of the society resides not in its "government," but in its individual members. Limited capacity is sometimes taken to reflect a "working memory" in such a system (e.g., Anderson, 1983), or in any case some sort of bottle-neck that forces the individual modules to compete or cooperate for access (Baars, 1983; Norman & Shallice, 1980; Reason, 1983, 1984; Jackendoff, 1987). In this book I work out one model of this kind.

Distributed models require a change in our usual way of thinking about human beings. We normally think of ourselves as guided by an executive "self"; intuitively we believe that "we" have control over ourselves. But distributed systems are strongly decentralized – it is the specialized components that often decide by their own internal criteria what they will do. This is comparable perhaps to a market economy, in which thousands of individual transactions take place without government intervention, although the marketplace as a whole interacts with global governmental influences. Distributed collections of specialized processors seem to have some distinct virtues (e.g., Greene, 1972; Gelfand, Gurfinkel, Fomin, & Tsetlin, 1971; Rumelhart, McClelland, & the PDP Group, 1986). A decentralized system does not *rule out* executive control, just as the existence of market forces in the economy does not rule out a role for government (9.0). But it limits the control of executives, and creates possibilities for a mutual flow of control between executives and subordinate elements. Details of processing are generally handled by specialized members of the processing society.

The Global Workspace model developed in this book is a distributed society of specialists that is equipped with a working memory, called a *global workspace*, whose contents can be broadcast to the system as a whole. The whole ensemble is much like a human community equipped with a television station. Routine interactions can take place without the television station, but novel ones, which require the cooperation of many specialists, must be broadcast through the global workspace. Thus novel events demand more access to the limited-capacity global workspace (5.0).

Notice that the recent theories propose an *architecture* for the whole cognitive system. In that sense they are more ambitious than the early models of short-term memory and selective attention. Perhaps the best-known architectural model today is Anderson's ACT*, which grew out of earlier work on semantic networks as models of knowledge and on production systems to model limited capacity mechanisms (Anderson, 1983). But similar architectures have been proposed by others.

In these models, conscious experience is often rather vaguely associated with limited-capacity mechanisms or working memory. Most of the architectural models do not suggest a functional reason for the rather astonishing fact of limited capacity. But explicit, running models of cognitive architectures do exist. That means we can go ahead in this book and discuss the issues without worrying too much about the formal specifics, which can be handled once the outlines of the theory are clear. This is not unusual in the natural sciences, where qualitative theory often precedes quantitative or formal theory (viz., Einstein, 1949). Indeed, Darwinian theory was purely qualitative in its first century of existence, and yet it revealed important things about the organization of life. Fortunately, we now have a number of computational formalisms that can be used to make the current theory more explicit and testable when that becomes appropriate.

1.3.7 The Global Workspace approach attempts to combine all viable metaphors into a single theory

The model we pursue in this book suggests that conscious experience involves a *global workspace*, a central information exchange that allows many different specialized processors to interact. Processors that gain access to the global workspace can broadcast a message to the entire system. This is one kind of cognitive architecture, one that allows us to combine many useful metaphors, empirical findings, and traditional insights regarding consciousness into a single framework. The word "global" in this context simply refers to information that is usable across many different subsystems of a larger system. It is the need to provide global information to potentially *any* subsystem that makes conscious experience different from the many specialized local processors in the nervous system.

Global Workspace (GW) theory attempts to integrate a great deal of evidence, some of which has been known for many years, in a single conceptual framework. Figure 1.4 shows the similarity between the three main constructs of GW theory – the global workspace, specialized processors, and contexts – and ideas proposed elsewhere. There is a clear similarity, although not an exact equivalence. Precision and coherence are the aims of the current theory; complete novelty may be less important.

So much for some ways of thinking about consciousness. One cannot think properly about conscious experience without some clear conception of *un*conscious events – the other side of the same coin. We turn to this issue now.

1.4   Unconscious specialized processors: A gathering consensus

Unconscious events are treated in this book as the functioning of specialized systems. The roots of this view can be found in the everyday observation that as we gain some skill or knowledge, it tends to become less and less conscious in its details. Our most proficient skills are

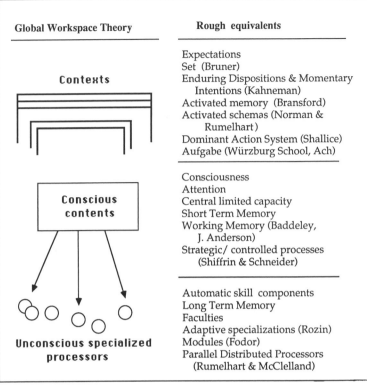

Figure 1.4. Similarities between GW terms and other widespread concepts. The concepts defined in this book are not new; they are modern variants of ideas that have been widely used elsewhere. However, they are specifically defined here in terms of unconscious and conscious functioning. This kind of definition has not been widely used in contemporary psychology, while the older psychology tended to be theoretically less precise than modern work. Notice that Global Workspace (GW) theory has only three main constructs: the *global workspace, unconscious specialized processors,* and *contexts.* Each of these has a graphic symbol associated with it, so that the theory can be expressed in intuitively obvious diagrams.

generally the least conscious. We will first explore the properties of unconscious *representations*; then see how representations are involved in unconscious information processing; this in turn leads to the notion of specialized unconscious *processors*.

1.4.1 There are many unconscious representations

A *representation* is a theoretical object that bears an abstract resemblance to something outside itself. In somewhat different terms, there is an abstract match or *isomorphism* between the representation and the thing that is represented. Human knowledge can be naturally viewed as a way of representing the world and ourselves. Instead of operating upon the world directly, we can try our ideas out on a representation of some part of the world, to predict its behavior. An architect's blueprint is a representation of a building, and one can investigate the effects of adding another story by calculating load factors on the structural supports shown in the blueprint. We can think of knowledge, percepts, images, plans, intentions, and memories as representations. Everyday psychology can be translated into these terms in a natural way.

Some psychologists prefer to speak of *adaptation* rather than representation (Grossberg, 1982). This approach has a long and honorable history with a somewhat different philosophical bent (e.g., Piaget, 1973). In practice, adaptation and representation are quite similar. Here we will use the term "representation" with the understanding that representations share many properties with adaptive systems.

What is the adequate evidence for the existence of a mental representation? In psychology we often infer that human beings have mentally represented an object if they can correctly detect *matches and mismatches* to the object at a later time. All psychological tasks involve some kind of selective matching of representations, conscious or not.

Recognition memory

Recognition memory provides one major class of cases in which people can spot matches and mismatches of previous events with impressive accuracy. In recognition studies subjects are given a series of pictures or sounds, and later are shown similar stimuli to see if they can tell old from new items. People are extremely good in this kind of task, often correctly recognizing more than 90 percent out of many hundreds of items a week or more afterwards (e.g., Shepard, 1967). There are indeed cases where recognition memory appears to fail, especially when the old and new stimuli are very similar. Nevertheless, even here it makes sense to suppose that the task involves a memory representation of the stimulus; the representation is just not completely accurate, it may be abstract, or it may be selectively stored and retrieved.

This brings us to the first, rather obvious class of unconscious representations. What happens to our memories of last week's stimuli before we see them again in a recognition test? According to the argument made above, we must be representing those memories somehow, otherwise we could not successfully detect matches and mismatches. The simplest supposition is that memories continue to be represented unconsciously. The remarkable accuracy of recognition memory indicates that human beings have a prodigious capacity for storing the things we experience, without effort. But of course most stored memories cannot be recalled at will.

Memory psychologists make a distinction between experiential, auto-biographical memories (*episodic*) and our memory for abstract rules (*semantic*) (Tulving, 1972). The reader is not conscious of the syntactic rules that are working right now to determine that the word "word" is being used as a noun rather than a verb. However, we do become conscious of events that match or mismatch those rules. Sentences that violate very subtle syntactic regularities are spotted instantly. Further, the evidence is good that people given artificial strings of symbols infer the underlying rules with remarkable facility, but without knowing consciously what those rules are (Franks & Bransford, 1971; Posner, 1982; Reber & Allen, 1978).

Thus the case of abstract rules shows that a great deal of knowledge involves abstract representations, which are known to *be* representations because they fit the match/mismatch criterion. Matches and mismatches are accurately "recognized," though people are not conscious of the syntactic representations themselves.

There is a third class of unconscious stimulus representations, namely the representation of predictable stimuli to which we are currently habituated. This example requires a little exposition.

Sokolov and the mental model of the habituated stimulus

A formal argument for unconscious stimulus representations has been given by the Russian physiologist Y. N. Sokolov (1963), working in the tradition of research on the Pavlovian "Orienting Response." The Orienting Response (OR) is a set of physiological changes that take place when an animal detects a new event. Any animal will orient its eyes, ears, and nose toward the new event, and at the same time a widespread set of changes take place in its body: changes in heart rate and breathing, in pupillary size, electrical skin conductivity, brain electrical activity, and in dilation and contraction of different blood vessels. We now know that a massive wave of activation goes throughout the brain about 300 millise conds after a novel event (Donchin, McCarthy, Kutas, & Ritter, 1978). All together this set of responses to novelty defines an Orienting Response. If the novel stimulus is repeated regularly over a period of time, the OR will gradually disappear – it habituates. Subjectively we lose awareness of the repeated, predictable stimulus.

Suppose the animal has habituated to a repeated one-second noise pulse, with two seconds of silence between noise bursts (Figure 1.5). Now we reduce the length of the silent period between the pulses, and suddenly

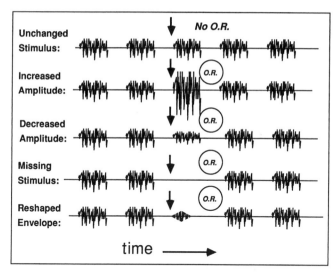

Figure 1.5. The Sokolov argument: Habituated stimuli are still represented in the nervous system. A repeated stimulus habituates rapidly, so that an animal will no longer orient to it. But after habituation, the Orienting Response (OR) will reappear when any parameter of the stimulus is changed. The figure shows several kinds of stimulus changes, including increase in amplitude, decrease in amplitude, total absence of the expected stimulus, and change in the amplitude envelope. Other parameters include location of the sound, repetition rate, spectral distribution, and association with a biologically significant stimulus such as food or shock. Because any change in the stimulus leads to another Orienting Response, Sokolov (1963) suggests that the nervous system must maintain an accurate representation of the habituated stimulus – otherwise changes could not be detected. In cognitive terms, this suggests that we maintain accurate internal representations of events that are so predictable that they have become unconscious.

the animal will orient again. We can increase *or* decrease the loudness of the stimulus, change its location in space, its pitch or spectral distribution, or other characteristics such as the rate of onset or offset. In each case, the change in stimulation will cause the animal to orient again to the stimulus, even after complete habituation of orienting. That is, the animal detects any kind of novelty. But how can the nervous system do this? Sokolov suggests that it can only do this as a result of some comparison process between the original stimulus and the new stimulus. (Indeed, "novelty" by definition involves a comparison of new to old.) But of course the original stimulus is long gone by the time the novel stimulus is given, so it is not available for comparison. Hence, Sokolov suggests, the nervous system must retain some model of the stimulus to which it has habituated. And since a change in *any* parameter of the stimulus will evoke a new OR, it follows that the stimulus representation must contain *all* parameters of the stimulus.

It is interesting to consider neurophysiological evidence about stimulus habituation from E. R. John's (1976) work with Event-Related Potentials (see 2.5). Prior to habituation, John and his co-workers have found, activity related to a repeated visual stimulus can be found throughout the brain. But once habituation takes place, it can only be found in the visual system. In our terms, the habituated stimulus appears to be processed, perhaps much as before, but it is not distributed globally (2.2). This finding is quite consistent with Sokolov's arguments. The fact that people become unconscious of a repetitive or predictable stimulus does not mean that the stimulus has disappeared; on the contrary, it continues to be processed in the appropriate input system.

Although Sokolov's arguments have been widely accepted in neurophysiology, in cognitive psychology they are not as well known as one might expect. This is curious, because the cognitive literature is generally quite receptive to compelling inferences based on well-established evidence. Many psychologists still consider habituation as a purely physiological effect without important psychological implications – perhaps due to "fatiguing" of feature detectors (e.g., Eimas & Corbitt, 1973) – in any case, as something nonfunctional. But Sokolov's argument suggests that the decline in orienting to redundant stimuli is something very functional for the nervous system.

In fact, Sokolov anticipated a "fatigue" explanation of habituation, and provided an interesting argument against it (Sokolov, 1963). Suppose there is some neural mechanism that is triggered by a repeated stimulus, such as the white noise burst described above. Now suppose that this mechanism – which might be a single neuron or a small network of neurons – declines over time in its ability to detect the stimulus, for reasons that have no functional role. Perhaps toxic metabolic by-products accumulate and prevent the "noise burst detector" from functioning properly, or perhaps some neurotransmitter becomes depleted. In any case, some "fatigue" affects the detector. If that were true, we might expect habituation of awareness, and that is in fact observed. But the pattern of *dis*habituation should be different from Sokolov's findings. A new Orienting Response might occur after habituation, but only if the stimulus were stronger in some way than the original stimulus – if the noise were louder or longer or more frequent. That is, the depleted and unresponsive detector might be triggered again by a *greater* stimulus. In fact, we find that a louder, longer, or more frequent stimulus does elicit an OR – but so does a softer, shorter, or *less* frequent noise burst. Indeed, an OR even occurs to a missing noise burst, which is the *absence* of an expected physical event! Thus release from habituation is not dependent upon the energy of the stimulus: It is dependent upon a change in *information*, not a change in *energy* as such (5.0). It follows that "fatigue" is not a plausible explanation for the universal fact of habituation of awareness under repeated or predictable stimulation. In support of this argument, recent work shows that the absence of an expected event triggers a great amount of activity in the cortical evoked potential (Donchin et al., 1978).

This argument can be generalized to another possible alternative explanation, a "general threshold" hypothesis. Suppose we deal with a repeated auditory stimulus by simply turning up our auditory threshold, much like the "filter" of early selective attention theory (Broadbent, 1958). This hypothesis would account for habituation and for dishabituation to *more* energetic input; but again, it would fail to explain why we become conscious again of a novel stimulus that is less energetic than the old stimulus.

We have noted that cognitive psychologists are generally willing to infer a mental representation whenever they find that people can retain some past event over time, as evidenced by their ability to accurately spot *matches* and *mismatches* with the past event. This is how we infer the existence of memories – mental representations of past events – based upon the impressive ability people show in recognition tasks. Formally, Sokolov's argument is exactly the same: It involves a kind of recognition memory. People or animals are exposed to a repeated stimulus, habituate, and respond accurately to matches and mismatches of the past event. But here we infer an *unconscious* kind of "recognition" process, rather than the recognition of a conscious stimulus.

Sokolov's argument has great significance for cognitive approaches to learning; indeed, one may say that the loss of consciousness of a predictable event *is* the signal that the event has been learned completely (5.0). Habituation of awareness is not just an accidental by-product of learning. It is something essential, connected at the very core to the acquisition of new information. And since learning and adaptation are perhaps the most basic functions of the nervous system, the connection between consciousness, habituation, and learning is fundamental indeed (see Chapter 5).

Section summary

The three classes of unconscious stimulus representations we have discussed – stored episodic memories, linguistic knowledge, and habituated stimulus representations – illustrate the main claim of this section, that there are indeed unconscious mental representations. There may be more than just these, of course. The next step suggests that there are many unconscious *processes* and even processors as well.

1.4.2 There are many unconscious specialized processors

A *process* involves changes in a representation. In mental addition, we may be aware of two numbers and then perform the mental process of adding them. A *processor* can be defined as *a relatively unitary, organized set of processes that work together in the service of a particular function* (Fodor, 1983; Rozin, 1976). A crucial claim in this book is that the nervous system contains many specialized processors that operate largely unconsciously.

One can think of these processors as specialized skills that have become highly practiced, automatic, and unconscious. Automatic skills are described as being "unavoidable, without capacity limitations, without awareness, without intention, with high efficiency, and with resistance to modification" (LaBerge, 1980). These are all properties of unconscious specialized processors, as we will see below.

1.4.3 Neurophysiological evidence

The neural evidence for specialized processors is extensive. Perhaps most obvious is the well-established fact that many small collections of neurons in the brain have very specific functions. Indeed, much of the cerebral cortex – the great wrinkled mantle of tissue that completely covers the older brain in humans – is a mosaic of tiny specialized areas, each subserving a specific function (Mountcastle, 1978; Rozin, 1976; Szentagotai & Arbib, 1975; see Chapter 3). These range from the sensory and motor projection areas, to speech production and comprehension, to spatial analysis, planning and emotional control, face recognition, and the like. Below the cortical mantle are nestled other specialties, including control of eye movements, sleep and waking, short-term memory, homeostatic control of blood chemistry, hormonal control of reproductive, metabolic and immune functions, pleasure centers and pain pathways, centers involved in balance and posture, breathing, fine motor control, and many more. Some of these specialized neural centers have relatively few neurons; others have many millions.

There is a remarkable contrast between the narrowness of limited-capacity processes and the great size of the nervous system – most of which operates unconsciously. The cerebral cortex alone has an estimated 55,000,000,000 neurons (Mountcastle, 1978), each with about 10,000 dendritic connections to other neurons. Each neuron fires an average of 40 and a maximum of 1,000 pulses per second. By comparison, conscious reaction time is very slow: 100 milliseconds at best, or 100 times *slower* than the fastest firing rate of a neuron. An obvious question is: Why does such a huge and apparently sophisticated biocomputer have such a limited conscious and voluntary capacity? (See 2.3.1, 10.01.)

Not all parts of the brain have specific assignments. For instance, the function of the cortical "association areas" is difficult to pinpoint. Most functions do not have discrete boundaries, and may be distributed widely through the cortex. Further, there is below the cortex a large *nonspecific* system, which we will discuss in detail in Chapter 3.

1.4.4 Psychological evidence

Psychologists have discovered evidence for specialized functional systems as well. Two sources of evidence are especially revealing: (a) the development of *automaticity* in any practiced task, and (b) the study of *errors* in perception, memory, language, action, and knowledge. Both sources of evidence show something of interest to us.

1 *The development of automaticity with practice.* Any highly practiced and automatic skill tends to become "modular" – unconscious, separate from other skills, and free from voluntary control (La Berge, 1974, 1980; Shiffrin & Schneider, 1977) – and any complex skill seems to combine many semiautonomous specialized units. In the case of reading, we have specialized components like letter and word identification, eye-movement control, letter-to-phoneme mapping, and the various levels of linguistic analysis such as the mental lexicon, syntax, and semantics. All these components involve highly sophisticated, complex, practiced, automatic – and hence unconscious – specialized functions.

Much research on automaticity involves perceptual tasks, which we will not discuss at this point. The reason to avoid perceptual automaticity is that perceptual tasks *by definition* involve access to consciousness (LaBerge, 1980; Neisser, 1967). Thus they tend to confuse the issue of *un*conscious specialized systems. Instead, we will focus on the role of automatic processes in memory, language, thought, and action. Perceptual automaticity will be discussed in Chapter 8, in the context of access-control to consciousness.

The best-known early experiment on automatic memory scanning is by Sternberg (1966), who presented subjects with small sets of numbers to hold in memory. Thus, they would be told to keep in memory the set "3, 7, 6," or "8, 5, 2, 9, 1, 3." Next, a number was presented that was or was not part of the set, and Sternberg measured the time needed to decide when the test stimulus belonged to the memory set. This task becomes automatic quite quickly, so that people are no longer aware of comparing every item in memory to the test item. Further, the time needed to scan a single item is much faster than conscious reaction time, suggesting again that memory scanning is automatic and unconscious. The big surprise was that reaction time to the test item did not depend on the position of the item in the set of numbers; rather, it depended only on the size of the whole memory set. Thus, if a subject were given the set "8, 5, 2, 9, 1, 3," and the test stimulus were "5," reaction time would be no shorter than when the test stimulus were the last number "3." This seemed most peculiar. In a 1964 conference N. S. Sutherland called it "extremely puzzling. On the face of it, it seems a crazy system; having found a match, why does the subject not stop his search and give the positive response?" (Sutherland, 1967).

Indeed it is rather crazy, if we assume that the subject is consciously comparing each number in memory with the test stimulus. Having found the right answer, it seems silly to continue searching. But it is not so unreasonable if the comparison process runs off automatically, without conscious monitoring or voluntary control. If the subject has available an unconscious automatic processor to do the job, and if this processor does not compete with other conscious or voluntary processes, little is lost by letting it run on by itself. More recent work by Shiffrin and Schneider (Schneider & Shiffrin, 1977; Shiffrin & Schneider, 1977) confirms that *voluntary* (controlled) search does not run on by itself. It terminates when the answer is found.

The automatic search process generally does not compete with other processes (Shiffrin, Dumais, & Schneider, 1981). It is unconscious, involuntary, and specialized. It develops with practice, provided the task is consistent and predictable. Further, and of great importance, separable components of automatic tasks often begin to behave as single units. That is, specialized functions seem to be carried out by "modular" automatic systems (see below). There is some question whether this is always true, but it seems to be true for most automatic processes (Treisman & Gelade, 1980).

Memory search is not the only process that has these properties. Much the same points have been made for the process of lexical access. In reading this sentence, the reader is using many specialized skills, among them the ability to translate strings of letters into meanings. This mapping between letter strings and meaning is called lexical access, though "lexico-semantic access" might be a more accurate term. A good deal of evidence has accumulated indicating that lexical access involves an autonomous processing module (Swinney, 1979; Tanenhaus, Carlson & Seidenberg, 1985). A typical experiment in this literature has the following format:

Subjects listen to a sentence fragment ending in an ambiguous word, such as

They all rose . . .

The word "rose" can be either a verb or a noun, but in this sentence context it must be a verb. How long will it take for this fact to influence the interpretation of the next word? To test this, one of two words is presented, either *flower*, or *stood*. Subjects are asked to decide quickly whether the presented word is a real English word or not. If the subjects make use of the sentence context in their lexical decision task, the verb "rose" should speed decisions for "stood," because the two words are similar in meaning and syntax; if the context is not used, there should be no time difference between the verb "stood" and the noun "flower." Several investigators have found that for the first few hundred milliseconds, the sentence context has no influence at all (Swinney, 1979; Tanenhaus, Carlson, & Seidenberg, 1985). Thus it seems as if lexical access is *autonomous* and *context-free* for a few hundred milliseconds. After this period, prior context does influence the choice of interpretation.

Lexical access seems to involve a specialized unconscious system that is not influenced by other processes. This system, which has presumably developed over many years of practice, seems to be "modular" (Tanenhaus, Carlson, & Seidenberg, 1985). It looks like another example of a highly specialized, unconscious processor that is separate both from voluntary control and from other unconscious specialists. Similar evidence has been found for the modularity of other components of reading, such as syntax, letter-to-phoneme mapping, and eye-movement control.

Notice how *un*consciousness and proficiency tend to go together. Specialized unconscious processors can be thought of as highly practiced and automatic skills. New skills are acquired only when existing skills do not work, and we tend to adapt existing skills to new tasks. Thus we usually have a *coalition* of processors, with mostly old subunits and some new components.

Automaticity often seems to be reversible; that is, just as predictability promotes automaticity, violations of predictability may re-create conscious access once again. We have already discussed the finding by Pani that practiced images, which disappear from consciousness when the task is easy, become conscious again when it is made more difficult. Probably subjects in Pani's imagery task could also use voluntary control to make the conscious images reappear. Although this is not widely investigated, informal demonstrations suggest that many automatized skills can become conscious again when they encounter some unpredictable obstacle.

Consider the example of reading upside-down. It is very likely that normal reading, which is mostly automatic and unconscious, involves letter identification and the use of surrounding context to infer the identity of letters. When we read a sentence upside-down, this is exactly what begins to happen *consciously*. For example:

> ˙ǝlʇʇoq ɹǝǝq ǝɥʇ uo ʞɹoɔ uʍop-ǝpᴉsdn ǝɥʇ ƃuᴉddod
> ʇᴉnb ǝʇᴉnb ʇou pᴉp ʎoq ɹǝdɐdsʍǝu pɐq ƃᴉq ǝɥʇ qoꓭ

This sentence was designed to have as many b's, d's, q's, and p's as possible, to create ambiguities that would be hard to resolve, and which therefore might need to be made conscious. In "newspaper" the reader may have used the syllable "news" to determine that the vertical stalks with circles were p's rather than b's, while the similar shape in "quite" may have been identified by the fact that q's in English are invariably followed by u's. This use of surrounding context is quite typical of the automatic reading process as well (Posner, 1982). It is well established, for example, that letters in a real-word context are recognized faster and more accurately than letters in a non-word context (Rumelhart & McClelland, 1982). The existence of deautomatization is one reason to believe that consciousness may be involved in debugging automatic processes that run into difficulties (Mandler, 1975a; see 10.3).

We turn now to another source of evidence for specialized unconscious processors, coming from the study of errors in perception, action, memory, and thought.

2 *Perceptual errors as evidence for specialized modules.* As we suggested above, perception is surely the premier domain of conscious experience. Nothing else can come close to it in richness of experience and accessibility. Ancient thinkers in Greece and India already argued for the five classical senses as separate systems that are integrated in some common domain of interaction. This is well illustrated by binocular interaction – "cooperation and competition" between visual input to the two eyes. Binocular interaction has been studied by psychologists for more than a century. Under normal conditions the slightly different perspectives from the two eyes fuse experientially, so that one sees a single scene in depth. This phenomenon led to the invention of the stereoscope, in which two separate slides, showing slightly offset images of the same scene, are presented to each eye. With increased disparity, the viewer is conscious of a very strong, almost surrealistic sense of depth, as if one could simply reach out and grasp the image. In the last century this dramatic effect made the stereoscope a popular parlor entertainment. But when the images in the two visual fields are incompatible, the two perspectives begin to compete, and one or the other must dominate. When they differ in time, space, or color, we get binocular

rivalry rather than binocular cooperation; fusion fails, and one image drives the other from consciousness. It is natural to think of all this in terms of cooperation or competition between two separable visual systems. Numerous other phenomena behave in this way, so that one can say generally that any two simultaneous stimuli can interact so as to fuse into a single experienced event; however, if the stimuli are too disparate in location, time of presentation, or quality, they will compete against each other for access to consciousness (Marks, 1978).

This analysis seems to emphasize the decomposability of perception. Historically there have been two contending views of perception: one that emphasized decomposability, and one that stressed the integrated nature of normal perception (Köhler, 1929; Mandler, 1983). The Gestalt psychologists were fervent advocates of the view that perception is not just the sum of its parts. In fact, these two conceptions need not be at odds. Modern theories involve both separate feature detection and integration (e.g., Rock, 1983; Rumelhart & McClelland, 1982). This book is based on the premise that perception and other conscious events are indeed decomposable, *and* that one major function of the system underlying consciousness is to unify these components into a single, coherent, integrated experience (Mandler, 1975a, b, 1983; Treisman & Gelade, 1980). Thus, as we pursue the issue of decomposable features here, we are by no means excluding the well-established Gestalt phenomena.

Clear evidence has emerged in recent decades for "feature detectors" in perception. The phonemes of English can be described by a small number of perceptual features, such as voicing, place, and manner. Thus the phonemes *b*, *d*, *g* are called "voiced," while *p*, *t*, *k* are "unvoiced." These are essentially perceptual features – they are not derived from analyzing the physical signal, but from studies of the experience of the speakers of the language. Linguists discover phonemes and their features by asking native speakers to contrast pairs of otherwise similar words, like "tore/door," "pad/bad," and so forth. At the acoustical and motor level these words differ in many thousands of ways, but at the level of phonemes there is a dramatic reduction for any language to an average of 25–30 phonemes; these in turn can be reduced to less than ten different feature dimensions.

A detailed study of sound and motor control in fluent speech shows that each feature is very complex, extremely variable between speakers, occasions, and linguistic contexts, and difficult to separate from other features (Liberman, Cooper, Shankweiler, & Studdert-Kennedy, 1967). For example, the *t* in "tore" is pronounced quite differently from the *t* in "motor" or in "rot." Yet English speakers consider these different sounds to belong to the same perceptual event. Confusions between phonemes in perception and short-term memory follow the features, so that *t*'s are confused with *d*'s far more often than they are confused with *l*'s (Miller, 1953). The complexity of phonemes below the level of perception implies that the neural detectors for these elements are not single neurons, but rather complex "processors" – populations of specialized neurons, which ultimately trigger a few abstract phonetic feature detectors.

Neurons that seem to act as feature detectors have been discovered in the visual system. The most famous work along these lines is by Hubel & Wiesel (1959), who found visual neurons in the cortex that are exclusively sensitive to line orientation, to a light center in a dark surround, or a dark center in a light surround. There are alternative ways to interpret this neurophysiological evidence, but the most widely accepted interpretation is that the neurons are feature detectors.

One argument against this approach is that features are demonstrably context-sensitive. For example, letters in the context of a word are easier to recognize than letters in a nonsense string (Rumelhart & McClelland, 1982). There are great numbers of demonstrations of this kind, showing that contextual information helps in detecting features at all levels and in all sensory systems (see Chapters 4 and 5). Thus features do not function in isolation. However, recent models of word perception combine features with contextual sensitivity, so that again, the ability to separate components and the ability to synthesize them are compatible with each other.

Some fascinating recent work shows that even "simple" visual percepts involve integration of different component systems. Treisman and Gelade (1980) give a number of empirical arguments for visual features, including the existence of perceptual errors in which features are switched. When people see rapid presentations of colored letters, they mistakenly switch colors between different letters (Treisman & Schmidt, 1982). In a very similar situation, Sagi and Julesz have shown that the location and orientation of short lines are often interchanged (1985). Analogous phenomena have been found in the auditory system.

All these facts suggest that perception can be viewed as the product of numerous highly specialized systems, interacting with each other to create an integrated conscious experience. Under some conditions this interaction seems to take up central limited capacity, a capacity that is closely associated with attention and conscious experience (see Chapter 2). For our purposes there are two cardinal facts to take into account: First, perceptual events result from decomposable specialized systems, or modules; and second, these systems interact in such a way that "the whole is different from the sum of its parts" (Köhler, 1929). One can point to several cases where such components seem to compete or cooperate for access to central limited capacity. These points can be generalized from perception to other psychological tasks, as we shall see next.

3 *Performance errors as evidence for specialized modules.* Slips are errors that we make *in spite of* knowing better. They are different from the mistakes that we make from ignorance. If we make a spoonerism, such as the Reverend Spooner's famous slip "our queer old dean" instead of "our dear old queen," the mistake is not due to ignorance – the correct information is available, but it fails to influence the act of speaking in time to make a difference. Thus slips of speech and action inherently involve a *dissociation* between what we do and what we know (Baars, 1985, in press, c). This is one reason to believe that slips always involve separable specialized processors.

Slips of speech and action generally show a pattern of decomposition along natural fault lines. Errors in speech almost always involve units like phonemes, words, stress patterns, or syntactic constituents – the standard units of language (Baars, in press, c; Fromkin, 1973, 1980). We do not splutter randomly in making these errors. This is another reason to think that actions are made up of these units, which sometimes fall apart along the natural lines of cleavage.

Action errors suggest the same sort of thing. For instance, many spontaneous action errors collected by Reason (1984) involve the insertion, deletion, or exchange of coherent subunits of an action. Consider the following examples:

1 "I went into my room intending to fetch a book. I took off my rings, looked in the mirror and came out again – without the book." (Deletion error)
2 "As I approached the turnstile on my way out of the library, I pulled out my wallet as if to pay – although no money was required." (Insertion error)
3 "During a morning in which there had been several knocks at my office door, the phone rang. I picked up the receiver and bellowed '*Come in*' at it." (Insertion error)
4 "Instead of opening a tin of Kit-E-Kat, I opened and offered my cat a tin of rice pudding." (Component exchange – a "behavioral spoonerism")
5 "In a hurried effort to finish the housework and have a bath, I put the plants meant for the lounge in the bedroom, and my underwear in the window of the lounge." (Component exchange)

In all five errors, action components are inserted, deleted, and exchanged in a smooth, normal, seemingly volitional fashion. This suggests that normal action may be organized in terms of such subunits – that is, actions may be made up of *modular* parts. Reason (1984) calls these modules the "action schemata," which, he writes, "can be independently activated, and behave in an energetic and highly competitive fashion to

---

1. Pragmatics: purposes of the speaker and listener.
2. Semantics: knowledge of the world.
3. Syntax: sequencing of meaning units.
4. Lexicon: identifying words and their meanings.
5. Morphemics: identifying meaningful affixes.
6. Phonemics: abstract classes of speech sounds.
7. Acoustics/Motorics: sound and speech control.

Figure 1.6. The standard linguistic hierarchy. The conventional structural hierarchy of linguistics suggests that there is a set of highly specialized and sophisticated but unconscious systems that control any level of language understanding and production. Thus pragmatics must include many motivational considerations for speaking or not speaking; semantics represents one's knowledge of the world; syntax is a remarkably complex system that controls the relationships between words and morphemes; and so on. Each linguistic level may be considered a specialized processor, and it may in turn consist of other specialized processors. Thus syntax, in many models, contains a Noun Phrase processor, which in turn may have a processor specialized in the very complex analysis of the English word "the" (see Winograd, 1972). Therefore the "language processor" consists of many levels, each of which has subsystems, which have their own subsystems, and so on. In technical language, the mental organization of language is *recursive*.

try to grab a piece of the action.'' That is to say, action schemata seem to compete for the privilege of participating in an action, to the point where they sometimes enter into the wrong context, as in errors (2)–(5) above. This claim is consistent with a widespread conviction that the detailed control of action is decentralized or "distributed," so that much of the control problem is handled by local processes (Arbib, 1980; Baars, 1980b, 1983; Greene, 1972; Gelfand, Gurfinkel, Fomin, & Tsetlin, 1971). It is also consistent with findings about the autonomy of highly practiced skills that have become automatized and largely unconscious. Normal actions, of course, combine many such highly practiced skills into a single, purposeful whole.

4 *Specialized modules in language processing.* It is widely believed that understanding a spoken sentence involves a series of structural levels of analysis, going from acoustic representations of the sound of the speaker's voice to a more abstract string of phonetic symbols; these symbol-strings specify words and morphemes, which are in turn codable in syntactic terms to represent the subject, predicate, and object of the sentence. This information is interpreted in the context of a complex representation of meaning, which permits inferences about the intentions of the speaker in saying the sentence (Figure 1.6). In recent years much progress has been made in understanding and simulating such fast,

symbolic, intelligent, rule-based systems (Jackendoff, 1987). Visual processing has been subjected to a similar analysis (e.g., Marr, 1982). In general, today the dominant approach to human language and visual processing involves a series of specialized modules, whose internal workings are to some extent isolated from the outside. Each level of analysis is very complex indeed. We have already considered lexical access, which involves all of the words in one's recognition vocabulary – perhaps 50,000 words for many people – plus the semantic relationships between them.

While the specialized levels are separable, they often need to work together in decoding a sentence, and not necessarily in a rigid, unvarying order. When a syntactic processor runs into an ambiguity it cannot resolve, it must be able to call upon the semantic processor for information (Reddy & Newell, 1974; Winograd, 1972). If we are given the ambiguous sentence "old men and women are delightful," we must use our best guess about the speaker's meaning to decide whether "old (men and women) are delightful" or "(old men) and women are delightful." Empirical evidence for this kind of cooperative interaction between different specialized systems has been found by Marslen-Wilson and Welsh (1978).

Thus the different specialized levels have a kind of separate existence; *and yet* they must be able to cooperate in analyzing some sentences as if they were one large, coherent system. This seems to be a general characteristic of specialized modules, that they can be decomposed and recomposed with great flexibility, depending on the task and context. Thus there may be different configurations of the linguistic hierarchy for speech analysis, speech production, linguistic matching tasks, etc.

We are certainly not conscious of such rapid and complex processes. Moreover, each of these specialized rule-systems must be *intelligent* in a reasonable sense of that word: It appears to be fast, efficient, complex, independent, symbolic, and functional. These are all aspects of what we usually call intelligence.

5 *Other sources of evidence for specialized processors.* Dissociation in memory offers additional evidence that specialized processors exist. There are many examples of dissociated access in memory, perhaps the most obvious is the "tip-of-the-tongue" phenomenon, in which a word that is readily available most of the time is frustratingly out of reach. There is some evidence that current states of mind, such as one's mood, will increase access to mood-relevant information and make it difficult to reach irrelevant material (Bower & Cohen, 1982). These differences can become extreme in hypnotic or post-traumatic amnesias, which do not involve a total *loss* of the original information, but a *loss of voluntary*

access to it (Jacoby & Witherspoon, 1982). Under some conditions these dissociated memories can be recovered. Indeed, most of our memory may consist of isolated islands of material.

One of the most interesting aspects of dissociation is the way in which automatic skills and islands of knowledge become unavailable to voluntary recall. Consider: In typing, which finger is used to type the letter *g*? Most people must consult their fingers to find out the answer, even if they have performed the action thousands of times; and indeed, in beginning to type, they may have known it quite voluntarily. As we gain automaticity in some skill, we also lose access to it in voluntary recall. Thus Langer and Imber found that after only a few trials of a letter-coding task, subjects reported a loss of consciousness of the task. Thereafter they could no longer report the number of steps in the task, and lost the ability to monitor their own effectiveness (Langer & Imber, 1979; see Chapter 7).

Finally, there is good evidence that knowledge is often fragmented. Cognitive scientists studying everyday knowledge have been surprised by the extent to which scientific reasoning by even very advanced students is lost when the same students are asked to explain everyday phenomena. This is well illustrated by a little puzzle presented by Hutchins (1980). Every educated person "knows" that the earth turns on its axis every day and travels around the sun during the year. Now imagine a man standing on top of a mountain at dawn, pointing at the sun just as it peeks above the eastern horizon. He remains on the same spot on the mountain all day, and at night as the sun is about to slip beneath the horizon in the West, he again points a hand, aimed exactly at the sun. Obviously we can draw one line from the man to the sun at dawn, and another from the man to the sun at sundown. The question then is: Where do the two lines intersect? Most people, including scientifically sophisticated people, seem to think the two lines intersect in the man, who has been standing on the same spot on the mountain all day. This answer is wrong: He has changed position, along with the mountain and the earth as a whole; he has moved even while standing still. It is the sun that has stayed in roughly the same position while the Earth turned, so that the two lines intersect in the sun only.

The fact that so many people cannot solve this little puzzle indicates that most of us have *two* schemata for thinking about the sun and the earth. When confronted with an educated question, we claim, certainly, that the earth rotates about its axis during the day. But when we take an earth-centered perspective we see the sun "traveling through the sky" during the day, and revert to a pre-Copernican theory. In this common-sense theory, the sun "rises" in the morning and "goes down" in the evening. There is nothing wrong with either perspective, of course. Each one serves us well very often. We only run into trouble when the two stories contradict each other, as they do in the little puzzle above. There is much more evidence along the same lines, that knowledge is actually quite fragmented, and that we switch smoothly between different schemas when it suits our purposes. (Notice, by the way, that the *contradictions* between the two accounts may cause us to make the problem conscious; without such contradictions we seem to go blithely along with several different schemas.)

In sum, there is evidence for separate functional units from neurophysiology, especially from the study of brain damage; and in psychology, from studies of the acquisition of automaticity of any practiced skill, of errors in perception, imagery, memory, action, language, and knowledge representation. All these sources of evidence suggest there are indeed many *intelligent, unconscious processors* in the nervous system.

1.4.5 General properties of specialized processors

Once having established the existence of specialized unconscious processors, we shall have very little to say about their inner workings. There is now a vast scientific literature about specialized processes in vision, language, memory, and motor control, which has made major strides in working out these details. In this book we cannot do justice to even one kind of unconscious specialist, and we will not try. Rather, we treat specialists here as the "bricks" for building an architecture of the nervous system, concentrating on the role of conscious experience in this architecture. Of course, we must give a general idea of what these bricks are like.

We can illustrate many elements that specialists have in common using the example of action schemata. Action schemata seem to be unitary at any one time. It makes sense to think that a complex action schema can often be called on *as a whole* to perform its function. In the act of leaping on a bicycle we cannot wait to gather the separate components of spatial orientation, control of the hands and feet, balance, and vision. Instead, we seem to call in an instant on a single "bicycle riding schema," one that will organize and unify all the components of bicycle riding.

However, in getting *off* the bicycle it makes sense to *decompose* the bicycle-riding schema, so that parts of it become available for use in standing, walking, and running. These other kinds of locomotion also require general skills like spatial orientation, motor control, balance, and vision. It makes sense to adapt general skills for use in a variety of similar actions. Further, if something goes wrong while we are riding the bicycle – if we lose a piece of the left pedal – we must be able to decompose the action-as-a-whole, in order to find the part of the bicycle-riding skill that must be altered to fix the problem.

Evidently we need two abilities that seem at odds with each other: the ability to call on complex functions in a unitary way, and *also* the ability to decompose and reorganize the same functions when the task or context changes. The first property we will call *functional unity*, and the second, *variable composition*. We will list these and other general properties next.

1   *Functional unity.* At any one time a coalition of processors that act in the service of some particular goal will tend to act as a single processor (Fodor, 1979; Rozin, 1976). That is, the coalition will have *cohesion* internally and *autonomy or dissociation* with respect to external constraints. This is sometimes called a high internal bandwidth of communication, and a low external bandwidth. Specialists are sometimes said to be *hierarchically* organized internally, though we will prefer the term *recursive*. That is, specialists are functionally nested or contained within other specialists. Presumably the bicycle-riding system contains a visual component, which in turn must have a control system for eye movements, and so on. These are defining properties of modularity.

2   *Distributed nature of the overall system.* If the nervous system can be thought to consist of large numbers of specialized processors, the details of processing are obviously not handled by some central control system, but by the specialists themselves.

3   *Variable composition.* Specialized processors are like Chinese puzzle boxes: They are *structured recursively*, so that a processor may consist of a coalition of processors, which in turn may also be a member of an even larger set of processors that can act as a single chunk. We should not expect to define a processor independently of task and context, though some tasks may be so common that they need generalized, relatively invariant processors.

4   *Limited adaptability.* Within narrow limits, specialized processors can adapt to novel input. One of the costs of specialization is that a syntax processor cannot do much with vision, and a motor processor is stumped when given a problem in arithmetic. But all processors must be able to change their parameters, and to dissociate and re-form into new processing coalitions (which then begin to behave as single processors) when conditions call for adaptation. We see this sort of reorganization when the visual field is experimentally rotated or transformed in dramatic ways,

when motor control is transformed by shifting from driving an automobile with a manual transmission to one with automatic transmission, or when a brain-damaged patient learns to achieve his goals by the use of new neuronal pathways (e.g., Luria, 1980). At a simpler level we see adaptation of specialized processors when a syllable like *ba* is repeated over and over again, and the distinctive-feature boundary between *ba* and *pa* shifts as a result (Eimas & Corbitt, 1973).

These points illustrate that processors may in part be *mismatch-driven.* That is to say, they must be able to adapt whenever the predictions they make about the world are violated, and it is even possible that many processors remain essentially passive unless such violations occur (see Chapter 5). We could speak of these processors as being mismatch-addressable.

5   *Goal-addressability.* While processors such as action schemata are unconscious and automatic, they appear to act *in the service of* goals that are sometimes consciously accessible. Indeed, action schemata can be labeled most naturally by the goal or subgoal which they appear to subserve. Performance error (1) in Section 1.4.4 is a failure of a goal that may be called "fetch book"; error (2) is an inappropriate execution of the goal "pull out wallet"; and so on. Each of these actions could be described in many different ways – in terms of physical movements, in terms of muscle groups, and so forth. But such descriptions would not capture the *error* very well. Only a description of the error in terms of goals met and goals unachieved reveals the fact that an error is an error. Thus, action schemata appear to be *goal-addressable*, though the goals are not necessarily conscious in detail. The fact that with biofeedback training one can gain voluntary control over essentially any population of neurons suggests that other functional processors are also goal-addressable (7.3).

6   *The unconscious and involuntary nature of specialized processors.* Control of specialized functions is rarely accessible to conscious introspection. Try wiggling your little finger. What is conscious about this? The answer seems to be, "remarkably little." We may have some kinesthetic feedback sensation; some sense of the moment of onset of the action; perhaps a fleeting image of the goal a moment before the action occurs. But there is no clear sense of commanding the act, no clear planning process, certainly no awareness of the details of action. Wiggling a finger seems simple enough, but its details are not conscious the way perceptual events are, such as the sight of a pencil or the sound of a

spoken word. Few people know where the muscles that move the little finger are located (they are not in the hand, but in the forearm). But that does not keep us from wiggling our fingers at will. No normal speaker of English has conscious knowledge of the movements of the jaw, lips, tongue, velum, glottis, and vocal cords that are needed to shape a single spoken syllable. It is remarkable how well we get along without retrievable conscious knowledge of our own routine actions. Greene (1972) calls this property *executive ignorance*, and maintains that it is true of many distributed control systems (see Chapter 7).

Section summary

We can sum up all these points by saying that specialists are *functionally unified* or *modular*. That means that detailed processing in the overall system is widely decentralized or *distributed*. Each module may be *variably composed and decomposed*, depending on the guiding goals and contexts. Specialized processors may be able to *adapt* to novel input, but only within narrow limits. Adaptation implies that specialized processors are sensitive to mismatches between their predictions and reality, that they are, in a sense, "mismatch-addressable." At least some specialists are also *goal-addressable*; perhaps all of them can be trained to be goal-directed by means of a conscious biofeedback signal. We are not conscious of the details of specialized processors, suggesting that executive control processes are relatively *ignorant* of specialized systems.

1.5 Some common themes in this book

The remainder of this book will be easier to understand if the reader is alert to the following themes.

1.5.1 Conscious experience reflects the operation of an underlying limited-capacity system

Conscious events always load nonspecific limited capacity, but not all limited-capacity events can be experienced consciously. There seem to be events that compete with clearly conscious ones for limited capacity, but which are not reportable in the way the reader's experience of *these words* is reportable. It appears therefore that conscious experience may be one "operating mode" of an underlying limited-capacity system; and that is indeed a reasonable way to interpret the Global Workspace architecture that we will develop in the next chapter. The question then is: "In addition to loading limited-capacity, what are the necessary conditions for conscious experience?'' We will suggest several during the course of this book, and summarize them in the final chapter.

1.5.2 Every conscious event is shaped by enduring unconscious systems that we will call "contexts"

This fundamental issue runs throughout this book. We treat a context as a relatively enduring system that shapes conscious experience, access, and control, without itself becoming conscious. The range of such contextual influences is simply enormous.

In knowing the visual world, we routinely assume that light shines from above. As a result, when we encounter an ambiguous scene, such as a photograph of moon craters, we tend to interpret them as bumps rather than hollows when the sun's rays come from the bottom of the photo (Rock, 1983). The assumed direction of the light is unconscious, of course, but it profoundly influences our conscious visual experience. There are many cases like this in language perception and production, in thinking, memory access, action control, and the like. The contrasts between unconscious systems that influence conscious events and the conscious experiences themselves provide demanding constraints on any theory of conscious experience.

Theoretically, we will treat contexts as coalitions of unconscious specialized processors that are *already committed* to a certain way of processing their information, and which have ready access to the Global Workspace. Thus they can compete against, or cooperate with, incoming global messages. There is no arbitrariness to the ready global access contexts are presumed to have. Privileged access to the Global Workspace simply results from a history of cooperation and competition with other contexts, culminating in a hierarchy of contexts that dominates normal access to the Global Workspace (4.3.2).

We may sometimes want to treat "context" not as a thing but as a relationship. We may want to say that the assumption that light comes from above "is contextual with respect to" the perception of concavity in photographs of the moon's craters (Rock, 1983) or that a certain implicit moral framework "is contextual with respect to" one's feelings of self-esteem. In some models context is a process or a relational event – part of the functioning of a network that may never be stated explicitly (Rumelhart & McClelland, 1982). In our approach we want to have contexts "stand out" so that we can talk about them and symbolize them in conceptual diagrams. There is no need to become fixated on whether context is a thing or a relationship. In either case contextual information is something unconscious that profoundly shapes whatever becomes conscious (4.0, 5.0).

1.5.3 Conscious percepts *and* images *are qualitative events, whereas consciously accessible* intentions, expectations, *and* concepts *involve nonqualitative contents*

As we indicated above (1.2.5), people report *qualitative* conscious experiences of percepts, mental images, feelings, and the like. In general, we can call these perceptual or imaginal. Qualitative events have experienced qualities like warmth, color, taste, size, discrete temporal beginnings and endings, and location in space. There is a class of representations that is not experienced like percepts or images, but which we will consider to be "conscious" when they can be accurately reported. Currently available beliefs, expectations, and intentions – in general, conceptual knowledge – provide *no* consistent qualitative experience (Natsoulas, 1982a). Yet qualitative and nonqualitative conscious events have much in common, so that it is useful to talk about both as "conscious." But how do we explain the difference?

Concepts, as opposed to percepts and images, allow us to get away from the limits of the perceptual here-and-now, and even from the imaginable here-and-now, into abstract domains of representation. Conceptual processes commonly *make use of* imagined events, but they are not the same as the images and inner speech that they may produce. Images are concrete, but concepts, being abstract, can represent the general case of some set of events. However, abstraction does not tell the whole story, because we can have expectations and "set" effects even with respect to concrete stimuli (e.g., Bruner & Potter, 1964; 4.0). Yet these expectations are not experienced as mental images. The opposition between qualitative and nonqualitative "conscious" events will provide a theme that will weave throughout the following chapters. Finally, in Chapter 7 we will suggest an answer to this puzzle, which any complete theory of consciousness must somehow address.

Both qualitative perceptual/imaginal events and nonqualitative "conceptual" events will be treated as conscious in this book. The important thing is to respect both similarities and differences as we go along, and ultimately to explain these as best we can (Chapters 4, 6, and 7).

1.5.4 Is there a lingua franca, *a trade language of the mind?*

If different processors have their own codes, is there a common code understood by all? Does any particular code have privileged status? Fodor

(1979) has suggested that there must be a *lingua mentis*, as it was called in medieval philosophy – a language of the mind. Further, at least one mental language must be a *lingua franca*, a trade language like Swahili, or English in many parts of the world. Processors with specialized local codes face a translation trade-off that is not unlike the one we find in international affairs. The United Nations delegate from the Fiji Islands can listen in the General Assembly to Chinese, Russian, French, or English versions of a speech; but none of these may be his or her speaking language. Translation is a chore, and a burden in other processes. Yet a failure to take on this chore presents the risk of failing to understand and communicate accurately to other specialized domains. This metaphor may not be far-fetched. Any system with local codes and global concerns faces such a trade-off.

We suggest later in this book that the special role of "qualitative" conscious contents – perception and imagination – may have something to do with this matter. In Chapter 2 we argue that conscious contents are broadcast very widely in the nervous system. This is one criterion for a *lingua franca*. Further, some conscious events are known to penetrate to otherwise inaccessible neural functions. For example, it was long believed that autonomic functions were quite independent from conscious control. One simply could not change heart rate, peristalsis, perspiration, and sexual arousal at will. But in the last decade two ways to gain conscious access to autonomic functions have been discovered. First, autonomic functions can be controlled by biofeedback training, at least temporarily. Biofeedback always involves conscious perceptual feedback from the autonomic event. Second, and even more interesting, these functions can be controlled by emotionally evocative mental images – visual, auditory, and somatic – which are, of course, also qualitative conscious events. We can increase heart rate simply by vividly imagining a fearful, sexually arousing, anger-inducing, or effortful event, and decrease it by imagining something peaceful, soothing, and supportive. The vividness of the mental image – its conscious, qualitative availability – seems to be a factor in gaining access to otherwise isolated parts of the nervous system.

Both of these phenomena provide support for the notion that conscious qualitative percepts and images are involved in a mental *lingua franca*. We suggest later in this book that all percepts and images convey spatio-temporal information, which is known to be processed by many different brain structures (6.5.2). Perceived and imagined events always reside in some mental place and time, so that the corresponding neural event must encode spatial and temporal information (Kosslyn, 1980). A spatio-temporal code may provide one *lingua franca* for the nervous system. Finally, we will suggest that even abstract concepts may evoke fleeting mental images (7.6.3).

*1.5.5 Are there fleeting "conscious" events that are difficult to
report, but that have observable effects?*

William James waged a vigorous war against the psychological unconscious, in part because he believed that there are rapid "conscious"
events we simply do not remember, and which in retrospect we believe
never to have been conscious. There is indeed good evidence that we
retrospectively underestimate our awareness of most events (Pope &
Singer, 1978). We know from the Sperling phenomenon (1.1.2) that people
can have fleeting access to many details in visual memory that they
cannot retrieve a fraction of a second later. Further, there are important
theoretical reasons to suppose that people may indeed have rapid,
hard-to-recall conscious "flashes," which have indirect observable effects (7.0). But making this notion testable is a problem.

There are other sources of support for the idea of fleeting conscious
events. In the tip-of-the-tongue phenomenon people often report a fleeting
conscious image of the missing word, "going by too quickly to grasp."
Often we feel sure that the momentary image *was* the missing word, and
indeed, if people in such a state are presented with the correct word, they
can recognize it very quickly and distinguish it from incorrect words,
suggesting that the fleeting conscious "flash" was indeed accurate
(Brown & McNeill, 1966). Any expert who is asked a novel question can
briefly review a great deal of information that is not entirely conscious,
but that can be made conscious at will, to answer the question. Thus a
chess master can give a quick, fairly accurate answer to the question,
"Did you ever see this configuration of chess pieces before?" (Newell &
Simon, 1972). Some of this quick review process may involve semicon-
scious images. And in the process of understanding an imageable sentence, we sometimes experience a fleeting mental image, flashing rapidly
across the Mind's Eye like a darting swallow silhouetted against the early
morning sky – just to illustrate the point.

One anecdotal source of information about conscious "flashes" comes
from highly creative people who have taken the trouble to pay attention
to their own fleeting mental processes. Albert Einstein was much interested in this topic, and discussed it often with his friend Max Wertheimer,
the Gestalt psychologist. In reply to an inquiry Einstein reported:

> The words or the language, as they are written or spoken, do not seem to play
> any role in my mechanism of thought. The psychical entities which seem to serve
> as elements in thought are *certain signs and more or less clear images which can
> be "voluntarily" reproduced and combined*. . . . This vague . . . combinatory
> play seems to be the essential feature in productive thought. . . . [These elements]
> are, in my case, of visual and some of muscular type. Conventional words or other
> signs have to be sought for laboriously only in a secondary stage, when the . . .

associative play is sufficiently established and can be reproduced at will. [But the initial stage is purely] visual and motor. (Ghiselin, 1952, p. 43; italics added).

About the turn of the century many psychologists tried to investigate the fleeting images that seem to accompany abstract thought. As Wood-worth and Schlossberg (1954) recall:

> When O's [Observers] were asked what *mental images* they had [while solving a simple problem] their reports showed much disagreement, as we should expect from the great individual differences found in the study of imagery. . . . Some reported visual images, some auditory, some kinesthetic, some verbal. Some reported vivid images, some mostly vague and scrappy ones. Some insisted that at the moment of a clear flash of thought they had no true images at all but only an awareness of some relationship or other "object" in [a] broad sense. Many psychologists would not accept testimony of this kind, which they said must be due to imperfect introspection. So arose the "imageless-thought" controversy which raged for some years and ended in a stalemate.

The possibility of fleeting conscious flashes raises difficult but important questions. Such events, if they exist, may not strictly meet our operational criterion of accurate, verifiable reports of experienced events. We may be able to test their existence indirectly with dual-task measures, to record momentary loading of limited capacity. And we may be able to show clear conscious flashes appearing and disappearing under well-defined circumstances. Pani's work (1982; 1.2.4) shows that with practice, mental images tend to become unconscious, even though the information in those images continues to be used to perform a matching task. Further, the images again become conscious and reportable when the task is made more difficult. Perhaps there is an intermediate stage where the images are more and more fleeting, but still momentarily conscious. People who are trained to notice such fleeting events may be able to report their existence more easily than those who ignore them – but how can we test the accuracy of their reports?

The evidence for fleeting glimpses of inner speech is weaker than the evidence for automatic visual images. Some clinical techniques based on the recovery of automatic thoughts are quite effective in treating clinical depression and anxiety (Beck, 1976). It is hard to prove, however, that the thoughts that patients *seem* to recover to explain sudden irrational sadness or anxiety, are *in fact* the true, underlying automatic thoughts. Perhaps patients make them up to rationalize their experience, to make it seem more understandable and controllable. In principle, however, it is possible to run an experiment much like Pani's to test the existence of automatic, fleetingly conscious thoughts.

In the remainder of this book we work to build a solid theoretical structure that strongly implies the existence of such fleeting "conscious" events. We will consequently predict their existence, pending the development of better tools for assessing them (7.0).

Should we call such quick flashes, if they exist, "conscious"? Some would argue that this is totally improper, and perhaps it is (B. Libet, personal communication). A better term might be *"rapid, potentially conscious, limited-capacity-loading events."* Ultimately, of course, the label matters less than the idea itself and its measurable consequences. This issue seems to complicate life at first, but it will appear later in this book to solve several interesting puzzles (Chapter 7).

1.6 Chapter summary and a look ahead

We have sketched an approach to the problem of understanding conscious experience. The basic method is to gather firmly established contrasts between comparable conscious and unconscious processes, and to use them to constrain theory. As we do this we shall find that the basic hypotheses used traditionally to describe the various aspects of conscious experience – the Activation Hypothesis, the Tip-of-the-Iceberg Hypothesis, the Novelty Hypothesis, and the Theater Hypothesis – are still very useful. All of the traditional hypotheses contain some truth. The whole truth may include all of them, and more.

In the next chapter we develop the evidence for our first approximation theory, Model 1 of the Global Workspace theory. After considering its neurophysiological implications in Chapter 3, we discover a need to add an explicit role for *unconscious contexts* in the shaping and direction of conscious experience (Chapters 4 and 5, Models 2 and 3). The discussion of unconscious guiding contexts leads to a natural theoretical conception of goal-directed activity and voluntary control (Chapters 6 and 7, Models 4 and 5), and finally to an integrated conception of attention, reflective consciousness, and self (Chapters 8 and 9). Chapter 10 sums up the adaptive functions of conscious experience, and the last chapter provides a short review of the entire book.

Part II

The basic model

In Chapter 2, we develop the basic theoretical metaphor of a global workspace operating in a distributed system of specialized processors. A first-approximation model (Model 1) based on these ideas is presented that fits a sizable subset of the evidence. The empirical constraints for Model 1 are provided by a contrastive analysis of the capabilities of comparable conscious and unconscious processes.

This simple model has only two theoretical constructs: a set of distributed specialized processors and a global workspace or "blackboard," which can be accessed by a consistent set of specialists and that can, in turn, broadcast information to all others. In spite of this simplicity, the model can explain all the contrastive facts detailed in this chapter. A number of additional findings support the hypothesis that conscious information may be broadcast very widely in the nervous system. We conclude by considering counterarguments and unanswered questions, specifying issues that must be addressed in later chapters.

Chapter 3 explores the natural neural interpretation of the global workspace metaphor found in the Extended Reticular-Thalamic Activating System (ERTAS) of the brain. Parts of the frontal and parietal cortex seem to control access to this system. We modify Model 1 to reflect changes suggested by the neuropsychology.

2 Model 1:
Conscious representations are *internally consistent* and *globally distributed*

> It seems that the human mind has first to construct forms independently before we can find them in things. . . . Knowledge cannot spring from experience alone, but only from a comparison of the inventions of the intellect with observed fact.
>
> *Albert Einstein,* 1949

2.0 Introduction

Almost everything we do, we do better unconsciously than consciously. In first learning a new skill we fumble, feel uncertain, and are conscious of many details of the action. Once the task is learned, sometimes after only a few repetitions, we lose consciousness of the details, forget the painful encounter with uncertainty, and sincerely wonder why beginners seem so slow and awkward. This pattern holds for everything from walking to knowledge of social relations, language acquisition, reading, and the skills involved in understanding this book.

These observations imply that we are unconscious of the complexity of whatever we know already. This is clearly true for high-level skills, like the reader's ability to process the syntax of a sentence. To grasp the meaning of a sentence, at least part of its syntax must be analyzed. The first small step in syntactic analysis involves assigning parts of speech to the words – nouns, verbs, pronouns, adjectives, and so on. Trying to do this deliberately, consciously, without paper and pencil, takes a great deal of time; it is a great burden on our immediate memory; it is prone to error and it interferes with other mental processes that are needed to understand the material. Conscious sentence parsing is hopelessly inefficient. But unconsciously we analyze hundreds of sentences every day, accurately and gracefully. This is true for all the skills that enable us to navigate through everyday life (La Berge, 1974; Langer & Imber, 1979; Pani, 1982; Shiffrin & Schneider, 1977). Any task improves with practice, and as it becomes more efficient it also becomes less consciously available. Thus anything we do well, we do largely unconsciously. But then what advantage is there to being conscious at all?

73

This chapter will focus on these kinds of questions, based on a contrastive consideration of the *capabilities* of conscious and unconscious functions. These capability contrasts (Table 2.1) provide the evidence for the core theoretical idea of this book: that conscious experience is closely associated with a *Global Workspace System*. A global workspace (GW) is an information exchange that allows specialized unconscious processors in the nervous system to interact with each other. It is analogous to a blackboard in a classroom, or to a television broadcasting station in a human community. Many unconscious specialists can compete or cooperate for access to the global workspace. Once having gained access, they can broadcast information to all other specialized processors that can understand the message.

The properties of a Global Workspace System fit the empirical capability contrasts very nicely, resulting in Model 1 (Figure 2.3). In this model, conscious events are simply those that take place in the global workspace; everything else in unconscious. We will have to modify this idea in future chapters, but the basic global workspace metaphor will serve us throughout the book.

Obviously Model 1 is only a first approximation, but a fruitful one. We explore its implications in some detail, looking at both input and output functions for the GW. For instance, does the claim that conscious contents are "globally distributed" mean literally that it is broadcast all over the central nervous system? We cite six sources of evidence in favor of this strong claim. Next, we point out that there may be systems that behave like Model 1, but which have somewhat different "hardware." Such functionally equivalent systems should not be excluded from consideration. Finally, we review similar proposals made in the cognitive and neurophysiological literature, make some testable predictions from the model, and point to some of its limitations – evidence that Model 1 cannot handle. These limitations suggest better models, which are developed in later chapters.

2.1 Contrasting the capabilities of conscious and unconscious processes

Table 2.1 presents our first major contrastive data set. Notice that we are comparing conscious process*es* with unconscious process*ors*. The reasons for that have been given in the previous chapter: There is good reason to think that unconscious functions are modular (1.4). Note also that the contrasts are not absolute. Conscious symbolic operations are not totally inefficient. Rather, in general the more efficiently some mental operation is handled, the more likely it is to be unconscious, and vice versa. We will now state each contrast formally, and discuss it in some detail.

Table 2.1. *Capabilities of comparable conscious and unconscious processes*

Capabilities of conscious processes	Capabilities of unconscious processors
1 Computationally inefficient: High number of errors, low speed, and mutual interference between conscious computations	1 Highly efficient in their own tasks: Low number of errors, high speed, and little mutual interference
2 Great range of different contents over time; great ability to relate different conscious contents to each other; great ability to relate conscious events to their unconscious contexts	2 Each specialized processor has limited range over time; each one is relatively isolated and autonomous
3 Have internal consistency, seriality, and limited capacity	3 Diverse, can operate in parallel, and together have great capacity

2.1.1 Conscious processes are computationally inefficient, but unconscious processors are highly efficient in their specialized tasks

Try to calculate (9 × 325)/4, doing each mental operation completely consciously. Or try to "diagram a sentence" consciously – assigning syntactic clause boundaries, word categories like noun, verb, adjective, etc., and deciding on the subject and object of the sentence. Probably no one can do even one of these symbolic operations completely consciously. Even linguists who have studied syntax for many years cannot parse a sentence consciously. The rare individuals who are extremely good at mental arithmetic have probably learned through long practice to do most computational steps automatically, with minimal conscious involvement.

Compared to similar unconscious processes, tasks performed consciously are slow, vulnerable to interference from other conscious or effortful mental processes, and hence prone to error. Consider each of these characteristics in turn:

The *speed* of conscious events is relatively slow. Simple reaction time (the time needed to give a single known response to a single known stimulus) is at best about 100 milliseconds (2.4.1). This is also the time region in which we experience perceptual fusion between physically different stimuli, and Blumenthal (1977) gives seven arguments in favor of the idea that the minimum "conscious moment" ranges around 100 milliseconds. In contrast, *un*conscious processes may take place at the speed of neural firing, ranging from 40 to 1000 times per second. In speech, when we say "bah," the vocal cords begin to vibrate before the lips open; when we say "pah" the order is reversed. The difference in this voice-onset time between "pah" and "bah" is about 20 milliseconds, much faster than conscious reaction time, and faster than the minimal integration time proposed by Blumenthal (1977). But of course we do not consciously control the details of the /pa/–/ba/ difference.

Conscious events are vulnerable to interference. Below we will make much of the remarkable fact that *any* conscious event can interfere with *any* other. Perceptual experiences in any sense modality interfere with those in any other. Any percept we experience will interfere with any mental image. Any mental image interferes with any simultaneous emotional or bodily feeling. Any of these experiences interfere with any voluntary, effortful action. And anything said in inner speech interferes with percepts, feelings, images, or mentally effortful actions. This fact is fundamental.

Unconscious processes, on the other hand, interfere with each less predictably. We have previously cited the lack of interference between automatic and voluntarily controlled skills (1.3.4) (Shiffrin, Dumais, & Schneider, 1981).

Finally, conscious events are prone to error. Even simple mental arithmetic is hard to do without error, much less conscious syntactic analysis, visual scene analysis, etc. This vulnerability to error is of great practical importance, since most airplane crashes, road accidents, and industrial disasters have a significant component of human error. Not all human errors are due to the limitations of consciousness – many are due to the rather different limitations of *un*conscious events, discussed in Chapter 1 and below (Reason, 1983, 1984). But conscious processing limitations are surely part of the problem.

By contrast to conscious limits, of course, unconscious processing of highly practiced, specialized functions is much more efficient.

Given this catalogue of woe about conscious processes, we may be tempted to ask, what good does it do? Should we give up consciousness if we had a choice? Or does it give the nervous system some selective advantage not provided by unconscious processes? The answer, fortunately, is yes. Consider the following points.

2.1.2 Conscious processes have a great range of
possible contents, but the range of any single unconscious
processor is limited

We can be conscious of an essentially endless range of possible contents: sensory and perceptual aspects of the world around us, internally generated images, dreams, inner speech, emotional feelings, pleasures, and pains. If we include conscious aspects of beliefs, concepts, and intentions, the range of possible contents becomes even greater. There is good evidence that we can gain a degree of conscious control over virtually any population of neurons, provided that we receive immediate conscious feedback from the neural activity (Chase, 1974; 2.5). Put all these things together, and it becomes clear that conscious contents can be involved in essentially *any* aspect of neural functioning. The range of conscious contents and involvements is simply enormous.

How do we know that *un*conscious processors tend to have limited range? One consideration is that specialization in general seems to lead to limitation. If there is an unconscious syntax processor, it is unlikely to be much good analyzing visual scenes. In Chapter 1 we cited several action errors collected by Reason (1983), as evidence for action schemata that are quite limited in their own ways, as shown by the stereotyped and mechanical quality of the errors. We can easily avoid these errors by remaining *conscious* of what we are doing. Langer and Imber (1979) have been able to induce mindless behavior by over-practicing people on a simple task, and found that once the task has been practiced to the point of being automatic and unconscious, the subjects can no longer accurately estimate the number of steps in the task. Further, subjects are much more willing than before to accept the false inference that they have performed poorly on the task, even when they have performed quite well! Obviously automaticity has its drawbacks.

These examples are revealing because they seem to show the functioning of unconscious components (specialized processors) without the intervention of conscious control. In each case, this functioning seems exceptionally "blind" because it seems to proceed in ignorance of apparently obvious changes in task and context. The overall pattern supports our basic contention that *unconscious processors have relatively limited range*.

The whole pattern makes sense if we consider the advantages and disadvantages of specialization. Clearly the main advantage of specialization is that one knows exactly what to do in a particular, routine situation. In computer language, one has a well worked-out *algorithm* for solving a particular problem. This off-the-shelf algorithm is unexcelled for its particular purpose, but it is likely to be useless for any other. The main drawback of specialization for routine tasks is a loss of *flexibility* in dealing with new situations.

Thus it seems that unconscious processors are excellent tools for dealing with whatever is known. Conscious capacity is called upon to deal with any degree of novelty. This leads directly to the next point.

2.1.3 Conscious processors have great relational capacity and context-sensitivity, but unconscious processors are relatively isolated and autonomous

The terms "relational capacity" and "context-sensitivity" are used here with very specific meanings. *Relational capacity* is used to refer to the ability to relate two conscious events to each other. Classical conditioning provides a good example. Here one conscious stimulus serves as a signal for another conscious stimulus – a bell may signal the coming of food, a light can signal an electrical shock, and so on. There is no natural connection between the bell and food, or between a light and shock. These relationships are arbitrary. Yet under the proper circumstances, any conscious stimulus can come to serve as a signal for the coming of a reinforcing stimulus.

What happens if one of the stimuli in classical conditioning is not conscious? Soviet researchers claim that Pavlovian association does not occur if the conditional stimulus has become habituated through repetition, so that it is no longer conscious (Razran, 1961). There is also good evidence to indicate that conditioning occurs in humans only when they have some consciously accessible idea of the relationship between the two stimuli. Dawson and Furedy (1976), in a brilliant series of experiments, used a tone in auditory noise to signal the coming of a moderate electrical shock. Ordinarily, people learn very rapidly that the tone signals shock, so that after several trials a rise in electrical skin-conductivity occurs as soon as the subject hears the warning tone. But now a different group of subjects was given the identical series of stimuli, and told a different story about the relationship between the tone-in-noise and the shock. The purpose of the experiment, they were told, was to see if people can detect a tone in background noise, and the function of the shock was only to mark the beginning of a new trial. (Subjects in experiments seem willing to believe almost anything.) Thus they were led to believe that *the shock may signal the coming of a tone,* not vice versa. Under these conditions classical conditioning of tone to shock never occurred, even with many repeated trials. Even though the subjects were conscious of both stimuli, they reinterpreted the relationship between tone and shock, and simply never learned that the tone signaled the coming of an electrical shock.

These findings suggest that for classical conditioning to occur, subjects must be conscious of *both* stimuli, and they must be conscious of the conditional relationship between the stimuli as well. If either of these components is lacking or unconscious, classical conditioning does not seem to take place. Only conscious functions seem to have the relational capacity to bring together two arbitrarily related stimuli; unconsciously we cannot apparently relate two novel, arbitrary stimuli to each other.

But consciousness has more than this kind of relational capacity; it also facilitates *context-sensitivity*.

"Context-sensitivity" is defined here as the way in which conscious events are shaped by unconscious factors. There are numerous examples of this (see Chapters 4 and 5). Perhaps the most obvious ones come from everyday examples of carrying out a routine action. When driving a car, we may take the same route every day, so that the predictable actions needed to drive become less conscious over time. If something new happens on the route from home to work, previously unconscious elements must become more conscious to adapt to the new situation. If we resolve one day to drive to the grocery store on the way home, we may suddenly find ourselves already home without having gone to the store, because we failed to be conscious of our goal at a critical intersection. Similarly, even if we know ahead of time that the road is blocked along our familiar route, that knowledge must become conscious in time to make the appropriate decisions to drive another way. In general, changes in context are not encoded automatically; they require consciousness. But once contextual information is encoded, it may control our routine actions and experiences without again becoming conscious.

Perception textbooks are filled with examples in which our conscious experiences are profoundly shaped by numerous unexpected unconscious factors (Gregory, 1966; Hochberg, 1964; Rock, 1983). For example, we live in a "carpentered" world, a world of rectangular surfaces and square corners. But we usually look at the surfaces aslant, so that our eyes receive *trapezoidal* projections, not rectangular ones (Figure 2.1). Each of these trapezoidal projections can result from an infinite set of rectangles or trapezoids, placed at different angles to the eye. What would happen if we were to look into a space that was made up of trapezoids, positioned in such a way as to cast the same retinal projections as a normal carpentered room?

Adelbert Ames (1953) first tried this experiment some fifty years ago, and found that people see the distorted space as a normal, rectangular room. The walls in a trapezoidal room are not of constant height, even though they seem to be constant, and it seems likely that the height of other objects is scaled relative to the nearest wall. What would happen if we observed someone walk back and forth in the Ames distorted room? The person is not changing height, while the walls, which seem of constant height, do change. Hence there is a perceptual conflict between the fact that human height does not change quickly, and the fact that walls are assumed not to change at all. The upshot is quite remarkable: People

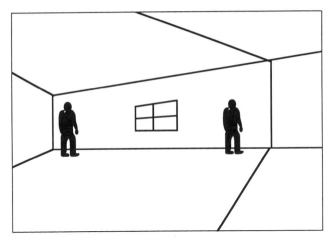

Figure 2.1. Trade-offs to maintain consistency in the Ames distorted room. The Ames distorted room provides one of many examples of trade-offs between competing factors to maintain internal consistency in conscious experience. The room appears to be rectangular, but is actually trapezoidal, and lower at one end than at the other. An individual walking back and forth in the room creates an internal conflict in the observer: Either the person is shrinking and growing, or the room must be distorted. Initially, the assumption of rectangularity is preserved, while the person is perceived to grow taller or shorter. If the observer then is allowed to toss a ping-pong ball against the opposite wall, perception is transformed; now the room is seen to be trapezoidal, and the person walking in it is experienced as constant in height (Allport, 1954). The pattern of trade-offs to maintain conscious consistency applies not just to vision, but to all conscious functions.

appear to grow and shrink dramatically as they walk to and from the observer (Figure 2.1).

As they walk toward the short end of the trapezoidal wall, their size in comparison to the perceived height of room may double, and as they walk toward the tall end of the trapezoid, they shrink in comparison. But why do we not see the room's actual proportions, and keep the perceived height of the people constant? For some reason the visual system seems "committed" to seeing the room as constant in height, and as a result, its only option is to interpret the person's height as changing. Clearly our conscious experience of the person in the Ames room is shaped by unconscious assumptions about the space in which he or she appears.

The pattern of trade-offs to maintain cognitive consistency applies not just to vision, but to all conscious functions. For example, one's consciously available idea of justice may be changed by seeing evil-doers escape punishment (Abelson, Aronson, McGuire, Newcomb, Rosenberg, & Tannenbaum, 1968). This tendency to maintain conscious consistency is also found in the well-known phenomenon of cognitive dissonance

(Festinger, 1957). Likewise, in visual imagery, if one imagines an elephant from a distance of 20 yards, and then a fly crawling on its ear, one will automatically "zoom in" on the fly; at that point, only a part of the elephant's ear is visible in the mind's eye. Thus, imaginary size and distance are kept in a consistent relationship (Kosslyn & Schwartz, 1981).

There are numerous other examples of this sensitivity of conscious contents to unconscious context. Our ability to comprehend a sentence in a conversation depends in great part on whether the new information in the sentence fits into what we take to be given in the conversation (Chafe, 1970; Clark & Haviland, 1977). But when we hear the new information, the givens are already unconscious; again, the unconscious context helps to shape the novel, conscious information. Our ability to learn any new information is critically dependent on prior, largely unconscious knowledge (e.g., Bransford, 1979).

Scholars who study changes or differences in knowledge are often acutely aware of the effects of unconscious presupposed context. An anthropologist studying a new culture is often forced to confront his or her own unconscious presuppositions, which may become conscious only in the encounter with a social world that violates them. And historians are well aware that each new age reinterprets the "same" past in accordance with its own presumptions, most of which are quite unconscious at the time they have this effect. Chapters 4 and 5 consider these context effects in detail.

All these examples indicate that unconscious expectations guide our conscious appreciation of the world. This is quite different from the "relational capacity" defined above, which involves relating two *conscious* events to each other. Context-sensitivity, as we use the term in this book, implies that all conscious experiences are constrained by unconscious context.

The contrasting claim about comparable unconscious events is that "unconscious processors are relatively isolated and autonomous." It is the unconscious processors that are presumably responsible for the very smooth and efficient actions cited in the action errors above, which are carried out perfectly well except for the fact that they are wildly inappropriate to the circumstances. These errors are often amusing because of the inappropriateness of the isolated action, which may be carried out perfectly even though its relevance and purpose are utterly lost.

Action errors all seem to involve either a failure to adjust to a change in the physical situation or a loss of the current task context. Getting up on a holiday and dressing for work is an error that involves a failure to access a new context. It seems that routine activities run off automatically, and adjusting to a new situation demands some conscious thought. Taking a can opener instead of scissors to cut some flowers seems to involve a loss of the current task context: We have "forgotten what we are doing."

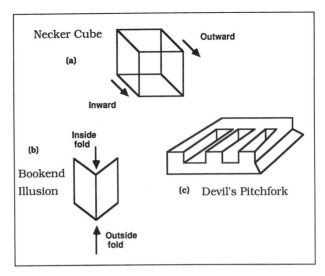

Figure 2.2. Conscious experiences are always internally consistent. These visual demonstrations seem to illustrate basic properties of conscious experience, which are not limited to vision: Very similar phenomena are found in all the senses, as well as in abstract knowledge. When a stimulus such as *a* or *b* has two different interpretations, only one can become conscious at a time, though there is evidence that the alternative interpretation continues to be represented unconsciously. Local ambiguity of this kind is extremely common in all sensory modalities, in language, abstract thought, etc. We seldom become aware of the numerous local ambiguities, because all input systems use context to resolve them (4.13). The "Devil's Pitchfork" is an "impossible" figure, one that has no single coherent interpretation; hence it is never experienced accurately as a whole. Typically, the experience of the impossible figure changes as the eye travels around it. All these facts suggest that conscious contents must be internally consistent.

2.1.4 Conscious experiences have internal consistency, but unconscious processors may be mutually contradictory

We have already pointed out (1.3.4) that selective attention always involves a densely *coherent* stream of events. We never mix up two streams of speech with different contents, or even with different vocal quality. It is generally true that conscious experiences are internally consistent. For example, the Necker Cube shown in Figure 2.2 can only be seen in one way at a time; each conscious interpretation is internally consistent. We never see a mix of the two conscious interpretations. For instance, we never see a corner in the front plane at a different depth than another corner in that plane, because to do so would violate the consistency constraint of a rigid, square cube.

These phenomena are well-known in perception, but they are not limited to perception. The same things are true at the conceptual level. Social psychologists for some decades have investigated cognitive consistency in value judgments and in person perception. Here, too, internal consistency is maintained (e.g., Abelson et al., 1968; Festinger, 1957). We cannot think of two alternative ideas at the very same instant, though we can consider two contradictory ideas one after the other. This becomes very clear when we consider ambiguous words: Most words have at least two different abstract, conceptual interpretations. It seems impossible for people to entertain two meanings of words like "turn," "look," or "book," at the same instant.

By contrast to conscious consistency, unconscious processors working at the same time may be mutually inconsistent. There is a great deal of evidence, for example, that the unconscious meaning of an ambiguous word is represented in the nervous system at the same time as the conscious meaning (Tannenhaus, Carlson, & Seidenberg, 1985). And the little puzzle discussed in section 1.4.1 about the man pointing at the sun at dawn and sundown also shows that we are perfectly capable of having two different and contradictory beliefs, as long as the contradiction does not become conscious (Hutchins, 1980). The effect of the puzzle is to make the contradiction conscious, and then we are in trouble. But unconscious contradictions are quite all right.

On to the next claim.

2.1.5 Conscious processors are serial, but unconscious processors can operate in parallel

There is much evidence for the seriality of conscious contents, but it is difficult to prove that the seriality is absolute. Conscious experience is one thing after another, a "stream of consciousness," as William James called it. Psychological theories that are largely confined to conscious processes, such as Newell and Simon's (1972) theory of human problem solving, postulate largely serial mechanisms. And, as Wundt observed in the 1880s, even two simultaneous conscious events are experienced either fused into a single experience or serially, one after the other. There is no such thing as true psychological simultaneity of two distinct events (Blumenthal, 1977).

Automaticity shows the close relationship between consciousness and seriality. As a skill becomes more and more practiced, it becomes less and less conscious; it can then also begin to operate independently from other processes, just as a parallel processor does (LaBerge, 1974, 1980; Shiffrin & Schneider, 1977; Sternberg, 1966). Conversely, when we interfere with an automatic skill so that it becomes "deautomatized," it will be more conscious, and it will be slower and more serial as well. However, at very fine time resolution, say the level of milliseconds, the seriality of conscious processes is not so clear. Just as a serial digital computer can simulate a parallel system simply by switching rapidly back and forth between different processes, so it is possible that some apparently parallel events are really controlled by a serial system (Anderson, 1983). For these reasons it is difficult to be absolutely sure about the seriality of consciousness. But it is clear that over a period of seconds and longer conscious events appear to be serial, while unconscious ones seem to work in parallel.

The claim here is that unconscious processors *can* operate in parallel, not that they must always do so (e.g., Banks & White, 1982; Sternberg, 1966). Indeed, if unconscious processors are required for a contingent series of decisions, it is hard to conceive how they could work in parallel: If A leads to B which leads to C, then A, B, and C must become available in that order. Thus the linguistic hierarchy discussed in a previous section may operate serially when there is no "top-down" information, even though the hierarchy is largely unconscious.

Further evidence for parallel unconscious processing comes from neurophysiology. As Thompson (1967) remarks, the organization and functioning of the brain "is suggestive of parallel processing." Many areas of the brain are active at the same time. Within the past few years, mathematical models of parallel processing have become available that cast light on the ways in which many of these neural systems could work, and several systems have been modeled in some detail (Grossberg, 1982; Rumelhart, McClelland, & the PDP Group, 1986).

Finally, there are some very important cases, like language comprehension, where evidence exists that unconscious language processors act in a "parallel-interactive" fashion (Marslen-Wilson & Welsh, 1978). Obviously when parallel processors interact with each other, they are no longer acting exactly in parallel (i.e., independently from each other). We suggest below that consciousness facilitates exactly this kind of parallel–interactive kind of processing.

But the simplest summary of the evidence is still the claim that conscious processes are serial, while unconscious processors can operate in parallel.

2.1.6 Conscious processes have limited capacity,
but unconscious processors, taken together,
have very great capacity

We have discussed (1.3.4) limited capacity in terms of three phenomena: (1) selective attention, in which one is conscious of only one of two demanding streams of information to the exclusion of the other; (2) dual-task paradigms, in which two conscious or voluntary tasks degrade each other; and (3) immediate memory studies, showing that only a very limited amount of novel or unorganized information can be retained. All three of these phenomena are associated with consciousness, though they are not identical to it.

There is one interesting counterargument to the notion of conscious limited capacity, and that is the case of a very rich perceptual scene. In looking at a football game with a stadium full of cheering sports fans, we seem to have an extremely complex visual experience, apparently full of detail, but apparently completely conscious. The key here is the internal organization of the football scene, the fact that each part of it helps to predict the rest. If instead we present people with an arbitrary number of small unrelated visual objects, and ask them to estimate the number in a single glance, visual perceptual capacity drops down again to about four to six items (Mandler & Shebo, 1982). In addition, we scan even a coherent scene with serial eye-movements, picking up a relatively small information with each fixation. Thus the complex scene is not necessarily in perceptual consciousness at any one time: We accumulate it over many serial fixations.

Thus conscious capacity does appear to be quite limited, as shown both by the selective attention experiments and by the limitations of short-term memory. What about the idea that unconscious processors "taken together have very great capacity"? This is obvious just from considering the size of the central nervous system. The cerebral cortex alone, taking up about half the volume of the cranium, contains on the order of 55 billion neurons, according to recent estimates (Mountcastle, 1978). Each neuron may have as many as 10,000 connections to other neurons. The interconnections between neurons are extremely dense – one can reach any neuron from any other neuron by passing through no more than six or seven intervening neurons. Each neuron fires on the average forty impulses per second, up to 1,000 when activated, and this activity continues in all parts of the brain, including those that are not currently conscious (Shevrin & Dickman, 1980).

This is by any standards a very large system. Viewed as an information processor, it is orders of magnitude larger than anything built so far by human beings. And clearly, most of its activities at any one moment are unconscious. Further, Long Term Memory, which has enormous capacity, is unconscious. The information-processing capacity of all the automatic skills learned over a lifetime is similarly great. And neurophysiologically, it is clear that the great bulk of brain activity at any single time is unconscious.

Why does this awesome system have such remarkable limitations of conscious capacity? There is something very paradoxical about these differences between conscious limitations and the huge unconscious processing capacity. Is this paradox a functional property of the nervous system, or is it somehow a mistake made by evolution? Later in this book we will suggest that humans have gained something valuable in return for our apparently limited conscious capacity (2.2, 10.0.1).

2.1.7 A summary of the evidence of Table 2.1

Before we begin to interpret the contrasts discussed so far, we will take a glance backwards. If one is willing to accept the vocabulary of information processing we apply here, speaking of conscious and unconscious "representations" and "processes," some facts can be established very clearly.

Conscious processes are computationally inefficient; they are relatively slow, awkward, and prone to error. But they involve an unlimited range of possible contents; any two conscious contents can be related to each other; and conscious contents are also profoundly shaped by unconscious contextual factors. Conscious experiences appear to be internally consistent; different ones appear serially; and there are rather narrow limits on our capacity to perform tasks that have conscious components.

On the other hand, unconscious processors seem to be highly efficient in their special tasks. Each unconscious processor seem to have a limited range, and it behaves relatively autonomously from the others. Unconscious processors are highly diverse and capable of mutual contradiction; can operate in parallel; and together have very great processing capacity.

In the following section we will suggest a theoretical metaphor to explain these observations. This metaphor greatly simplifies the diverse facts described above, combining them into only a few basic theoretical properties. Further, it suggests a functional interpretation for these facts, a selective advantage for having this kind of nervous system.

2.2   The basic model: A global workspace (blackboard) in a distributed system of intelligent information processors

In recent years computer scientists, psychologists, and some neuroscientists have become increasingly interested in distributed information-processing systems – systems that are really collections of intelligent, specialized processors. These systems are a hot topic of research in artificial intelligence (e.g., Erman & Lesser, 1975; Reddy & Newell, 1974), cognitive psychology (Rumelhart, McClelland, & the PDP Group,

1986), and neuroscience (Arbib, 1980; Grossberg, 1982; Mountcastle, 1978). They have been used to model the visual system, human memory, control of action, and speech perception and production. In a distributed system, numerous intelligent specialists can cooperate or compete in an effort to solve some common problem. Together, several specialists may perform better than any single processor can. This is especially true if the problem faced by the distributed system has no precedent, so that it must be handled in a novel way.

In a true distributed system there is no central executive – no single system assigns problems to the proper specialists, or commands them to carry out some task. For different jobs, different processors may behave as executives, sometimes handing off executive control to each other in a very flexible way. Control is essentially decentralized. The intelligent processors themselves retain the processing initiative – they decide what to take on and what to ignore. In a later chapter we will argue that the nervous system does have components that act as executives. But these executives operate in a fundamentally decentralized environment, much as a government may operate to regulate a market economy, which is still fundamentally decentralized.

But even without a true executive, a distributed collection of processors still needs some central facility through which the specialists can communicate w:th each other. This kind of central information exchange has been called a "global workspace," "blackboard," or "bulletin board" (Erman & Lesser, 1975; Hayes-Roth, 1984; Reddy & Newell, 1974). A "workspace" is just a memory in which different systems can perform operations, and the word "global" implies that symbols in this memory are distributed across a variety of processors (Figure 2.3). Each processor may have local variables and operations, but it can also be responsive to global symbols. This is discussed in more detail below.

Analogies will be used throughout this book. To make things a bit more comprehensible, we may speak of the global workspace as a television station, broadcasting information to a whole country. There is one especially apt analogy: a large committee of experts, enough to fill an auditorium. Suppose this assembly were called upon to solve a series of problems that could not be handled by any one expert alone. Various experts could agree or disagree on different parts of the problem, but there would be a problem of communication: Each expert can best understand and express what he or she means to say by using a technical jargon that may not be fully understood by all the other experts. One helpful step in solving this communication problem is to make public a *global* message on a large blackboard in front of the auditorium, so that in principle anyone can read the message and react. In fact, it would only be

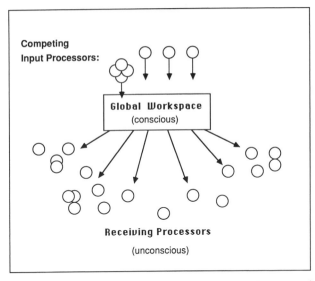

Figure 2.3. Model 1. A global workspace in a distributed system. A first-approximation Global Workspace model, showing the role of conscious limited-capacity mechanisms. The assumption is that the nervous system can be treated as a collection of specialized unconscious processors, including perceptual analyzers, output systems, action schemas, syntax systems, planning and control systems, etc. In general, these specialists are highly efficient in their own domains, but not outside of them. The system is fundamentally decentralized or "distributed." Interaction, coordination, and control of the unconscious specialists requires a central information exchange – a "global workspace." Input specialists can cooperate and compete for access to the workspace. In this case, a coalition of four input processors cooperates to place a global message. Once there, the message is broadcast to the system as a whole. This model accounts for the contrastive evidence shown in Table 2.1. (All future theoretical claims will be shown in this graphic format.)

read by experts who could understand it or parts of it, but one cannot know ahead of time who those experts are, so that it is necessary to make it potentially available to anyone in the audience.

At any time a number of experts may be trying to broadcast global messages, but the blackboard cannot accommodate all of the messages at the same time – different messages will often be mutually contradictory. So some of the experts may compete for access to the blackboard, and some of them may be cooperating in an effort to broadcast a global message. (Indeed, one effect of a global message may be to elicit cooperation from experts who would not otherwise know about it. Coalitions of experts can be established through the use of the blackboard.)

This sort of situation is common in human society. It describes fairly well the case of a legislature or a committee, or even a large scientific conference. Clearly this "system architecture" has both advantages and disadvantages. No one is likely to use it when the problem to be solved is simple and well understood, or when quick action is required. But it is not a bad way to do things when cooperation between otherwise separate knowledge sources is required, so that all viewpoints must be heard, when there is time to agree or disagree over possible solutions, and when the costs of making a mistake are greater than the benefits of a quick, makeshift action.

Given this brief description, we can now go back to the facts about conscious and unconscious processes shown in Table 2.1 to see if we have a theoretical metaphor that can simplify and make sense of those facts.

2.3   How the theoretical metaphor fits the evidence of Table 2.1

If we assume, as a first approximation, that messages on the blackboard are conscious and that the experts in the assembly hall correspond to unconscious processors, the fit between the model and the contrastive analysis in this chapter is quite close.

Take the first point of Table 2.1: Conscious processes are computationally inefficient. Committees and legislatures are not notoriously efficient in getting things done, because every action requires at least the tacit consent of many separate individuals. If something is to be done efficiently it is better done by a hierarchical organization like a bureaucracy, an army, or a police force. Committees and legislatures have some virtues, but speed and efficiency are not among them.

This point applies also to global processes in a large, distributed nervous system. Any global message is likely to involve a set of cooperating processors, and at least tacit cooperation from other processors that could interrupt the first set. This is very useful in dealing with a novel problem, one that does not have a known algorithm for its solution. Information from many knowledge sources may be combined to reach a solution. For example, Reddy and Newell (1974), and Erman and Lesser (1975) developed a distributed system called Hearsay to deal with the very difficult problem of speech recognition. A good deal is known about the ways in which sound waves can represent English phonemes – but not enough to determine the right phoneme for every sound. Indeed, as we have suggested above, it is may be that speech is simply locally ambiguous, so that there is no unique phonetic solution for every acoustical waveform. For this reason, Hearsay used a number of distributed specialists called "knowledge sources" cooperating and competing by means of the global workspace to arrive jointly at the best phonetic description of the sound.

In the rapidly developing field of machine speech recognition, the Hearsay system was quite good for its time: It was able to understand almost 1,000 words spoken by any male speaker in a normally noisy room, using an ordinary microphone. This was quite a bit better than most comparable systems were doing at the time.

The subsequent history of the Hearsay project is rather interesting. In working with the various expert knowledge sources used by Hearsay, the researchers discovered a way to improve the acoustic processor so that it could do predictive tracking of acoustical formants, the regions of the highest acoustical energy in the frequency spectrum. In other words, they discovered a successful algorithm that made it possible for the acoustical processor to solve problems that previously required cooperation from other processors, like syntax and semantics. Once this became clear, the team was able to dispense with the distributed architecture of Hearsay, since cooperative computation was less necessary. They developed a new system called Harpy based on the improved acoustical processor, which could do the same job in a more specialized way (Erman & Lesser, 1975). But from our point of view, Hearsay is actually more interesting as a psychological model than the specialized Harpy. Hearsay did not fail; rather, it succeeded as a development system, a stepping stone to a specialized algorithm for translating sounds into phonetic code.

There is a nice analogy between this history and the development of new human skills. When people start learning some new task, doing it takes a great deal of conscious processing. Apparently many functionally separate processors need to cooperate in new ways in order to perform the task. Over time, however, simpler means are found for reaching the same goal, and control over the task is relegated more and more to a single specialized processor (which may take components from existing processors). Thus the distributed "committee system" *should be* surpassed in the normal course of events by the development of a new expert system. This is certainly what we would expect to happen as a new skill becomes automatic and unconscious.

Thus the first point in Table 2.1, the computational inefficiency of consciousness, fits the model we are considering. Computations carried out entirely through the medium of the global workspace demand the tacit or active cooperation of all relevant processors. Naturally such a process takes much more time than a comparable process that is done exclusively by an expert system prepared to solve the problem by itself. But what about the contrasting point about unconscious processors? According to Table 2.1 "unconscious specialists are highly efficient in their own tasks." This is already assumed in the model we are discussing here, so this point also fits the model.

What about the second point in Table 2.1? "Conscious processes have great range, but unconscious processors have relatively limited range." If blackboard messages correspond to conscious contents, then they must range as widely as do the distributed processors that are able to place a message on the blackboard. Thus the range of messages in the global workspace is very great, while the range of information processed locally by any individual processor must be more restricted.

Further, conscious processes have great relational capacity and context sensitivity. Relational capacity is defined as the ability to relate different conscious contents to each other. Obviously, several blackboard messages could be related to each other, especially if some expert were alert to such relationships, and if several messages occurred close together in time. (We will defer discussion of context sensitivity, the shaping of conscious contents by unconscious factors, until Chapter 4.) Contrastively, on this point, unconscious processors are "relatively isolated and autonomous." This is assumed, of course, in the very nature of a distributed system. So far, the fit between the model and the data to be explained is very close.

What about the internal consistency of conscious contents? This fits well also, because blackboard messages require at least tacit cooperation from the audience of experts. If some global message immediately ran into powerful competition, it could not stay on the blackboard. And what about the contrastive point that unconscious processors are highly diverse? This, too, is already inherent in the idea of distributed system of expert systems. So far, so good.

Table 2.1 further claims that conscious processes are serial. This follows directly from the requirement that they be internally consistent – different messages, those which cannot be unified into a single message, can only be shown one after the other. Thus we cannot see two objects occupying the same location in space at the same time, as we would have to, to interpret the Necker Cube in two different ways simultaneously. The blackboard portion of the system is therefore forced into seriality. But unconscious processors "can operate in parallel." This, too, is already inherent in our model.

Finally, "conscious processes have limited capacity." This feature also flows from the internal consistency requirement. If any global message must be internally consistent, one must exclude irrelevant or contradictory messages that may come up at the same time. Such irrelevant or contradictory messages are likely to exist somewhere in some of the distributed processors, and are therefore a part of the system. But they cannot gain access to the blackboard, unless they can drive off the current message, or unless it leaves the blackboard of its own accord. Hence unconscious processors, taken together, have very great capacity and can be doing many things locally at the same time, provided these local processes do not require access to the global workspace.

In conclusion, we can now replace all of the facts described in Table 2.1 with a rather simple model: the idea of a set of specialized processors, each well equipped to handle its own special job; all the specialists can communicate with the other through a global workspace. In this way they can cooperate and compete with each other, to strengthen or weaken a global message.

Like consciousness itself, this system works best when routine tasks are directly delegated to the best expert that is ready to solve it, and the use of the blackboard is reserved for just those problems that cannot be solved by any expert acting alone. When the cooperating processors discover a single algorithm able to solve the problem, that algorithm can again be handled by a single expert, freeing up limited global capacity for other unsolved problems.

2.3.1 When is a Global Workspace system useful?

The main use of a GW system is to solve problems that any single expert cannot solve by itself – problems whose solutions are *under*determined. Human beings encounter such problems in any domain that is novel, degraded, or ambiguous. This is obvious when we are faced with novelty: If we are just learning to ride a bicycle, or to understand a new language, we have inadequate information by definition. Further, if the information we normally use to solve a known problem becomes degraded, determinate solutions again become indeterminate. So much is clear. What may not be so obvious is that there are problems that are inherently ambiguous, in which all the local pieces of information can be interpreted in more than one way, so that we need to unify different interpretations to arrive at a single, coherent understanding of the information.

This kind of inherent ambiguity is often found in language processing and even in visual perception (e.g., Marr, 1980; Rock 1983). We discuss the prevalence of local ambiguity in the world of perception, action, language, and thought in Chapter 4. Briefly, the argument is that any highly localized, restricted amount of information tends to have more than a single interpretation. Since we often must deal with local, restricted information, ambiguities must be resolved by reference to new and unpredictable information. The global workspace architecture is designed precisely to allow resolution of ambiguity by unpredictable knowledge sources.

A further use of a global workspace is to *update* many specialized processors at the same time. Updating is necessary not merely to remember where one's car is parked, but also to track changes in social relations, perceptual conditions, and the like. There is good evidence that social perception can be changed by a single conscious experience (Levicki, 1986) and, similarly, phoneme perception is known to be changed by recent experiences (Eimas & Corbitt, 1973).

2.3.2 Cooperative computation: An illustration

We can illustrate this process in a slightly fanciful way by imagining the different language experts communicating to analyze a children's language game, based on a junctional ambiguity, "I scream, you scream, we all scream for ice cream." Suppose that the sound is consciously perceived, and globally displayed, as the following string:

AYSKREEMYOOSKREEMWEYALSKREEMFRAYSKREEM

This is quite realistic, because there are no physical gaps between most words in ordinary speech. (Most of the word boundaries we *seem* to hear are perceptual, not physical.) Now let us imagine a conversation between several experts trying cooperatively to understand this string.

LEXICAL PROCESSOR: Looking at the first syllable, I can make out a couple of possibilities. The phoneme A could be the exclamation "ah!"; AY could be "I", AYS could be "ice"; AYSK is not in my lexicon, nor is AYSKR.

SYNTACTIC PROCESSOR: If the first syllable is the start of an exclamation "ah!", I predict another exclamatory word, or the beginning of a new sentence. If it is "I", I predict a verb phrase with an active first-person verb, or much less probably a subordinate clause. If the first syllable is "ice" it would be an unusual way to start a sentence, though it could be a generic noun. Highest probability: "I."

LEXICON: OK, let's assume it's "I." Next syllable, SKREE or SKREEM. "Scree" is very rare, "scream" is possible.

SYNTAX: "Scream" is an active, first-person verb, as predicted. Most likely, the next word will be the preposition "at," which will start a noun phrase with the object of the verb.

SEMANTICS: "I scream" is indicative of excitement, usually due to fear.

LEXICON: Assuming the analysis is on the right track so far, the next syllable is YOO ("you") or YOOS ("use"), but not YOOSK or YOOSKR.

SYNTAX: Surprise! Neither "you" nor "use" is the expected preposition "at"; therefore I'm changing my prediction about a coming noun phrase. "I scream" must be treated as a separate clause, or we're doing this all wrong. If so, then "you" could start the next clause, with the optional copula "and" being understood. If so, we should get a verb phrase next, with an active first-person verb.

LEXICON: OK, let's assume it's "you"; then the next syllable is SKREE or SKREEM as before. "Scree" is rare, "scream" is predicted.

SYNTAX: "You scream" is a well-formed formula.

SEMANTICS: "I scream, you scream" indicates a lot of excitement, probably due to fear.

PRAGMATICS: What is this speaker trying to tell me? I am not screaming.

COUNTERFACTUAL ASSERTION: Look out for possible joke or language game.

LEXICON: Next syllable is WE, WEY, WEYA, or WEYAL – only "we" is in my vocabulary. We and WEY could be alternative strings for the same word, since WE is followed by a vowel, and Y is often used as a transition before a vowel.

SYNTAX: I'm beginning to see a pattern here. We could be getting a series of clauses consisting of subject–predicate pairs, strung together without copulas. If so, I predict the next word will be another first-person action verb.

SEMANTICS: If so, the next verb should have something to do with excitement, possibly fear. "I scream, you scream, we . . . what?"

LEXICON: Assuming we are OK so far, next syllable is YAL or AL. "All" is in my vocabulary.

SEMANTICS: OK, "all" makes sense after the plural "we."

SYNTAX: Not quite what I expected, but it could be part of the subject noun phrase. Next, I predict a verb phrase with an active first-person verb.

SEMANTICS: OK, that fits "we."

LEXICON: Looking for parallels as suggested, the next word SCREEM is "scream" again. This is getting boring.

SYNTAX: Just as I expected.

SEMANTICS: Just as I expected. "I scream, you scream, we all scream." More excitement, possibly fear.

PRAGMATICS: Don't trust the predictions too much. Watch out for a tricky language game!

LEXICON: Next syllable could be FRA, FRAY, or if the vowel is reduced, FOR. "Fry" and "for" are in my vocabulary.

SYNTAX: I vote for "for," now expecting an object noun phrase.

SEMANTICS: Finally, we find out what this is all about. "We all scream for . . ." what?

LEXICON: Same string as before A, AY, or AYS. Predict AY on the basis of previous pattern.

SYNTAX: Sorry, "I" is not an object noun.

LEXICON: Well, going back a bit, "for" could mean "because," but that is archaic and unlikely. How about "ice"?

SYNTAX: OK, let's try it. If there is any more to this sentence, I predict it will be the remainder of the object noun phrase.

LEXICON: Assuming we are OK so far, the next syllable is KREE, or KREEM; only KREEM is in my vocabulary as "cream."

SEMANTICS: "I scream, you scream, we all scream for ice cream." "Ice cream" is a food-stuff much appreciated by young humans, who stuff it in a hole in the middle of their faces. Previous use of "scream" three times could be indicative of excitement about ice cream, though the style is distinctly hyperbolic. Note repetition of the same pattern three times.

LEXICON: No, four times, given the phonetic identity of KREEM, and the fact that the string AYSKREEM has two distinct readings.

PRAGMATICS: See, told you, it's a language game. Presumably humorous.

FACIAL PROCESSOR: Please initiate a small smile.

Notice how the cooperating and competitive hypotheses generated by these very different expert systems help to solve quite a complex problem. The sameness of "I scream" and "ice cream" never presented any real problem to this system, because syntax predicted "I scream" for the first occurrence of AYSKREEM; similarly, syntax predicted a noun phrase like "ice cream" for the second occurrence. The Hearsay system used a global workspace to communicate hypotheses back and forth, but more direct channels might also be used. The advantage of a global workspace is that it permits rule-systems *whose relevance cannot be known ahead of time* to participate in solving the problem. The more novelty and ambiguity there is to be resolved, the more useful it is to have a global workspace.

Notice that the conscious outcome of this process is not a simple fusion of elementary features, but rather an intelligent *construction* of the input that goes beyond any input component and beyond any single processor (Mandler, 1983, 1984; Marcel, 1983a, see. 1.3.5).

2.3.3 Spreading activation and inhibition to carry out cooperative and competitive processing

There are several ways to carry out this notion of cooperative processing in detail. One method that is currently very promising involves the spread of activation in a network (e.g., Rumelhart & McClelland, 1982). Processing in the GW model can also use activation; in practice, this means assigning a number to different potentially conscious messages to show the likelihood of their becoming conscious. In the example above, the acoustic processor can display its hypothesis on the global workspace. Syntax, semantics, the lexicon, and others can then add or subtract activation from this hypothesis. If the activation falls below a certain level, or if some alternative gathers more activation, the current acoustic hypothesis fades from the GW and is replaced by a more popular one. This is processing as a popularity voting contest.

We have previously suggested that high activation may be a necessary but not sufficient condition for conscious experience (1.3.1). We can now add the idea that activation may be contributed by many cooperating processors, adding to the vote for the current content, to keep it on the blackboard.

2.4   Input properties of the global workspace

We can suggest a few input properties of the conscious global workspace. First, we emphasize, as in Chapter 1, that relatively long-lasting conscious contents seem heavily biased toward perception and imagery (and imagery resembles perception). Further, it seems that the minimal conscious integration time is approximately 100 milliseconds. The details follow.

2.4.1 *Conscious experience has a strong perceptual bias*

Consciousness is not identical to perception, but perception is certainly the premier domain of detailed conscious experience. In later chapters we will argue that conscious access to abstract concepts, and even conscious control of action, may be mediated through rapid, quasi-perceptual events (7.0). If that is true, then the "language" of GW input systems may be perceptual (1.2.4).

2.4.2 *The conscious moment: Temporal limits on conscious stimulus integration*

Several temporal parameters are associated with conscious experience. Short Term Memory seems to involve maximum retrieval times on the order of ten seconds without rehearsal (Simon, 1969), and there is evidence for an 0.5-second lag time between sensory input and conscious appreciation of a stimulus (Libet, 1978, 1981; Figure 2.4). Here we are mainly concerned with the "cycle time" of the conscious component, presumably the global workspace. Most of the evidence for such a cycle time comes from studies of perceptual integration. Blumenthal (1977) presents a remarkable synthesis of the vast perceptual literature on the psychological moment. He argues that "Rapid attentional integrations form immediate experience; the integration intervals vary from approximately 50 to 250 milliseconds, with the most common observation being about 100 milliseconds."

Blumenthal's excellent summary of the evidence for this integration interval is worth quoting in full:

    1 *Time–Intensity Relations.* Within the integration interval there is a reciprocity of time and experience. A mental impression is integrated and formed over this duration. Several faint stimuli occurring within the interval may be summed to the mental impression of one intense stimulus. If events should somehow be cut off midway through the integration, our impression of them will be only partially or incompletely formed.

    2 *Central Masking.* When two or more events that cannot be easily integrated occur within an integration interval, the process may develop or form impressions for some events and reject others.

3   Apparent Movement. Two spatially as well as temporally separate
    stimuli that fall within an integration interval may again be fused, or
    integrated, to a unitary impression. Because of their spatial separation,
    however, they will be experienced as one object in motion between the
    two locations.
4   *Temporal Numerosity and Simultaneity.* In any sequence of rapidly
    intermittent events, intermittency can be experienced at rates no faster
    than approximately 10 events per second. This is a limit on the rate of
    human cognitive performances in general.
5   *Refractory Period and Prior Entry.* Sometimes when two events occur in
    the same integration interval and are neither fused nor masked, one
    event will be delayed and integrated by a succeeding pulse of attention.
    It will thus appear to be displaced in time away from its true time of
    occurrence. If two responses must be made, one to each of two rapidly
    successive events, the second response is delayed for the duration of a
    rapid integration interval.
6   *Memory Scanning.* Impressions that are held in Short Term Memory can
    be scanned no faster than the rate determined by the attentional
    integration process. In searches of logically structured information held
    in long-term memory, the scan through chains of associations proceeds
    at the rate of the attentional integration process – about 75–100 msec for
    each node in the chain.
7   *Stroboscopic Enhancement.* In an otherwise unstructured stimulus envi-
    ronment, an intermittent stimulus (such as a flashing light) that pulses at
    a rate of about 10 per second can drive the rapid attentional integration
    process to exaggerated levels of constructive activity so as to produce
    hallucinatory phenomena.

The most straightforward interpretation of these findings is that perceptual specialists can cooperate and compete within the rough 100-msec
period, but that longer intervals between them do not allow them to
interact to create a single, integrated experience.

There is a problem with 100-msec period: Some competition for access
to limited capacity mechanisms takes much longer than that. For example, we may have conscious indecision, considering this side and that of
a difficult question. Such indecision may take seconds, minutes, or hours;
it does seem to involve a kind of slow competition for access to conscious
experience (7.0). Usually after a decision is made, only one perspective
will continue to have access to consciousness. One hundred milliseconds
is an absurdly short time to allow two different thoughts to compete for
access to consciousness, or to decide between two different courses of
action. We will suggest in Chapters 4 and 5 that these kinds of competition
for limited capacity involve competition between the *contexts* of immediate experience, rather than between instantaneous qualitative conscious
events.

It is good to put this in a larger perspective. Figure 2.4 presents a
number of time parameters associated with conscious experience.

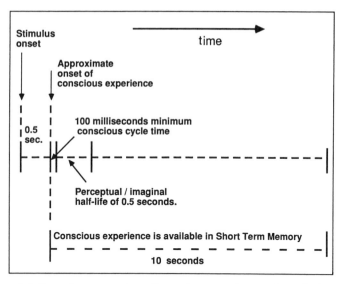

Figure 2.4. Some time parameters of conscious experience and recall. A proto-typical conscious experience may start with a perceptual stimulus, which may take as long as 0.5 seconds to become conscious (Libet, 1978). Neurophysiolo-gical findings indicate that this period can be further subdivided into an early stage, focused on the more concrete properties of the stimulus and lasting about 200 msec. and a later, abstract stage that peaks at about 300 msec. Minimum duration of a conscious experience (cycle time) may be about 50–250 msec modally about 100 msec according to estimates by Blumenthal (1977) and others, based on perceptual fusion time. A rapid, isolated conscious event has a half-life of approximately 0.5 seconds, depending upon a number of factors. If it fits within Short Term Memory limits, it can still be retrieved for about 10 seconds, according to estimates by Simon (1969). This time can be extended if the conscious event is refreshed by rehearsal.

2.4.3 The Threshold Paradox

The reader may already have noticed a problem with our approach so far. Namely, in order to recruit a coalition of specialized processors to work on some global message, we must broadcast it. But it needs the help of other systems to become a global message in the first place. How then can a message gain access to the global workspace if it does not already have a set of other systems supporting it? How does it cross the threshold of conscious access? This is not unlike the problem faced by a budding young artist or writer. In order to get public interest, one needs to show that the work has appeal. But one cannot show that unless the work has been shown to the public.

   This Threshold Paradox may be quite serious for our model, and may demand some change. In general, there are two solutions. First, it may be that there is a hierarchy of workspaces of increasingly global reach. At lower levels there may be broadcasting across some systems, but not all; at higher levels, there may be truly global broadcasting. This would allow new messages to recruit an increasing number of supportive systems, until ultimately it is broadcast globally. We can call this the Waiting Room Hypothesis, as if there were a series of waiting rooms, each closer to the global broadcasting facility. In the same way the budding artist can show his or her work to increasingly large and influential groups of people, who then may make it possible to come closer and closer to true public acceptance.

   There is another option. It is conceivable that all systems clamoring for conscious access may receive momentary global access, but for too short a time to be reported consciously. Each instant of access may allow the recruitment of additional supportive systems. The more systems are recruited, the more likely it is that the message will remain on the global workspace long enough to be perceived and recalled as a conscious event. In this way a new message may gain more and more support, and increase its likelihood of being held long enough to be reportable. This may be called the Momentary Access Hypothesis.

   The Threshold Paradox leads to a theoretical choice-point that we cannot entirely resolve at the present time. Indeed, both options may be true. They are both consistent with the finding that conscious access may take as long as 0.5 seconds (Libet, 1978, 1981). We will suggest in Chapter 3 that the neurophysiological evidence supports a "snowballing" development of access to consciousness, rather than an instantaneous process. The temporal factor may seem to support the Momentary Access option, but in fact the Waiting Room option presumably takes time as well. We do not have the evidence at this point to choose between them.

2.5   Output properties of the global workspace: How global is global?

Once a specialized system gains access to the global workspace, what does it gain? In everyday language the word "global" means "worldwide" or "relating to the whole of something," but in computational parlance its meaning is more specific. A *global variable* is one that is defined for all subsystems of a larger system, as opposed to *local* variables, which are only defined for a single subsystem. If the entire system has three parts, a global variable can be recognized in all three. Thus access to a global workspace implies access to the larger system as a whole.

Things get a lot more interesting if we consider that the nervous system has a very large number of processors, many of which can themselves be decomposed into subproccessors. A truly global variable in the nervous system might be distributed in principle to all levels of all processors, perhaps down to the level of single cells. Thus one question we can ask is, "How widely is global information distributed"? Is it made available to just a few specialists? Or is there evidence that in the nervous system, "global information" is really broadcast throughout?

Several sources of evidence suggest that conscious events have very wide distribution in the nervous system. Consider:

1 Any *conscious or effortful task competes with* any other.

We can call this the "any" argument. Perceiving a single star on a dark night interferes with the voluntary control of a single motor unit in one's thumb; the consciousness of the letters in this sentence will interfere with conscious access to the meaning of this chapter. Indeed, being conscious of *any* stimulus in *any* sense modality interferes with consciousness of *any* other stimulus, and also with conscious access to *any* voluntary act or conceptual process. When these same events are unconscious and involuntary they usually do not interfere at all. If we believe that the nervous system consists of many specialized systems that decide by their own criteria what information to process, it follows that even relatively small systems – like those needed to see a single star on a dark night or to control a single muscle fiber – must somehow have access to the conscious system.

One can extend the "any" argument to other cases. Psychophysicists have used the technique of "cross-modality matching" for decades now, showing that any stimulus in any modality can be compared in intensity with any other stimulus in any other modality – and the result is not chaos, but some of the most elegant and mathematically regular data found in psychological research (Stevens, 1966). Research on classical conditioning indicates that within wide biological limits (Garcia & Koelling, 1966) very many different stimuli can come to signal the appearance of a great variety of other stimuli, even if there is no natural connection between them. The strength of classical conditioning is greatly increased when there is a natural, biological connection between the conditioned and unconditioned stimulus. But the fact that classical conditioning can occur at all between a tone and shock, which are not biologically related, suggests a capacity for some arbitrary connections. In the following subsection, we will explore in detail the related finding that one can apparently gain novel voluntary control, at least temporarily, of *any* neural system with the help of biofeedback training (Chase, 1974). In humans, *any* stimulus can serve as a signal to perform *any* voluntary act. In language comprehension, when one encounters ambiguities – which are rife at every level of language – influences from almost *any* contextual factor can serve to resolve *any* ambiguity (4.0) – and so on. The *any* argument applies in a number of domains, and always implies the existence of some integrative capability, one that allows very different specialized systems to interact.

If the brain equivalent of a global workspace is truly global, it should be true that any brain event that is conscious or under conscious control can interact with any other event, no matter how different. It seems difficult to explain this without something like a truly global workspace. Consider now the case of biofeedback training.

2   Conscious feedback can be used to gain a degree of voluntary control over essentially *any* *neural event*.

It is not emphasized often enough that biofeedback training *always* involves conscious information. To gain control over alpha waves in the EEG, we sound a tone or turn on a light whenever the alpha waves appear; to gain control over muscular activity we may play back to the subject the sound of the muscle units firing over a loudspeaker; and so on (Buchwald, 1974; Chase, 1974). This is not to say, of course, that we are conscious of the details of action – rather, we must be conscious of some feedback from the action to establish voluntary control. In terms of the Global Workspace theory, establishing biofeedback control requires that we "broadcast" the conscious feedback in some way.

With conscious feedback people can gain at least temporary control over an extremely wide range of physiological activities with surprising speed. In animals, biofeedback control has been established for single neurons in the hippocampus, thalamus, hypothalamus, ventral reticular formation, and preoptic nuclei (Olds & Hirano, 1969). In humans large populations of neurons can also be controlled, including alpha waves in the EEG, activity in the sensorimotor cortex, evoked potentials, and the lateral geniculate nucleus (Chase, 1974). In the human voluntary muscle system, single motor units – which involve only two neurons – can come under conscious control with half an hour of training, and with further biofeedback training subjects can literally learn to play drumrolls on single spinal motor units! (Basmajian, 1979). Autonomic functions like blood pressure, heart rate, skin conductivity, and peristalsis can come under temporary control; more permanent changes in autonomic functions are unlikely, because these functions are typically controlled by interlocking negative feedback loops, producing a system that tends to resist change. But in the central nervous system (CNS), as Buchwald

(1974) has written, "There is no question that operant conditioning of CNS activity occurs – in fact, it is so ubiquitous a phenomenon that there seems to be no form of CNS activity (single-unit, evoked potential, or EEG) or part of the brain that is immune to it."[1]

This is what we would expect if conscious feedback were made available throughout the brain, and local distributed processes "decided" whether or not to respond to it. We may draw an analogy between biofeedback training and trying to locate a child lost in a very large city. It makes sense initially to search for the lost child around home or school, in a *local* and *systematic* fashion. But if the child cannot be found, it may help to broadcast a message to all the inhabitants of the city, to which only those who recognize it as personally relevant would respond. The message is global, but only the appropriate experts respond to it. Indeed, it is difficult to imagine an account of the power and generality of biofeedback training without some notion of global broadcasting.

> 3   *Event-Related Potential studies show that conscious*
> *perceptual input is distributed* everywhere *in the brain until*
> *stimulus habituation takes place.*

There is direct neurophysiological evidence for global broadcasting associated with consciousness. E. R. John has published a series of experiments using Event-Related Potentials (ERPs) to trace the neural activity evoked by a repeated visual or auditory train of stimulation – that is, a series of bright flashes or loud clicks (Thatcher & John, 1977). Thus a cat may have a number of recording electrodes implanted throughout its brain, and a series of light-flashes are presented to the cat (which is awake during the experiment). Electrical activity is monitored by the implanted electrodes and averaged in a way that is time-locked to the stimuli to remove essentially random activity. In this way, remarkably simple and "clean" average electrical traces are found amid the noise and complexity of an ordinary EEG.

John's major finding of interest to us was that electrical activity due to the visual flashes can initially be found everywhere in the brain, far beyond the specialized visual pathways. At this point we can assume that the cat is conscious of the light flashes, since the stimulus is new. But as the same stimuli are repeated, habituation takes place. The electrical activity never disappears completely, as long as the stimuli are presented, but it becomes more and more localized – until finally it is limited only to the classical visual pathways. These results are strikingly in accord with

---

1   Some researchers treat biofeedback as a type of operant conditioning. In GW theory, operant conditioning is the acquisition of novel voluntary actions (Chapter 7).

our expectations. According to Model 1, prior to habituation, the information is conscious and globally distributed. But after habituation, it ceases to be conscious and becomes limited only to those parts of the brain that are limited to visual functions. Only the specialized input processor is now involved in analyzing the stimulus.

> 4   *The Orienting Response, closely associated with conscious surprise at novelty, is known to involve* every *major division of the nervous system.*

First, we know that any novel stimulus is likely to be conscious, and that it will elicit an Orienting Response (OR) (e.g., Sokolov, 1963). The OR is probably the most widespread reflexive response of all. It interrupts alpha activity in the EEG, it dilates or contracts blood vessels all over the head and body, it changes the conductivity of the skin, causes orienting of eyes, ears, and nose to the source of stimulation, triggers changes in autonomic functions such as heart-rate and peristalsis, evokes very rapid pupillary dilation, and so on. In recent years it has been found to have major impact on the cortical-evoked potential (Donchin, McCarthy, Kutas, & Ritter, 1978). All these changes need not be produced by a globally broadcast message, but the fact that they are so widespread, both anatomically and functionally, suggests that something of that sort may be going on.

> 5   *The reticular-thalamic system of the brain stem and midbrain is closely associated with conscious functions.*

It is known to receive information from *all* input and output systems, connects to virtually *all* subcortical structures, and projects diffusely from the thalamus to *all* parts of the cortex. Thus it can broadcast information to the cortex.

This system is explored in detail in the Chapter Three.

> 6   All *aspects of a conscious event seem to be monitored by unconscious rule systems, as suggested by the fact that errors at* any *level of analysis can be caught if we become conscious of the erroneous event.*

This may seem obvious until we try to explain it. Take a single sentence, for example, spoken by a normal speaker. We very quickly detect errors or anomalies in pronunciation, voice-quality, location, room acoustics, vocabulary, syllable stress, intonation, emotional quality, phonology, morphology, syntax, semantics, stylistics, discourse relations, conversational norms, communicative effectiveness, or pragmatic intentions of the speaker. Each of these aspects of speech corresponds to a very complex, highly developed rule system, which we as skilled speakers of the language have learned to a high level of proficiency (Clark & Clark, 1977). The complexity of this capacity is simply enormous. Yet as long as we are conscious of the spoken sentence we bring all these different knowledge sources to bear on it, so that we can automatically detect violations in *any* of these rule systems. This implies that the sentence is somehow available to all of them. But if we are not conscious of the sentence, we do not even detect our own errors (MacKay, 1981). Again, there is a natural role for global broadcasting in this kind of situation.

In sum, how global is global? The previous six arguments suggest that conscious events can be very global indeed.

2.6   Further considerations

Below I explore further ramifications of Model 1. There are several models that behave much like the Global Workspace System, and these must be considered. I have derived some testable predictions from Model 1 and suggested some further questions it may answer and some that it fails to handle. Some of these puzzling questions may be answered by more advanced models developed in later chapters.

2.6.1 Functional equivalents of a Global Workspace System

While we will continue to speak of a global workspace in this book, there are other systems that behave in much the same way: They are *functionally equivalent*. Our previous analogy of an assembly of experts, each one able to publicize his or her ideas by writing a message on a blackboard for all to see, is much like a global workspace in a distributed system of specialized processors. However, if we take away the blackboard and instead give each expert a megaphone loud enough to be heard by all the others, with the megaphones wired together in such a way that turning on any megaphone turns off all the others, only one expert can broadcast a message at any moment. *Functionally* this is equivalent to the blackboard system (see Figure 2.5).

We suggest in this book that consciousness is associated with a global workspace *or its functional equivalent*. How this system is realized in detail remains to be seen. One way to emphasize this is to say, following the title of this chapter, that consciousness is characterized by at least two properties: Conscious contents are *internally consistent* and *globally distributed*. If we state things at this level of abstraction, we can avoid becoming committed to any particular "hardware" instantiation.

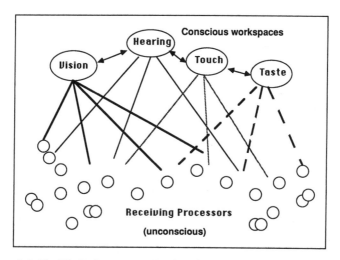

Figure 2.5. The Mind's Senses as a global workspace equivalent. Many different systems may behave like a global workspace. One of these GW equivalents is shown here as a mutually inhibiting group of Mental Senses. The Mind's Eye is the domain of visual imagery (Kosslyn, 1980), and by analogy one may speak of the Mind's Hearing, Touch, or Taste. Each of these defines a domain of conscious experience, which often tends to exclude the others. If each Mental Sense is able to broadcast globally, but acts to inhibit the others from doing this at the same time, only one Sense can distribute a message at any time. Functionally, this system behaves very much like the single global workspace shown in Model 1.

2.6.2 The Mind's Eye, Mind's Voice, and Mind's Body as aspects of a global workspace

Figure 2.5 shows one kind of functional equivalent to the global workspace system, in which the mind's senses are global workspaces, wired so that only one can work at a time. As we have noted, the mind's senses can be treated as workspaces (2.6.2). Inner speech has long been associated with Short Term Memory or "working memory" (Baddeley, 1976).

Note however that we have some voluntary control over visual imagery, and especially over inner speech. Voluntary control is something a theory of conscious experience should tell us about (Chapter 7). Certainly we cannot take voluntary control for granted, or presuppose it in a theory of mental imagery. Further, current models of mental imagery have little to say about consciousness as such (but see Pani, 1982). They typically do not account for habituation and automatization. Nevertheless, Figure 2.5 suggests one attractive instantiation of the global workspace notion.

2.6.3 What is the global code?

We have previously raised the question of a mental *lingua franca,* a common language of mental functioning that may operate across many systems. Such a common code seems plausible to make a GW system work, though it may not be absolutely necessary, since one could broadcast local codes through a global workspace.

One possibility is that input into the GW may be perceptual or quasi-perceptual, as we suppose in Model 1, and that processors in the "audience" respond only to the most general aspects of these global messages, namely their spatio-temporal properties. Thus a motor control program may be able to recognize at least the spatio-temporal aspects of a rich perceptual scene, enough to know that "something of interest is happening at 12 o'clock high at this very moment." The motor program could then cause other receptors to orient to the stimulus, thereby helping to make better information available to all relevant parts of the system. The idea that the *lingua franca* may be a spatio-temporal code is consistent with the fact that many brain structures are sensitive to spatio-temporal information. Further, we know that biofeedback training, which can be done with any specialized system, always involves temporal near-simultaneity between the biofeedback event and the conscious feedback signal. This is consistent with the notion of global temporal coding.

2.6.4 A theoretical choice-point: Are there separate Global Input Processors, or can any element in the nervous system gain access to the global workspace?

One difficult question is whether we should divide the set of distributed specialists into Global Input and Receiving Processors. There are arguments on either side of this question, and some versions of it are very difficult to resolve with our current techniques. For example, one may argue that the apparently unique role of perception and imagery suggests that input to the global workspace must be perceptual or quasi-perceptual in nature (2.4.1). In that case, there is a separate set of Global Input Processors, namely perceptual and imaginal processors. Given the arguments from the biofeedback literature (2.4.5), essentially all other neuronal units may then act, under the right conditions, as Global Receiving Processors, which can receive but not place global messages. This seems rather straightforward; but the question becomes much more complex when we take into account the fact that many of these Global Receiving Processors have conscious perceptual consequences. Thus muscular control systems give immediate perceptual feedback because the perceptual world changes as they change. Similarly, it may be argued that there are subtle and difficult-to-report mental images associated with many nonperceptual abstract concepts (Holender, 1986; James, 1890/1983, Ch. X; see 1.5.5, 6.5.2, 7.6.4). If this is possible, then the question becomes extremely difficult to test at the present time, and we are better off defining a *theoretical choice-point* here, to be resolved at some future time.

2.6.5 Other related models

Ideas related to the GW system have been discussed for some time. In Chapter 1 we pointed out that Aristotle's common sense has much in common with the global workspace. More recently, Lindsay and Norman (1977), among others, have pointed to the global workspace architecture as a psychological model. Recent work on formal models of distributed systems also has explored a global workspace architecture (McClelland, Rumelhart, & the PDP Group, 1986, Chapter 10). Others refer to the "spotlight of consciousness" (e.g., Crick, 1984).

A GW is a natural domain for interaction between otherwise separate capacities. The relationship between conscious experience and integration between separable aspects of experience has been noted by Treisman and Gelade (1980) (above), as well as by La Berge (1974; 1980), Mandler (1983), Marcel (1983a, b), and others.

There are fewer sources for the somewhat surprising notion that conscious experiences may be broadcast everywhere in the nervous system. E. R. John's "statistical model of learning" seems to be closely related to this (1976). Neurophysiologists have long known about diffuse and nonspecific anatomical areas, and some neuroanatomists have explicitly related the brain stem reticular formation to Aristotle's "common sense," (see Chapter 3). Gazzaniga (1985) has recently proposed that consciousness serves as a publicity organ in the brain. Curiously enough, he also suggests that its primary function is post-hoc rationalization of past events. This seems an unduly limited view of the functions of consciousness (see Chapter 10).

The closest models are those which relate conscious experience to limited capacity mechanisms in parallel distributed systems. Reason (1984) and Norman and Shallice (1980) have proposed systems along these lines. Similarly, John Anderson (1983) suggests that the "working memory" in his ACT* system, currently the most detailed architectural model, is closely related to conscious experience.

2.7   Testable predictions and counterarguments

2.7.1 Testable predictions from Model 1

Many of the empirical studies we have cited can be further developed to test aspects of Model 1. We will focus here on a few possibilities. Note that many of these are phrased in terms of measures of limited capacity, rather than of conscious experience as such. This is because Model 1 states some but not all of the necessary conditions for conscious experience; but it is a model of limited capacity. Thus we will phrase predictions in terms of limited capacity *or* conscious experience at this point.

The global workspace as a domain for novel interactions
One core concept is that novel interactions between routine processors require the global workspace. Sophisticated processing may go on much of the time without conscious or limited-capacity processors, but *novel* processes are presumably unable to proceed in this way. One experimental prediction, then, is that novel word-combinations cannot be processed unconsciously, while routine ones can. We will discuss the issue of novelty and informativeness in Chapter 5, and suggest some experimental predictions there.

Testing global interaction and broadcasting
Biofeedback training may provide an excellent experimental paradigm for investigating the claims about global interaction and broadcasting. It is quite a strong claim that any part of the nervous system can in principle interact with any other, given the global workspace as a mediator; but this result is predicted by Model 1. Because any global message should interfere with any other, and because biofeedback allows us to control a repetitive neural event, perturbations in the control of a biofeedback-controlled tracking task may be used to monitor global-workspace activity. It is well established that people can learn to control a single muscle fiber, controlled by two spinal neurons, separately from all the others with a brief period of biofeedback training. Typically, the feedback is provided by a "click," consisting of the amplified electrical signal from the muscle unit played over a loudspeaker. Indeed, Basmajian (1979) has shown that one can learn to play drum rolls on a single motor unit! If subjects can be trained to emit a steady stream of motor pulses, at a rate of perhaps 5 Hz, one could investigate the interaction of this marker stream with other conscious or voluntary events, such as the detection of a perceptual signal, the comprehension of a sentence, and the like as long as the control was not entirely automatic. Any conscious or limited-capacity event should interfere with the control over the motor unit.

The minimum integration time of conscious experience

Evidence for perceptual fusion has been cited above to support the possibility of a rather brief 100-millisecond cycle time for the global workspace. One might use biofeedback training to investigate this temporal interaction window. For example, in motor unit training, a discrete and covert neural event (the motor spike) is amplified and fed back through loudspeakers to create a discrete conscious event (the auditory click). It would be easy to delay the click for 50, 100, 200, and 300 msec to measure the allowable lag time between the two. An approximate 100-millisecond upper limit would be very interesting. If the 100-millisecond cycle time is approximately correct, biofeedback training should not be possible past this conscious exposure time.

The same suggestion may be made on the input side. The work of Treisman and her colleagues (Treisman & Gelade, 1980; Treisman & Schmidt, 1982) and Julesz (Sagi & Julesz, 1985) suggests that one can easily specify separable features in visual perception. What would happen if one were to delay one feature 50 msec before others became available? If the notion of a minimal cycle time were valid, there should be integration with short temporal disparities, with a rapid loss of integration beyond some "magic number" around 100 msec.

Does composition, decomposition, and reorganization of processors take up limited capacity?

We claimed in Chapter 1 that many slips of speech and action show a momentary separation of otherwise integrated action schamata. Does such separation take place when limited capacity is overloaded? And if one reintegrates the fragmented schema, does that require limited capacity? Model 1 would certainly suggest that reintegration between otherwise separate systems makes use of the global workspace. In recent years it has become possible to trigger a variety of predictable slips of speech and action in the laboratory (e.g., Baars, 1980). We have not at this point investigated the question of limited-capacity loading in errors, but it may provide a fertile domain for testing GW theory.

There are numerous other cases of reorganization of coalitions of processors. Speaking and listening probably involve different configurations of overlapping sets of processors – both involve lexical access, syntax, and semantics. Presumably, switching from speaking to listening should require at least a momentary load on limited capacity.

2.7.2 More questions for which Model 1 suggests answers

Along similar lines, the creation of new specialized modules, perhaps from previously available separate automatic systems, should take up limited capacity and may have testably conscious aspects (e.g., Case, 1985).

Parallel error detection by many unconscious systems
A related question is whether error detection in performance involves parallel monitoring systems (7.3.2). Notice that the reasons why an error *is* an error are not conscious ordinarily, and that, like other specialized processors, error detectors should be able to operate in parallel unless they are contingent on each other. If monitoring systems operate in parallel, "looking at" a globally displayed event, then the time needed to detect two simultaneous errors in some conscious material should take no longer than detecting only one. The work of Langer and Imber (1979) indicates that error detection becomes quite poor when some skill becomes automatic: The less conscious it is, the more difficult it is to monitor. Of course, automatic skills can "deautomatize" when they encounter difficulties (4.1.4). That is, aspects of these skills can become conscious once again. Any experiment on error detection in automatic skills must deal with this complication. However, deautomatization presumably takes more time, and the skill should degrade when it becomes more conscious. Thus, one could monitor whether some automatic skill continues to be automatic and unconscious during the experiment (e.g., Marslen-Wilson & Welsh, 1978).

A functional explanation for limited capacity
Limited capacity is a prominent and surprising feature of human psychology, but we seldom ask *why* it exists. Would it not be wonderful to be able to do half a dozen things at the same time? Why has evolution not resulted in nervous systems that can do this? Model 1 suggests an answer. If it is important for information to be available at one time *to the system as a whole,* global information must necessarily be limited to a single message at a time. There is only one "system as a whole," and if all of its components must be able to receive the same message, then only one message at a time can be broadcast. There are many reasons for making information available to the system as a whole, notably the case where a problem cannot be solved by any single known specialist. The knowledge required to solve the problem may reside somewhere in the system, but in order to reach it, the problem must be made available very widely. Notice that this suggests a purely *functional* explanation of limited capacity.

Of course, global broadcasting is expensive. If some problem can be assigned to a specialized processor, it is efficient to do this and not take up the limited resources of the global workspace.

Organization versus flexibility

Other facts about human psychology also fall into place with Model 1. For example, cognitive psychologists over the past few decades have become convinced of the importance of organization in perception and memory. There are numerous powerful demonstrations of the effects of organization (e.g., Bransford, 1979; Mandler, 1967; Rock, 1983). It is easier to remember something if we learn a set of regularities that apply to it; indeed, we cannot remember or even perceive utterly disorganized information. Even "random" noise has specifiable statistical properties.

The trouble with this is that organization tends to commit us to a particular way of doing and viewing things. Organization often creates rigidity. Most of the time it is appropriate for adults to analyze language in terms of meaning, but there are times (in proofreading, for example) when we must switch from a meaning analysis to a spelling analysis; this switch often leads to problems. The famous "proofreader illusion" shows that we often miss errors of spelling and vocabulary when we focus on meaning. What kind of a system architecture is needed to reconcile the value of organization with the need for flexibility? In terms of Model 1, it should be a system in which specialized processors can be decomposed and rearranged when the demands of the task change. This is very difficult to do with other conceptions of organization in memory.

Some of the best demonstrations of flexibility in the nervous system come from the area of conditioning. Originally, conditioning theorists believed that any arbitrary relationship between stimuli and responses could be connected, and they proved that under surprisingly many circumstances a tone can indeed come to signal a shock, and the like. This is the very opposite of the powerful organizational effects found by cognitive psychologists: There is no natural connection between tones and shocks or many of the other standard stimuli used routinely in conditioning studies. Indeed, when conditioning occurs between ecologically related stimuli and responses, the effects found are far stronger than when biologically arbitrary stimuli are used (Garcia & Koelling, 1966). Nevertheless, it is striking that biologically arbitrary connections can be made at all in a system that is so strongly affected by nonarbitrary, organized, and biologically significant relationships.

Biofeedback training provides an excellent example. When it was first discovered, physiologists and psychologists were surprised that autonomic functions such as heart rate, skin conductivity, blood vessel dilation and contraction, and the like were affected by biofeedback (at least in humans). As the word "autonomic" suggests, these activities were thought to be free from conscious control. It now appears that just about any neural system can be responsive to conscious biofeedback control, although autonomic functions seem to resist permanent retraining (Chase, 1974).

To account for this high degree of flexibility we favor something like Model 1, in which routine organization of information and control can be accessed quickly, but which also allows for movement between different levels of organization, for reorganization of modules in different ways, and for the creation of entirely new, organized coalitions of processors.

How can people talk about their conscious experiences?

Finally, how is it that people can talk about the things they experience consciously? And how can they act upon conscious information? This if after all, our first operational definition of conscious experience, and at some point our model should be able to connect to it (see Chapter 7 and 9). We can already suggest part of the answer. Speech requires a coalition of specialized processors. Since all such processors can receive information from the global workspace, we can explain in general terms how it is that speech processors can describe and act upon conscious contents. Speech systems in the global "audience" can presumably receive the relevant information; but this does not explain how these linguistic systems organize a coherent speech act to describe the global information. Nevertheless it is a step in the right direction (8.5.4).

Presumably the same point applies to other voluntarily controlled systems. Instead of asking people to say "there is a banana" when we present a banana, we can ask people to raise their fingers or blink their eyes for bananas, and not for anything else. All of these voluntarily controlled systems must presumably have access to global information provided by the conscious stimulus.

Surprise as a momentary erasure of the global workspace

We know that surprise triggers all the measures of the Orienting Response, that it loads limited capacity, creates massive neural activity, and tends to cause a loss of current conscious contents. One obvious explanation is that surprise serves to erase the Global Workspace, thereby allowing the new and surprising information to be distributed for widespread cooperative analysis (Baars, in press, b; Grossberg, 1982; Luborsky, in press). This is indeed part of the story that seems to follow from the theory developed so far, though we will have more to say about this in Chapters 4 and 5.

Consciousness and executive control

We are not claiming, of course, that consciousness is an executive; in the society metaphor, it resembles a broadcasting station rather than a government. However, governments can use broadcasting facilities to exercise control, and presumably executive processors may use consciousness to try to control other processors. In this connection Shallice (1978) suggests that consciousness has to do with the selection of a "Dominant Action System," an idea that has obvious similarities with our Model 2 and 3 (see Chapters 4 and 5). However, action is not the only thing that is selected in consciousness – conscious experience is as selective for perception as it is for action – and Shallice still leaves unexplained why a Dominant Action System would bother to dominate conscious capacity. What is the pay-off for actions and goals to become conscious (2.3.1)? Nevertheless, the general concept of a Dominant Action System is extremely valuable, and we propose a generalization from Shallice's idea in Chapters 4 and 5, called a Dominant Goal Context. This is where we introduce executive control systems as goal contexts that shape and control access to conscious contents, though they are not themselves conscious.

Consciousness and repression

Some readers will no doubt wonder how we can possibly discuss our topic in any depth without dealing with the Freudian unconscious, surely the most influential idea of this kind in this century. The general answer is that Freud's work *presupposed* a cognitive theory of conscious and unconscious processes, one we need to work out explicitly (Erdelyi, 1985). Like most nineteenth-century thinkers, Freud tended to take the existence of conscious experience for granted. He treated it as equivalent to perception, and did not discuss it in much detail. The great surprise at the end of the 19th century was the extraordinary power of *un*conscious processes, as shown, for example, in post-hypnotic suggestion and the relief of hysterical symptoms after emotional expression of traumatic memories (Baars, 1986a; Ellenberger, 1970). Freud has nothing to say about unconsciousness that is due to habituation, distraction, or hypnotic dissociation – those phenomena are all quite obvious to him, and require no explanation. He is really concerned with the *dynamic* unconscious, the domain in which wishes and fears are purposefully kept unconscious, because their becoming conscious would lead to intolerable anxiety. The dynamic unconscious is a conspiratorial unconscious, one that aims to keep things from us. It is closely associated with primary process thinking, the magical thinking displayed by young children, in dreams, and in some mental disturbances. But these phenomena presuppose a more general understanding of consciousness and its functions (see Chapters 8 and 9).

Our aim in this book, therefore, is to try to build a solid cognitive foundation from which such phenomena can be understood. In later chapters we make some suggestions for specific ways in which psychody-namic phenomena can be explored empirically, and how they may be modeled in a general cognitive framework (7.8; 8.4).

However, these is an interesting relationship between our basic meta-phor and the repression concept of psychodynamic theory. The global workspace is a publicity device in the society of processors – after all, global messages become available to potentially *any* processor, just as published information becomes available to potentially any reader. Freud originally used the opposite metaphor to explain repression, that is, motivated *un*consciousness: the idea of newspaper censorship. As he wrote in *The Interpretation of Dreams* (1900, p. 223):

> The political writer who has unpleasant truths to tell to those in power . . . stands in fear of the censorship; he therefore moderates and disguises the expression of his opinion. . . . The stricter the domination of the censorship, the more thorough becomes the disguise, and, often enough, the more ingenious the means employed to put the reader on the track of the actual meaning.

For Freud, the dynamic unconscious exists because of censorship. Would it follow then that making things conscious is the opposite of censorship, namely publicity? Repression is presumed to be a censoring of anxiety-provoking information, but Freud apparently did not pursue the question, "What is the censored information hidden *from*?" We might speculate that it is sometimes desirable to conceal information from global publicity, because some processors in the system might react to it in an unpredictable way, challenging established control mechanisms. For someone on a diet, it may be useful to exclude from consciousness seductive advertisements for delicious food; conscious contemplation of the food may lead to a loss of control. In the same sense a politician might wish to hide a scandal from publicity, because some political forces might react to this information in an uncontrollable way. In both cases, limiting publicity is a useful device for maintaining control.

There are many ways for information to become unconscious. These mechanisms are not inherently purposeful. Habituation, forgetting, and distraction are not conspiratorial devices to hide a stimulus from con-scious experience. However, mechanisms like distraction may be *used by* some specialized systems in a purposeful way to help control the system as a whole (Chapters 7, 8, and 9).

Experimental psychologists have had great empirical difficulties in assessing the existence of repression (Baars, 1985; 1986a; Erdelyi, 1974, 1985). The points we are making here do not solve these empirical problems, but it is pleasing to find that this very influential conception of the psychological unconscious may fit our analysis quite readily.

2.7.3 Some counterarguments

Model 1 is clearly incomplete. Worse than that, it seems to contradict some empirical findings, and certain powerful intuitions about conscious experience. It clearly needs more development. Consider the following four counterarguments.

> *1   The model does not distinguish between conscious experience and other events that load limited capacity.*

So far, Model 1 suggests a way of thinking of the limited capacity part of the nervous system, the part that presumably underlies conscious experience. But in fact there are events that load limited capacity that are *not* consciously experienced (see Chapters 4–7). One counterargument to Model 1 is simply that it does not distinguish between conscious experience and other limited capacity-loading events. Later models will correct this deficiency.

> *2   The idea that we are conscious of only a single internally consistent event at any time seems counterintuitive to some people.*

In reading this sentence, the reader is presumably conscious of the printed words as well as inner speech. Most experiences, at least in retrospect, seem to combine many separable internal and external events. But of course at any single instance, or in any single 100 millisecond cycle of the global workspace, we may only have one internally consistent object of consciousness; multiple events may involve rapid switching between different conscious contents, just as a visual scene is known to be integrated over many rapid fixations of the eyes. We can call this the *bandwidth question:* In any single integration period of the global workspace, can more than one internally consistent message gain access? Again, this is a difficult question to decide with certainty at this point, so we will call this another *theoretical choice-point:* We will assume for the sake of simplicity that only one global message exists in any psychological instant, and that the sense we have of multiple events is a *retrospective* view of our conscious contents. Normal conscious experience may be much like watching the countryside flash by while sitting in a train; when we reflect metacognitively on our own experience, we can see parts of the train that have just gone by, as if it has gone around a curve so that we can view if from the outside. Presumably in retrospect we can observe much more than we experience in any instant.

3   The 100-millisecond global integration time is much too
short for many integrative processes involving consciousness.

A single coherent conscious content is presumably at least 100 msec long. Though it may last as long as a second or two, longer than the minimum conscious integration time, even that is not long enough to think through a difficult problem, to integrate information from two domains in memory, or to do many other things that people plainly do consciously. Even if we assume that people can voluntarily "refresh" a conscious content by mentally rehearsing it, for example, there are surely structures that can gain access to consciousness that last longer than we are likely to voluntarily rehearse a thought. Attitudes, for example, may last an adult lifetime, and attitudes surely must affect one's conscious thoughts, images, and feelings. We need something else to bridge the gap between evanescent conscious contents and long-term knowledge structure. In Chapter 4 we introduce a new construct to fill this need, called a "context," defined as a representation that shapes and evokes conscious experiences, but that is not itself conscious.

4   The Threshold Paradox: At what point does a global
message become conscious?

If it takes global broadcasting to become conscious, and if newly global systems need to broadcast in order to recruit support for staying on the global workspace, there is a paradox, a kind of catch-22: In order to be global long enough to be perceived as conscious, a system must first be globally broadcast. I suggested above (2.4.3) that this problem may be fixed in two ways: by having an increasingly global hierarchy of work-spaces or by allowing momentary access to all potential contents – long enough to broadcast a recruiting message to other systems, but not long enough to be recalled and reported as conscious. This Threshold Paradox is a counterargument, but one that does seem to have a possible solution.

2.7.4 Other unanswered questions

There are several questions that we have not yet touched on, which a complete theory must address. Some obvious ones are:

1   Why do we lose consciousness of habituated stimuli and automatic skills (Chapter 5)?
2   Why are we unconscious of local perceptual contexts that help to shape our conscious percepts and images (Chapter 4)?
3   Why are we unconscious most of the time of the *conceptual* context, the presuppositions that form the framework of our thoughts about the world (Chapters 4 and 5).

4 Does the common idea that we have "conscious control" over our actions have any psychological reality? Is there a relationship between consciousness and volition (Chapter 7)?

5 What if anything is the difference between consciousness and attention (Chapter 8)?

For some questions we have no ready answers. For example:

6 How does the item limit of Short Term Memory fit in with a globalist conception of consciousness? We know that with mental rehearsal people can keep in mind 7 plus or minus 2 unrelated items – words, numbers, or judgment categories. But that fact does not "fall out of" the GW framework in any obvious way.

7 Why do perceptual and imaginal processes have a unique relationship to consciousness? What is the difference between these "qualitative" and other "nonqualitative" mental contents (Chapters 4 and 7)?

8 We are never conscious of only single features or dimensions, such as specialized processors presumably provide, but only of entire objects and events, that is, internally consistent and complete *combinations* of dimensional features. Why is that?

Finally:

9 When we say that "I" am conscious of something, what is the nature of the "I" to which we refer? Or is it just a meaningless common-sense expression (Chapter 9)?

Obviously there is still much to do.

2.8 Chapter summary

We have explored the first detailed contrastive analysis of conscious and unconscious phenomena. Conscious processes were said to be computationally inefficient, but to have great range, relational capacity and context sensitivity. Furthermore, conscious events have apparent internal consistency, seriality, and limited capacity. In contrast to all these aspects of conscious functioning, unconscious process*ors* are highly efficient in their specialized tasks, have relatively limited domains, are relatively isolated and autonomous, highly diverse, and capable of contradicting each other; they can operate in parallel, and, taken together, unconscious processors have very great capacity.

There is a remarkable match between these contrasts and a system architecture used in some artificial intelligence applications, called a global workspace in a distributed system of specialized processors. This organization can be compared to a very large committee of experts, each speaking his or her specialized jargon, who can communicate with each other through some global broadcasting device, a large blackboard in front of the committee of experts, for example. If we pretend for the time being that global messages are conscious and specialized experts are unconscious, the whole contrastive analysis of Table 2.1 can be seen to flow from this model. Model 1 yields a great *simplification* of the evidence.

Encouraged by this apparently helpful model, we considered some issues in more detail. How global is global broadcasting? We presented six arguments in favor of the idea that conscious (global) information is truly distributed throughout the nervous system. We pointed out that there may be several different way to implement Model 1, ways that are "functionally equivalent." Several authors have made similar claims; this work is acknowledged here. We ended the chapter by setting forth predictions that flow from Model 1 and pointing out some of its deficiencies.

The upshot is a major simplification of the evidence in terms of a straightforward model (Figure 2.3). As the title of this chapter indicates, conscious experience seems to involve mental representations that are globally distributed throughout the nervous system and that are internally consistent. This is clearly not the whole story. In later chapters we will discover that Model 1 needs additional features to accommodate further contrastive analyses. Notably, Chapter 3 suggests the existence of feedback from the input and output processors to create a stable coalition of processors that tends to support one conscious content over another. In Chapter 4 we are compelled to create a role for *context* in our model – to represent the fact that conscious experience is always shaped and directed by an extensive unconscious framework. Later in the book we will find that the theory leads in a natural way to a new theoretical perspective on intentions, voluntary control, attention, and self-control.

3   The neural basis of conscious experience

3.0   Introduction

In this chapter we apply the contrastive analysis strategy to the neural basis of conscious experience. That is, we look for populations of neurons that control the difference between conscious and unconscious states – most obviously sleep, waking, and coma. These neural structures behave in several ways like the Global Workspace model we have developed so far.

There is a curious traditional dichotomy between psychologists and neuroscientists in the way they tend to regard the nervous system. By and large, neuroscientists tend to see a gigantic assemblage of complex neurons, extremely densely interconnected, operating in parallel and at a fairly fast rate (e.g., Thompson, 1967). Psychologists have traditionally seen a very different system. Their nervous system was slow, appeared to do comparatively simple tasks with high error rates, and seemed to operate serially, performing only one task at a time (e.g., Atkinson & Shiffrin, 1968; Broadbent, 1958; Newell & Simon, 1972; Norman, 1976). Naturally there are exceptions to these generalizations. Over the past decade psychologists have increasingly explored parallel or parallel-interactive processes, while some neuroscientists have been studying relatively serial aspects such as event-related potentials (e.g., Anderson, 1983; Donchin, McCarthy, Kutas, & Ritter, 1978; Hinton & Anderson, 1981). Nevertheless, over the broad sweep of the last hundred years of research, the dichotomy between these two views of the nervous system appears to hold to a remarkable degree.

I am most grateful to several neuroscientists and psychologists who have provided valuable comments on the ideas presented in this chapter, especially David Galin, Benjamin Libet, and Charles Yingling (University of California, San Francisco), Paul Rozin (University of Pennsylvania), Michael A. Wapner (California State University, Los Angeles), Theodore Melnechuk (Western Behaviorial Sciences Institute), Arnold Scheibel (University of California, Los Angeles), and James Newman.

119

In fact neither extreme is wrong, though both are incomplete. Viewed at the level of neurons, a structure such as the cerebral cortex is indeed immensely complex, containing by recent estimates 55,000,000,000 neurons, each firing off an electrochemical pulse 40–1000 times per second, with rich subcortical and contralateral connections, and all apparently active at the same time (Mountcastle, 1978). But when we look at the same system functionally, through input and output performance, it appears to solve simple problems (especially novel ones) at a rate slower than 10 Hz, it makes numerous errors, it tends to serialize even actions that seem superficially executable in parallel, and its efficiency in learning new facts and strategies seems relatively unimpressive.

The difference is, of course, that most psychologists work with the limited capacity component of the nervous system, which is associated with consciousness and voluntary control, while neuroscientists work with the "wetware" of the nervous system, enormous in size and complexity, and unconscious in its detailed functioning. But what is the meaning of this dichotomy? How does a serial, slow, and relatively awkward level of functioning emerge from a system that is enormous in size, relatively fast-acting, efficient, and parallel? That is the key question.

One guise in which this puzzle appears is the issue of "attention" versus "cortical arousal." Both of these concepts have been associated with conscious processes, but in quite different ways (Scheibel, 1980). The psychologist can easily find *selectivity* in human information processing, so that the great array of potential stimulation is reduced to just one stream of information at a time. From William James to the present, psychologists have thought of attention and consciousness in terms of selectivity, a *reduction* in complexity. The neuroscientist, however, looking at the nervous system more directly, finds plentiful evidence for system-wide *cortical arousal* associated with wakefulness and orienting to novel stimuli, but much less evidence for selectivity. Cortical arousal involves widespread desynchronization in the EEG. That is to say, when novel stimuli "catch the attention" of an animal, regular, relatively slow brain waves are interrupted by fast, irregular, low-voltage activity suggestive of increased information processing. This implies not a reduction but an *increase* in complexity at the neural level. Thus attention and arousal seem to be quite different things, and tend to be treated as separate though somehow related topics.

This chapter pursues the hypothesis that the split between psychologists and neuroscientists in looking at the nervous system reflects the global-workspace architecture. One advantage of the GW model is that it predicts *both* selectivity and widespread activation, so that it reconciles these apparently contradictory views within a single framework (Baars, 1987).

3.1   The neurophysiological fit with Model 1

3.1.1 The nervous system as a parallel distributed system

The various parts of the nervous system operate all at the same time, and to a degree independently from each other (Thompson, 1976). Further, there is extensive evidence that anatomical structures in the brain often subserve very specialized functions (e.g., Geschwind, 1979; Luria, 1980). Under these circumstances it is natural to think of the brain as a parallel distributed system, and several interpreters of brain function have done so. Arbib has for some years argued that motor systems should be viewed as collections of multiple specialized processors, operating independently of each other to a considerable degree (e.g., Arbib, 1980), and recently a number of neuroscientists have interpreted the columnar organization of the cerebral cortex in terms of distributed "unit modules" (Mountcastle, 1978). Rozin (1976) has interpreted the evolution of intelligence as an increase in the accessibility of specialized functions, which originally developed as very specific evolutionary adaptations. In more highly evolved nervous systems, he suggests, specialized functions can become available for new adaptive purposes. All these contributors support the idea of the nervous system as a parallel distributed system. Thus Mountcastle (1978) writes:

> The general proposition is that the large entities of the nervous system which we know as the dorsal horn, reticular formation, dorsal thalamus, neocortex, and so forth, are themselves composed of local circuits. These circuits form modules which vary from place to place . . . but which are at the first level of analysis similar within any large entity. . . . The closely linked subsets of several different large entities thus form precisely connected, distributed systems; these distributed systems are conceived as serving distributed functions. (p. 36)

Mountcastle also interprets the cerebral neocortex as such a collection of specialized distributed processors. The cortex is really a huge layered sheet folded into the upper cranium. Seen in cross-section, this sheet consists of many microscopic columns of cells:

> The basic unit of operation in the neocortex is a vertically arranged group of cells heavily interconnected in the vertical axis . . . and sparsely connected horizontally.

> I define the basic modular unit of the neocortex as a minicolumn. It is a vertically oriented cord of cells . . . (which) contains about 110 cells. This figure is almost invariant between different neocortical areas and different species of mammals, except for the striate cortex of primates, where it is 260. Such a cord

of cells occupies a gently curving, nearly vertical cylinder of cortical space with a diameter of about 30 microns. . . . The neocortex of the human brain . . . contains about 600 million minicolumns and on the order of 50 billion neurons. (p. 38)

Next, Mountcastle suggests that these minicolumns of cells are gathered together into *cortical columns*, which constitute the basic "unit modules" of the cerebral cortex:

It is possible to identify within the neocortex a much larger processing unit than the minicolumn. The diameters or widths of this larger unit have been given as 500 microns to 1,000 microns for different areas. . . . This larger unit may vary in its cross-sectional form, being round, or oval, or slablike in shape. . . . One can estimate that the human neocortex contains about 600,000 of these larger [cortical columns], each packaging several hundred minicolumns. The calculations . . . are given to indicate order of magnitude only.

Thus a major problem for understanding the function of the neocortex . . . is to unravel the intrinsic structural and functional organization of the neocortical module.

That module is, I propose, what has come to be called the *cortical column*.

Unlike Mountcastle, who defines a module anatomically, I would like to view the basic units as functional (Luria, 1980). These approaches are not contradictory, of course, because functional units must ultimately make use of anatomical units. But there is a difference of emphasis. To mark the difference, I will call these specialized distributed units "processors" rather than "modules."

3.1.2 The Reticular-Thalamic Activating System: Evidence for a global workspace in the nervous system

What part of the brain could carry out the functions described by Model 1? We can specify some of its properties:

First, it should be associated with conscious functions like wakefulness, focal attention, habituation, and indeed all the facts described in the contrastive analyses in this book.

Second, it should fit the model developed in Chapter 2. On the *input side*, many systems should have access to the presumed global workspace, and incompatible inputs should compete for access. On the *output side*, it should be able to distribute information to many specialized parts of the nervous system. Since a great many parts of the nervous system seem to be specialized in some way, GW output should be able to reach essentially everywhere.

There is an anatomical and functional system in the brain stem and forebrain that is known to have close relationships with consciousness, in the sense that people gain or lose consciousness when it is activated

(Dixon, 1971; Hobson & Brazier, 1982; Magoun, 1962; Scheibel & Scheibel, 1967). This structure includes the classic Reticular Formation discovered by Moruzzi and Magoun (1949), which receives information from all major structures within the brain, including all sensory and motor tracts, and permits very close interaction between all these sources of information. It extends well upward to include the nonspecific nuclei of the thalamus. It makes functional sense to include in this larger system the Diffuse Thalamic Projection System, which sends numerous fibers to all parts of the cortex (Figure 3.1). It is possible that cortico-cortical connections should also be included. We will refer to this whole set of anatomical structures as the *Extended Reticular-Thalamic Activating System* (ERTAS).

The results of a great deal of research done since the late 1940s is summarized in Table 3.1.

The lower component of this system, the Reticular Formation of the brainstem and midbrain, was described by one of its codiscoverers as follows:

Within the brain, a central transactional core has been identified between the strictly sensory or motor systems of classical neurology. This central reticular mechanism has been found *capable of grading the activity of most other parts of the brain* . . . it is proposed to be subdivided into a grosser and more tonically operating component in the lower brain stem, subserving global alterations in excitability, as distinguished from a more cephalic, thalamic component with greater capacities for fractionated, shifting influences upon focal regions of the brain.

In its ascending and descending relations with the cerebral cortex, the reticular system is *intimately bound up with and contributes to most areas of nervous activity*. It has to do significantly with the *initiation and maintenance of wakefulness*; with the *orienting reflex* and *focus of attention*; with *sensory control processes* including habituation . . .; with *conditional learning*; through its functional relations with the hippocampus and temporal cortex, with *memory functions*; and through its relations with the midline thalamus and pontile tegmentum, with the cortex and *most of the central integrative processes* of the brain. (Magoun, 1962, p. 10) (Italics added)

The fact that the Reticular Formation involves wakefulness, the orienting response, focus of attention, and "most of the central integrative processes of the brain" certainly suggests that it may be a part of what we are looking for. Other neuroscientists associate parts of this system with the capability of "altering the content of consciousness" (Livingston, 1958, p. 178), and with "general alerting" and "focused attention" (Lindsley, 1958, p. 515). The Reticular Formation, which is part of the Extended Reticular-Thalamic System we are considering here, thus easily meets our first criterion, that our neuronal candidate should be closely associated with conscious experience.

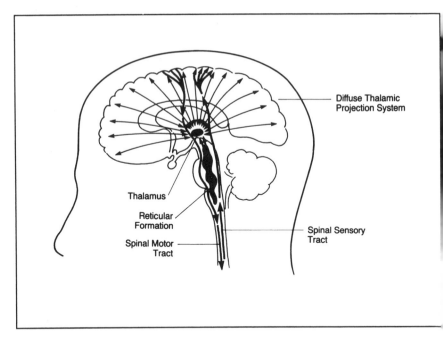

Figure 3.1. The ERTAS: A neural global workspace? Brain structures most closely associated with conscious experience include the Reticular Formation of the brain stem and midbrain, the outer shell of the thalamus, and the set of neurons projecting upward diffusely from the thalamus to the cerebral cortex. Together these structures can be labeled the "Extended Reticular-Thalamic Activating System" (ERTAS), since stimulation of a number of neurons throughout this system causes cortical activation. The ERTAS as a whole can be interpreted as a functional global workspace, or perhaps as an increasingly global set of workspaces (see Model 1A, Figure 3.2). ERTAS has many properties reminiscent of global workspaces, including connections in both input and output with all sensory and motor systems and with almost all areas of the brain; the existence of competition between different inputs; and the possibility of global broadcasting of information through the Diffuse Thalamic Projection System. It is possible that other brain structures also serve the function of global broadcasting, including the corpus callosum connecting the two hemispheres, and the tertiary cortico-cortical fibers that connect distant parts of the cortex.

Neurophysiological evidence that specialists can cooperate and compete for access to a central integrative "blackboard"

The Reticular Formation is called "reticular" (i.e., network-like) because the neuronal axons in this system are usually very short, suggesting a great amount of interaction between adjacent neurons. Further, it receives input from all sensory and motor systems, as well as from other major structures in the brain. Through its connections with the thalamus, it can send information to, and receive it from, all areas of the cortex. If

Table 3.1. *Neural contrasts*

Conscious	Unconscious
Stimulation of the reticular formation and outer thalamus	Rapid lesioning of the reticular formation, the outer thalamus, and the thalamo-cortical projection system

the ERTAS corresponds to our "blackboard," different specialized systems can have access to it.

Aristotle's "common sense" was supposed to be a domain of integration between the different senses. In fact, anatomists who have studied the Reticular Formation have pointed to its resemblance to Aristotle's concept. Scheibel and Scheibel (1967) point out that "Anatomical studies of Kohnstamm and Quensel, which suggested pooling of a number of afferent and efferent systems upon the reticular core, led them to propose this area as a 'centrum receptorium,' or 'sensorium commune' – a common sensory pool for the neuraxis."

Moreover, and of a great significance to our discussion, these authors note that "the reticular core mediates specific delimitation of the focus of consciousness *with concordant suppression of those sensory inputs that have been temporarily relegated to a sensory role*" (p. 579) (italics added). Along similar lines, Gastaut (1958) describes the brain stem reticular formation as an area of "convergence . . . where signals are concentrated before being redistributed in a divergent way to the cortex." Thus different sensory contents can suppress each other, as we would indeed expect of input to a global workspace. This meets our second requirement, that different specialized processors can compete for access to the ERTAS.

> *Neurophysiological evidence that integrated, coherent information can be broadcast by the Reticular-Thalamic System to all parts of the nervous system*

As we noted above, we are including in the term *Extended Reticular-Thalamic Activating System* the diffuse thalamic projection system, a bundle of neurons that projects upward like a fountain from the thalamus to all parts of the cortex. It contains both specific and nonspecific projections, and both kinds usually contain feedback loops going in the opposite direction as well. The thalamic portion of this system may "broadcast" information from the Reticular System to all parts of the brain. We have already discussed evidence from evoked potentials that indicates that nonhabituated stimuli are indeed broadcast nonspecifically throughout the brain (Thatcher & John, 1977) (2.5). In one scenario, one sensory projection area of the cortex could provide input to the Extended Reticular-Thalamic Activating System. If this input prevails over competing inputs, it becomes a global message that is widely distributed to other areas of the brain, including the rest of the cortex. Thus one selected input to the ERTAS is amplified and broadcast at the expense of others (3.1.3).

We can therefore suggest that the ERTAS underlies the "global broadcasting" function of consciousness, while a selected perceptual "processor" in the cortex supplies the particular *contents* of consciousness to be broadcast. (These are typically perceptual contents, because the ERTAS receives collateral pathways from all sensory tracts; and of course, we have previously remarked on the favored relationship between conscious experience and perception). These conscious contents, in turn, when they are broadcast, can trigger motoric, memory, and associative activities.

There is independent evidence that cortical activity *by itself* does not become conscious (Libet, 1978, 1981; Magoun, 1962; Shevrin & Dickman, 1980). We would suggest that any cortical activity must trigger ERTAS support in a circulating flow of information before it can be broadcast globally and become conscious (e.g., Scheibel, 1980; Shevrin & Dickman, 1980). Dixon (1971, 1981) has also argued that a circulating flow of information between the reticular formation and the cortex is required before sensory input becomes conscious.

3.1.3 One possible scenario

There are probably several ways to gain access to the brain equivalent of a global workspace. In one scenario, two perceptual inputs arrive in the cortex at the same time through the direct sensory pathways and begin to compete for access to the limited-capacity system – presumably the thalamus and reticular formation. Suppose the two inputs are auditory and visual, respectively, so that we get stimulus competition (Figure 3.2). One may be a speech sound in the left ear, and the other a falling glass in the right visual field. It has been known for at least a century that two simultaneous, incompatible events do not become conscious at the same time (e.g., Blumenthal, 1977; Wundt, 1912/1973). In our scenario, only one of the two can be broadcast at any moment, because they conflict in spatial location and content, so that the two simultaneous cortical events cannot be fused into a single, consistent conscious event. One of the two may be favored because of readiness in the receiving

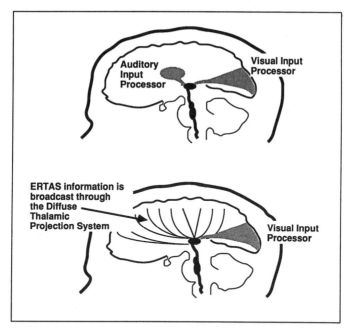

Figure 3.2. One possible scenario: Cortical centers competing for access to ERTAS. In this scenario the primary sensory projection areas of the cortex compete for access to the ERTAS. This is consistent with evidence found by Libet (1978) that cortical access time in the somatosensory areas is very fast, while conscious detection time is as slow as one-half second. It is therefore likely that the cortical sensory areas analyze a stimulus very early on, and that different cortical analyzers may then compete for ERTAS access. The winning stimulus representation may then loop downward to the thalamus through two-way thalamo-cortical connections and be broadcast diffusely to the cortex and other parts of the brain.

specialized processors to support it. For instance, we may be alert to the possibility of the glass falling; in that case, the specialized processors involved with moving a hand to catch the falling glass would trigger quickly to help direct consciousness to the visual stimulus, and away from the auditory input. Possibly there is rapid alternation between the visual and auditory stimulus, so that each is broadcast for 100 msec to recruit additional processors. Receiving processors may then support the visual message over the auditory one. But glasses fall quickly; losing a few hundred milliseconds will probably cause us to miss the falling glass; and competition for access to consciousness inevitably slows down effective action.

This scenario has the following features. First, there is competition between perceptual systems for access to the global workspace. Only one input can win, and it is the one that garners most support from potential receiving systems, especially those that are ready for and "interested in" the winning system. "Winning" means that one system gains access to the thalamus and perhaps to the reticular formation, allowing a general broadcasting of some central aspects of the winning system – its spatio-temporal properties, its significance, its relevance to current goals, etc. Probably some receiving processors gain more information from the global message than others. There is probably a circulating flow of information between the winning input system, the global workspace, and the receiving processors, each component feeding back to the others, so that there is for some time a self-sustaining loop of activated systems (see Figure 3.3). This flow may allow more direct local channels to be established between the perceptual input and some receiving systems; over time, this local flow of information may allow the creation of a new, efficient specialized "falling glass detector," which operates independently of the global workspace.

3.2   Extensions suggested by the neurophysiology

While the neurophysiology seems compatible with the GW model, it also suggests some additions to the model.

1   The outer thalamus as a common sensory mode

The outer layer of the thalamus, the *nucleus reticularis thalami*, is thought to contain a body-centered spatiotemporal map, that can "gate" different inputs before cortical activation occurs (Scheibel, 1980). Thus auditory signals to the right rear of the body may be coded in one place, and visual signals in the same location may converge on the same area. This suggests the existence of a kind of *lingua franca* in which the outer thalamus may act as a common sensory mode. The thalamic centers have much more specificity in this sense than the lower reticular centers.

2   The brainstem reticular formation as a mode switch

What then, is the role of the Reticular Formation (RF), especially the brain stem components that are known to be involved in sleep, waking, and coma? The RF may act as a "mode switch" on the system that does more specific selection. If we use the searchlight metaphor of consciousness, the RF nuclei may act as a dimmer switch to increase or decrease the amount of light, but not to direct it to any particular object. Sleep, waking, and dreaming can be plausibly described as different "operating modes" of the nervous system.

3   Locations of some specialized capacities

Perceptual–imaginal systems as GW input. A large part of the cortex is devoted to perceptual analysis, especially vision, and this may be one reason for the predominance of perceptual/imaginal input to consciousness. It seems likely that imagery also makes use of these perceptual systems, using stimulation of internal origin. Thus some of the input specialists would seem to be located in the sensory projection areas of the cortex.

Clearly voluntary decisions can affect conscious contents, and these are not perceptual for most people, so that it is possible that nonperceptual events can gain global access. Alternatively, it is possible that these nonperceptual systems make use of perceptual/imaginal processors to gain access to the system underlying consciousness.

Short Term Memory and the hippocampus. There is now good evidence that the hippocampus, a structure that surrounds the thalamus, is closely associated with the transfer of Short Term Memory information to Long Term Memory (e.g., Milner, 1959). Clearly Short Term Memory is intimately associated with consciousness, and if the hippocampus contains such a system, it is presumably one of the recipients of global broadcasting (Winson, 1985).

Voluntary speech control and the rehearsal component of Short Term Memory. Similarly, voluntary control of speech is clearly involved in short-term rehearsal, as in memorizing a telephone number. Speech production is one of the few functions that is quite well lateralized to the left hemisphere (Springer & Deutsch, 1981), in particular to Broca's area. It seems likely that this system is involved in mental rehearsal, which is after all mental speaking; rehearsal really acts to refresh conscious access to immediate memory. Therefore this rehearsal system would also seem to provide input to the GW. However, voluntary control in general is more associated with the frontal cortex, so that this functional system may include both frontal areas and Broca's area.

4   Spatiotemporal coding as a lingua franca

We have claimed that perception and consciousness have a special relationship, in the sense that all qualitative experiences are perceptual or quasi-perceptual (like imagery or inner speech). All perceptual experiences involve spatiotemporal information, of course, and the neurophysiology indicates that a great many neural systems can process spatiotemporal information. This suggests that spatiotemporal coding may be the *lingua franca* that is broadcast through the neural equivalent of a global workspace.

5   *Globally broadcast information may feed back to its sources*

If broadcasting is truly global, the systems that provide global input should also receive their own results, just as a television playwright may watch his own play on television. Such a circulating flow back to the source is postulated in certain cognitive theories. It is known to have a number of useful properties. For example, McClelland and Rumelhart (1981) have shown that a circulating flow in an activation model of word recognition helps to stabilize the representation of the word.

6   *Receivers of global information may feed back their interest to the global workspace*

The physiological evidence discussed above suggests that global *output* flows in two directions as well. There are anatomical connections that allow feedback from the cortex back to the thalamus. Such feedback loops are extremely common in the nervous system. Most sensory systems allow for a flow of information "top down" as well as "bottom up." In the optic nerve a substantial proportion of the neurons go from the higher visual centers outward to the retina – in the "wrong" direction. This anatomical evidence may mean that receiving systems, those that take in globally broadcast information, may be able to feed back their interest to the global workspace, thus strengthening or weakening any particular global message. One can make an analogy to the well-known Nielsen Ratings for television programs in the United States. Each program is continuously sampled to see how many viewers are watching it, and programs of low popularity are quickly dropped. In Chapter 5 I will suggest that this kind of popularity feedback may explain such phenomena as habituation and the development of automaticity with practice.

7   *Other anatomical systems may facilitate global broadcasting*

The Diffuse Thalamic Projection System (Figure 3.1) is not the only projection system that may be used to broadcast information. There are long tertiary cortical neurons that connect frontal to other areas of the cortex, and cross-hemispheric fibers that connect the two halves of the cortex through the corpus callosum. All such transmission pathways may be involved in global broadcasting.

8   Cyclical snowballing rather than immediate broadcasting

The neurophysiology suggests that broadcasting may not be an instantaneous event, but a "snowballing" recruitment of global activation supported by many systems that may feed back on each other. For example, Libet's work indicates that it may take as long as a half second for cortical activity to become conscious (Libet, 1978, 1981). This is much longer than a single-broadcast message would take, and suggests a circulating flow between cortical and subcortical areas, building upon itself until it reaches a threshold. Thus we must not take the broadcasting metaphor too literally: A relatively slow accumulation would accomplish much the same functional end. This kind of snowballing would also explain the role of the anatomical feedback loops described above.

9   Attention: Control of access to the global activating system

In Chapter 8 we will draw a distinction between consciousness and *attention* in which the latter serves to control access to consciousness. Such attentional systems have been found in the parietal and frontal cortex (e.g., Posner, 1982). Possibly the frontal components are involved in voluntary control of attention, which can often override automatic attentional mechanisms.

3.2.1 Changes suggested by the neurophysiology

Figure 3.3 is a modified version of Model 1, with feedback loops from the global message to its input sources and from the receiving processors back to the global message. We will explore additional evidence for these feedback loops in Chapter 5.

3.3   Recent refinements of the neurophysiological evidence

The above interpretation of the neurophysiology resembles earlier models of the Reticular Formation (RF), which we treat here as a subset of the more broadly defined ERTAS (Lindsley, 1958; Magoun, 1962; Moruzzi & Magoun, 1949). Arguments for a central role in conscious experience of the RF have come under some criticism (e.g., Brodal, 1956; Thompson, 1967). Some of these criticisms serve to qualify our conclusions, though they do not contradict them decisively.

First, as more detailed studies have been performed using long-term implanted electrodes, a number of specific components have been found in the RF, so that the bald statement that the RF is nonspecific is not quite true (Hobson & Brazier, 1982). We should be careful not to refer to the whole RF and thalamus as subserving these functions, but only to nuclei

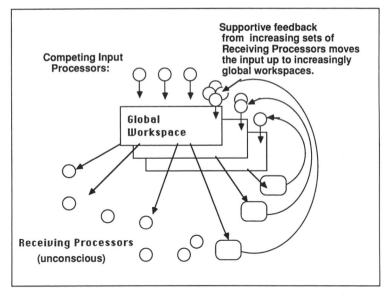

Figure 3.3. Model 1A. Some changes in the theory suggested by the neurophysiology. One implication of the neural structures involved in conscious experience is that there is a two-way flow of information between the ERTAS system – the neural equivalent of a global workspace – and both input and receiving processors. One possibility, shown here, is that receiving processors can support the successful input coalition in much the way a human audience can feed back its appreciation for some particular performer. The neurophysiology is also consistent with the idea that there may be a set of workspaces available to an increasingly wider audience, and that a given input must cycle for some time, gathering support from input and receiving systems, before it becomes fully conscious. (For the sake of simplicity, only a single global workspace will be shown in future diagrams).

and networks within these larger anatomical structures. Second, under some circumstances one can show that lesioned animals with little or no surviving RF tissue show relatively normal waking, sleeping, orienting, and conditioning. It is possible that the outer layer of the thalamus may be able to replace RF functions, especially if the lesions are made gradually, so that there is time for adaptation to take place. Third, it is clear that a number of other parts of the brain are involved in functions closely related to conscious experience, such as voluntary attention; the sense of self; voluntary control of inner speech, imagery, and skeletal musculature; and control of sleep and waking. We must be careful therefore not to limit our consideration to just the extended reticular-thalamic system; surely many other systems act to contribute to, control, and interact with any neural equivalent of a global workspace.

Brain duality

Before concluding this chapter, we should mention the puzzling role of brain duality. The human brain has a major division down the midline, extending far below the great cortical hemispheres into most subcortical structures, including the thalamus and even the brainstem reticular formation. This suggests that duality may be an "architectural" feature of the nervous system. But Model 1 has no place for duality; it emphasizes unity rather than duality.

Brain duality is a fundamental fact of nervous system anatomy. In the intact brain, it is not clear that it has major functional implications; most of the evidence for brain lateralization in normal people shows only very short time delays between left- and right-sided functioning. The corpus callosum, which connects the two hemispheres, is estimated to add perhaps 3 msec of transmission time to interactions between the two sides – not enough to make much of a difference (D. Galin, personal communication, 1986). Still, this massive anatomical feature must be functional in some sense, and it is curious that our architectural approach to the nervous system has no obvious role for it. It is possible that its role is primarily developmental, and that in the intact adult brain its effects are more difficult to observe (e.g., Galin, 1977).

Some qualified conclusions

Even with these qualifications, the evidence is strong that parts of the Extended Reticular-Thalamic Activating System are necessary for the conscious waking state, whereas the cortex and perhaps other parts of the brain provide the *content* of conscious experience. This evidence can be naturally interpreted in terms of the GW model, derived from purely cognitive evidence. Contributions from both the ERTAS and cortex are presumably required to create a stable conscious content. The evidence comes from numerous studies showing a direct relationship between the ERTAS and known conscious functions like sleep and waking, alertness, the Orienting Response, focal attention, sharpening of perceptual discriminations, habituation of orienting, conditioning, and perceptual learning. Further, there is evidence consistent with the three major properties of Model 1: First, major brain structures, especially the cortex, can be viewed as collections of distributed specialized modules; second, some of these modules can cooperate and compete for access to the ERTAS; and third, information that gains access may be broadcast globally to other parts of the nervous system, especially the huge cortical mantle of the brain.

Thus substantial neurophysiological evidence seems to be consistent with Model 1, with one addition: There is evidence of a feedback flow from cortical modules *to* the ERTAS, suggesting that a circulating flow of information may be necessary to keep some content in consciousness. In addition, global information may well feed back to its own input sources. Both kinds of feedback may serve to strengthen and stabilize a coalition of systems that work to keep a certain content on the global workspace. These modifications have been incorporated into Model 1A (Figure 3.3).

3.4 Chapter summary

Let us review where we have been. First, many neuroscientists suggest that the nervous system is a distributed parallel system, with many different specialized processors. A constrastive analysis of neurophysiological evidence about conscious versus unconscious phenomena focused on the well-known Reticular Formation of the brainstem and midbrain, on the outer layer of the thalamus, and on the diffusely projecting fibers from the thalamus to the cortex. Several established facts about the nervous system suggest that we may take the notion of *global* broadcasting quite seriously, that conscious information is indeed very widely distributed in the central nervous system. At least parts of the ERTAS system bear out our expectations regarding a system that can take input from specialized modules in the brain and broadcast this information globally to the nervous system as a whole.

Part III

The fundamental role of context

The next two chapters explore the role of *contexts* – unconscious systems that evoke and shape conscious experience. Chapter 4 maintains that context effects are pervasive in all psychological domains. We survey the extensive evidence for this claim, the various kinds of contexts, and the ways in which they may interact. In a sense, contexts can be thought of as information that the nervous system has *already* adapted to; it is the ground against which new events are defined. Consciousness always seems to favor novel and informative messages. But recognizing novelty requires an implicit comparison to the *status quo*, the old knowledge that is represented contextually.

Chapter 5 develops the notion that all conscious events provide *information* by reducing uncertainty within a stable context. Repeated events tend to fade from consciousness, yet they continue to be processed unconsciously. To be conscious, an event must be novel or significant; it must apparently trigger widespread adaptive processing in the nervous system. One result of this view is an interpretation of *learning* as a change in context, one that alters the way the learned material is experienced. Numerous examples are presented.

4   Model 2:
Unconscious contexts shape
conscious experience

4.0   Introduction

Imagine stepping on a small sailboat on a fine, breezy day, and setting off for a short sail. The weather is fair, and as you set sail from the harbor the water becomes choppy but not uncomfortable. At first, the horizon seems to swing up and down, but you quickly realize that it is the boat that is moving, not the horizon. As you gain your sea legs, the world becomes much steadier. On the way home the movements of the boat seem almost placid, though the force of the wind and the waves has not changed. Your sailboat is tied up to the dock, and as you step back on dry land, the horizon suddenly seems to sway, and you must steady yourself; but very quickly the world becomes stable again.

   This common experience sums up the topic of this chapter and the next. As we walk, run, turn, sit, dance, or climb on dry land, specialized components of the nervous system make running predictions to compensate for our changing relationship to gravity and to the visual surroundings. The world is experienced as stable only when this remarkable feat of prediction is successful. These contextual orientation predictions are entirely unconscious, but they profoundly influence our conscious experience. As long as they are successful, they give no sign of their existence. That may change for a time when we step on a small sailboat, but in a curious way: We still do not experience the change in the *framework* of our experience, we just notice an instability in the *entire perceptual field*. Stepping on the sailboat we experience the novel, unpredictable movements of our body as a change in the world, even though we know full well that the world has not changed; only our relationship to it has. The real world is not swaying with the motion of the deck. We experience the same sensation for a moment when we step back on dry land after

---

The notion of a context as developed in this chapter and the next owes much to many fruitful discussions with Michael A. Wapner.

"gaining our sea legs": unconsciously we now predict a regular yawing and rolling, so that the relationship between reality and expectation has once more gone awry. This experience of an unstable world causes the contextual orientation system to revise its predictions again, and since we are experienced land walkers, we soon regain our equilibrium.

The system that computes our orientation to gravity and the visual world is part of the *context* of our experience. We continually benefit from a host of such contextual processes without experiencing them as *objects* of conscious experience. Their influence can be inferred from many sources. The example of the sailing trip involves a perceptual-motor context, but much the same argument can be made for the contexts of thinking, belief, and communication (4.2). A great deal of the research literature in perception and cognition provides evidence for the pervasive influence of unconscious contexts (e.g., Bransford & Franks, 1976; Levicki, 1986; Rock, 1983).

Context is a key idea in this book. Chapter 2 defined context-sensitivity as the way in which unconscious factors shape our conscious experience. Chapter 5 will suggest that habituated or automatized processes do not disappear, but become part of a new context that will shape later conscious experiences. A *context* is thus *a system that shapes conscious experience without itself being conscious at that time.*[1] It is a close modern relative of "set" and "adaptation level" in perception (Allport, 1954; Bruner, 1957; Helson, 1964; Uznadze, 1966), and of various proposals for knowledge structures and "frames" in cognitive science (Clark & Carlson, 1981; Minsky, 1975). Contexts include currently unconscious *expectations* that shape conscious experiences, and currently unconscious *intentions* that shape voluntary actions (see 6.0 and 7.0). The observations supporting this idea were well known to prebehavioristic psychologists in Europe and the United States, including Wundt, James, the Würtzburg School, Brentano, Gestalt psychologists, and the psychologist Narziss Ach (Blumenthal, 1977; Murray, 1983; Rapaport, 1951). There is nothing really new here, except for a modern theoretical framework – and the fact that modern psychology has neglected this evidence for so long.

The word "context" is often used in current psychology to mean the

---

1   We may sometimes want to treat "context" not as a thing but as a relationship. The assumption made by the visual system that light comes from above may be said to be "contextual with respect to" the perceived concavity of moon craters (Rock, 1983); likewise, an implicit moral framework may be "contextual with respect to" one's feelings of self-esteem. There is no need to become fixated on the question whether context is a thing or a relationship. In either case, contextual information is something unconscious and stable that profoundly shapes whatever becomes conscious.

physical surround, but in this book it only refers to the *inner* world that shapes our experience. After all, the physical environment affects our experiences and actions only if it is represented in the inner world. Thus the context-in-the-world inevitably shapes our experience by way of the context-in-the-head. Further, the inner context preserves important information from the past, which is not available from our current surroundings at all. It makes more sense, therefore, to locate the psychological context inside the nervous system.

Contexts are similar to "activated knowledge structures," "mental representations," "semantic networks," "frames," "schemas," "scripts," "plans," "expectations," and other kinds of knowledge representation that are widely discussed in the cognitive sciences (Bransford, 1979; Helson, 1964; Mandler, 1975a; Miller, Gallanter, & Pribram, 1960; Minsky, 1975; Piaget, 1952; Rumelhart & Norman, 1977). We will borrow freely from this literature. But why add one more term to the current rash of words that mean much the same thing? The reason is simple. For us, the word "context" is not just any mental representation: It is an *unconscious* representation that acts to influence another, conscious representation. This special meaning is not captured by any of the other terms.

This chapter will look into some of the characteristics of stable contexts. We begin with a survey of the great amount of evidence for contextual knowledge, specify some common properties of contexts, and explore the interaction between conscious contents and unconscious contexts.

4.1 Sources of evidence on contexts

Contexts are a bit tricky to think about, because by definition we do not experience them directly. For this reason, we begin with four pervasive sources of evidence for unconscious contexts that shape conscious experience:

1 the existence of *priming effects*, where one conscious experience alters the processing of another, although the first experience is gone by the time the second arrives;
2 the universal phenomenon of *fixedness*, where one cannot escape the influence of unconscious contextual assumptions that stand in the way of solving a problem, or of perceiving an alternative;
3 the case of top-down contextual influences, which *change our conscious* experience of any event that is ambiguous, unknown, degraded, fragmentary, isolated, unpredictable, or partly forgotten;
4 the case of *strong violations* of contextual expectations, which can cause a part of the unconscious context to become conscious and reportable.

Table 4.1. *Contrasts between a conscious experience and its unconscious contexts*

Conscious	Unconscious
1 Percepts, images, inner speech, and bodily feelings Immediately accessible concepts	1 Contextual factors that shape and evoke these conscious events Conceptual presuppositions
2 Input that can be interpreted within a currently dominant context	2 "Acontextual" input for which context is not currently dominant
3 Previously unattended events interrupting the attended stream (e.g., the subject's name)	3 Unattended events that affect the interpretation of attended events (e.g., disambiguating words)
4 Strong violations of unconscious contexts (decontextualization)	4 Weak violations of unconscious contexts (e.g., proofreader effect)

Table 4.1 summarizes the contrast between conscious and unconscious phenomena connected with context.

We will give examples of each case.

4.1.1 Priming effects: Conscious experiences generally improve receptivity to related conscious experiences

When one experience affects the likelihood of a similar experience, we can say that the first event has "primed" or shaped the context for the second event. This is a phenomenon of extreme generality. Blumenthal quotes Fraisse (1963), for example:

"When I listen to speech, I perceive the clause being pronounced by the speaker, but I interpret it in accordance with all the sentences which I no longer perceive and of which I have only retained a general idea. When I listen to music, I perceive again and again a short, rhythmic structure, but this is integrated with a melodic whole to which it owes its affective resonance." (Blumenthal, 1977, p. 88)

Music and speech are indeed very good examples. Psycholinguistic research has now amassed extensive evidence for widespread discourse relations that are necessary to understand even a single word in a conversation, although those relationships are of course not focally conscious (Clark & Carlson, 1981; Clark & Clark, 1977; see 4.1.3). Similarly, in a piece of music the key, the initial statement of the themes, their development and variations, all must shape the way we experience a single phrase in the middle of a symphony, but none of that is conscious when we have that experience.

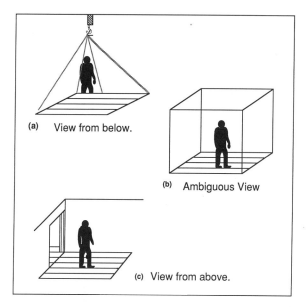

Figure 4.1. Priming effects: Conscious events increase access to similar events. One of many hundreds of demonstrations of priming effects, the ambiguous Necker cube allows one to interpret the middle figure (*b*) as seen either from above or below. Which interpretation will be chosen is influenced by previous conscious experiences. The construction worker being lifted on a platform by a crane (*a*) provides one imaginable framework in which we view from below a person standing on a floor. Viewing *a* for a little while will tend to prime the view from below, whereas contemplating *c* will tend to prime the view from above. Since we more commonly experience the top view (*c*), there is an overall bias toward it, which may be considered a long-term priming effect.

Figure 4.1 gives an example of a short-term priming effect. The middle Figure (*b*) is an ambiguous Necker cube. By paying attention to Figure *a* for several seconds and then going back to *b*, we tend to interpret the ambiguous figure as if we are looking at the bottom of the cube. The experience of Figure *a* structures the experience of *b*, even though *a* is not conscious when it does so. Now, if we pay attention to Figure *c* for a while, we are more likely to see the ambiguous cube from the top.

We can easily show linguistic priming. Compare the next two examples, in which the first word primes an interpretion of the second:

volume: book

versus

arrest: book.

The conscious interpretation of "book" will differ depending upon the prime.

In general, a conscious priming event:

1 decreases reaction time to similar conscious events;
2 lowers the threshold for related material that is near the perceptual threshold, or is ambiguous, vague, fleeting, degraded, badly understood, or isolated from its surround. Indeed any task that has an unconscious *choice-point* in the flow of processing is sensitive to priming for the relevant alternative (Baars, 1985);
3 a prime increases the likelihood of similar events emerging in memory through free association, cued recall, and recognition tasks; and
4 finally, a conscious prime increases the probability of actions and speech related to the priming stimulus (Baars, 1985; see 7.4).

Priming effects are ubiquitous in sensation, perception, comprehension, and action. In an older psychological vocabulary, priming creates set (Ach, 1905/1951; Bruner, 1957; Luchins, 1942). Indeed, the Psychophysical Law, the oldest and one of the best-established findings in psychology, states that the experienced intensity of any stimulus depends on the intensity of preceding stimuli. This can be thought of as a temporal priming effect with universal application.

Priming effects are not always momentary; they can last at least as long as a conversation (Foss, 1982), and we suggest below that some contexts triggered by conscious experiences may last for years (9.2.1). So we are not talking merely of momentary events. Even a single conscious experience may trigger a short-term change in context (Levicki, 1986); in the case of traumatic experiences the effects can last for years (Horowitz, 1975a,b).

Generally the word "priming" is used to refer to those cases where our perception of an event *is improved by* earlier similar experiences. There are also cases of *contrast*, where an earlier event causes the later one to be perceived in an opposite way. For example, Uznadze (1966) showed that sometimes the perceived weight of a rubber ball will be *increased*, and sometimes it will be *decreased* by earlier exposure to another weighted ball. All these effects can be treated as context effects by our definition, since the observer is not conscious of the influence of the earlier event *at the time* the later one becomes conscious. But we will focus on the more common case, where later processes are facilitated by an earlier conscious experience.

The similarity of the prime and the primed event can be either perceptual or conceptual. The similarity between "book" and "volume" in the example above is not perceptual but semantic or conceptual; the similarity between the two views of the Necker cube in Figure 4.1 is more perceptual.

The predictions made about contexts throughout this book can often be tested with priming tasks. This is one reason to emphasize the role of priming.

4.1.2 Fixedness: Being blind to "the obvious"

The four sentences below are normal, coherent English sentences:

1   The ship sailed past the harbor sank.
2   The building blocks the sun shining on the house faded are red.
3   The granite rocks by the seashore with the waves.
4   The cotton clothing is made of grows in Alabama. (Milne, 1982, p. 350)

On first reading these sentences, most of us feel stuck; they do not cohere, they do not work somehow. We may be driven to try rather farfetched ideas to make sense of them: Maybe sentence (1) is really two conjoined clauses, such as "The ship sailed past *and* the harbor sank?" But harbors do not sink, so that interpretation does not work either. If we truly believe that these are normal English sentences, the experience of trying to understand them can be intensely frustrating and annoying.

What is going on? Consider the following *context* for sentence (1):

A small part of Napoleon's fleet tried to run the English blockade at the entrance to the harbor. Two ships, a sloop and a frigate, ran straight for the harbor while a third ship tried to sail *past* the harbor in order to draw enemy fire. The ship sailed past the harbor sank.

If you have just encountered sentence (1) for the first time, this little story should help solve the problem. "Oh! You mean 'The ship (comma) sailed past the harbor (comma) *sank!*' But that's dirty pool!" Not so; the sentence is really quite normal, as we can see when it is put in context.

We could, of course, insert the subordinate clause marker "which" to create

(1') The ship *which* sailed past the harbor sank;

but this use of "which" is optional in English, though we tend to insert it when needed for clarity.

The problem we encountered with sentence (1) is one kind of *fixedness*. We approach sentences in English with the contextual assumption that the first verb will be the main verb, barring contrary semantic or syntactic information (viz., Milne, 1982). If "sailed" is assumed to be the main verb, then we do not know what to do with the verb "sank." But "sailed" may also be the verb of a *subordinate clause*, as in the following examples:

a   The ship *sailed* by the commodore *was* a beautiful sight.
b   The ships *sailed* at Newport *are* racing sloops.
c   To my surprise, a ship *sailed* by a good crew *sank*.

Here the main verbs always come later in the sentence. The trouble with sentence (1) is that we tend to become committed to one syntactic interpretation before all the evidence is in, and we may find it impossible to back away from it. In the most general terms, we are captured by one unconscious interpretation of the beginning of the sentence. We are *fixated by the wrong syntactic context.*

Fixedness can be found in all kinds of problem solving. It is found in vision, in language perception, in solving puzzles, in science, literature, politics, and warfare (Bruner & Potter, 1964; Duncker, 1945; Levine, 1971; Levine & Fingerman, 1974; Luchins, 1942). American policy during the Vietnam war may have been an example of fixedness, since it followed certain assumptions about international relations that were widely accepted at that time, across the political spectrum. In retrospect, some of those assumptions are questionable. But that is just the point about fixedness: Seen in retrospect or from "the outside," it is hard to believe that the fixated person cannot see the "obvious" solution. But *within* the fixating context the solution is not obvious at all: It is literally impossible to perceive.

Yet fixedness is a completely normal part of learning. Whenever we try to learn something before we have the knowledge needed to make sense of the material, we may find ourselves interpreting it in the wrong context. McNeill (1966) cites the example of a mother trying to teach her child something about English negation – a bit prematurely:

CHILD: Nobody don't like me.
MOTHER: No, say "Nobody likes me."
CHILD: Nobody don't like me.
MOTHER: No, say "Nobody likes me."
(*Eight repetitions of this dialogue*)
MOTHER: No, now listen carefully, say, "Nobody likes me."
CHILD: Oh! Nobody don't likes me.

A year later the same child would laugh at the error, but when the dialogue was recorded he was not prepared to perceive the difference. In learning, as in life, readiness is all.

A major point is to realize that our notion of "fixedness" depends critically on having an outside point of view in which the mistake *is* a mistake. That is to say, as adults we can find the above example comfortably amusing, because we know the right answer. But for the child the error is no error at all. The "flawed" sentence is not experienced as erroneous; in terms of the child's internalized rules, it is not an error at all.

Selective attention as a contextual fixedness effect
One powerful implication is that "fixedness" exists in states of mind we consider to be perfectly correct. For example, one can plausibly argue that selective attention is a fixed state of mind – after all, in shadowing speech in one ear we are utterly oblivious to the unattended stream of

speech, as much as the child in the language example is oblivious to the "correct" sentence. Thus the remarkable ability of one stream of speech to capture our conscious experience to the exclusion of any other looks like a contextual fixedness effect. Notice that structural similarities between the two streams of speech will cause leakage between them; that is, when they share context, the "unconscious" stream tends to affect the conscious stream (e.g., Norman, 1976). Normally we can hear the acoustical qualities of the unattended ear, perhaps because these qualities match the acoustical contexts of the attended ear. After all, the attended ear must detect a range of sounds as well. Further, when the semantic context of the attended involves an ambiguous word like "bank," it is open to influences from the unattended ear to the extent those influences are consistent with the semantic ambiguity (MacKay, 1973). In Table 4.1 this point is made by listing "acontextual" information on the unconscious side of the contrastive table. When there is potentially conscious input, but the right context is not brought to bear on it, it does not become conscious.

Similarly, in absorbed states of mind – in reading an engrossing novel or watching an entrancing motion picture – we are deaf and blind to the world. In absentminded states we are likewise captured by one train of thought to the exclusion of others (Reason, 1983). One plausible supposition is that all these states are initiated, shaped, and bounded by powerful context hierarchies that permit no interruption for the time being.

Only a change in the fixating context, or giving up on the task, can release us from fixedness. Above, this change in context is created by the little story about Napoleon's ships running the English blockade. This creates a new context that works, but that no doubt has its own fixating properties. This is the normal case, of course: We may change to a more effective context, but we cannot undo context as such. Inevitably we are condemned to both its advantages and drawbacks.

The existence of fixedness provides extensive evidence for the power of contexts. Next, we consider the case in which context actually enters into conscious experience.

4.1.3 Top-down influences and the pervasiveness of ambiguity

Many domains of experience are full of local ambiguities. This is obvious in some cases, and not so obvious in others. Among the obvious examples, there many times when information about the world is degraded, inadequate, or forgotten, such as when listening to a conversation in a noisy room, trying to see an oncoming bus at a great distance, or walking through a dark room at night. In all these cases we rely more than usual on the inner context to constrain conscious experience. In the social realm, it is terribly important for us to know other people's minds – their intentions, beliefs, and attitudes toward us. But we cannot read their minds directly. The evidence we have is ambiguous, and hence vulnerable to our own goals and expectations, wishes, and fears. We often make inferences about other people's minds with a degree of confidence that is simply not justified by the evidence (Nisbett & Wilson, 1977). In this case, inner context controls our experience far too often. Political convictions show this even more graphically. A glance at the editorial pages of a newspaper shows how people with different convictions use the same events to support opposite beliefs about the world, about other people, and about morality. Or take the domain of "the future": Human beings are intensely concerned about the future, and we often have strong beliefs about it, even when future events are inherently probabilistic (Tversky & Kahneman, 1973). The evidence is inadequate or ambiguous, and hence we rely more and more on internal contextual constraints.

These examples are fairly obvious, but there are many ambiguous domains in which we experience events with great confidence, though careful experiments show that there is much more local uncertainty than we realize. There is extensive evidence that our own bodily feelings, which we may use to infer our emotions, are often ambiguous (Schachter & Singer, 1962; Valins, 1967). Further, our own intentions and reasons for making decisions are often inaccessible to introspection, or at least ambiguous (Nisbett & Wilson, 1977) (see Chapters 6 and 9). Our memory of the past is often as poor as our ability to anticipate the future, and it is prone to be filtered through our present perspective (Bransford, 1979; Mandler, 1984). Historians must routinely cope with the universal tendency of people to reshape the past in light of the present, and lawyers actively employ techniques designed to make witnesses change their memory of a crime or accident (see Bransford, 1979).

Even perceptual domains that seem stable and reliable are actually ambiguous when we isolate small pieces of information. Every corner in a normal rectangular room can be interpreted in two ways, as an outside or an inside corner. To see this, the reader can simply roll a piece of paper into a tube, and look through it to any right-angled corner of the room. Every room contains both two- and three-dimensional ambiguities in its corners, much like the Necker cube and book-end illusions (Figure 2.1). Similarly, the experienced brightness of surfaces depends upon the brightness of surrounding surfaces (Gelb, 1932; Gilchrist, 1977). Depth perception is controlled by our contextual assumptions about the direction of the incoming light, about the shape and size of objects, and the like

(Rock, 1983). These ambiguities emerge when we isolate stimuli – but it is important to note that in normal visual perception, stimulus input is often isolated. In any single eye-fixation we only take in a very small, isolated patch of information. Normal detailed (foveal) vision spans only 2 degrees of arc; yet when people are asked about the size of their own detailed visual field, they often believe it must be about 180 degrees. Even the visual world, which seems so stable and reliable, is full of local ambiguities (Marr, 1982).

Language, as we have seen, provides a great many examples of ambiguity. Indeed, every level of linguistic analysis has its own kind of ambiguity. Thus,

1   Ambiguities of sound. The English /l/ is perceived as either /r/ or /l/ by Japanese speakers, while the unaspirated /k/ (as in "cool") is freely exchanged by English speakers with the aspirated /kh/ (as in "keel"). In Arabic this difference marks very different words. Most English speakers simply do not hear the tones that are critical in languages like Chinese. Further, there are many identical strings of sounds in every language that are divided up differently, as in "ice cream" and "I scream" in English. We typically become conscious of these ambiguous sound sequences only in learning a new language.
2   Morphemic ambiguity. The final /s/ in English has four different morphemic interpretations. It can be plural ("the books"), third person singular verb ("he books the tickets"), possessive ("the book's cover"), or plural possessive ("the books' covers").
3   Lexical ambiguity. A glance at the dictionary should convince anyone that each word has more than one meaning. More common words tend to have more meanings.
4   Syntactic ambiguity. There are numerous syntactic ambiguities. The best-known ones are the surface and deep-structure ambiguities of Chomskyan theory (Chomsky, 1957, 1965). Thus, "old men and women" is a surface ambiguity that involves grouping: One can have "old (men and women)," or "(old men) and women." Sentences like "Flying planes can be dangerous" and "They are eating apples" have ambiguities that cannot be represented in a single tree diagram; they involve ambiguity in underlying subjects and objects.
5   Discourse ambiguity. Consider the following example:
    a The glass fell off the table.
    b It broke.
    b' It was always a little unstable.
    The referent of "it" changes between (b) and (b'). It can only be determined by an appeal to context, and to our knowledge about glasses and tables. Such ambiguities are extremely common.
6   Referential ambiguity. This occurs when we refer to "that chair" in an auditorium full of chairs, or to "that book" in a library.
7   Semantic ambiguity. All too often, concepts do not relate clearly to other concepts. What really is consciousness? What is an atom, or a physical force, or a biological species? All unresolved scientific questions involve deep semantic ambiguity.

8   Topical uncertainty and ambiguity. Consider the following paragraph
(from Bransford, 1979, p. 134):

> The procedure is actually quite simple. First you arrange items into
> different groups. Of course one pile may be sufficient depending upon
> how much there is to do. If you have to go somewhere else due to lack
> of facilities that is the next step; otherwise, you are pretty well set. It is
> important not to overdo things. That is, it is better to do too few things
> at once than too many. In the short run this may not seem important but
> complications can easily arise. A mistake can be made as well. At first,
> the whole procedure will seem complicated. Soon, however, it will
> become just another facet of life. It is difficult to foresee any end to the
> necessity for this task in the immediate future, but then, one never can
> tell. After the procedure is completed one arranges the materials into
> different groups again. Then they can be put into their appropriate
> places. Eventually they will be used once more and the whole cycle will
> have to be repeated. However, that is part of life.

> Confused? Here is the context: The paragraph is about washing
> clothes. If you read it again, it will be much more comprehensible, details
> will clarify in experience, and memory for the material will improve
> greatly.

What is the point of this litany of ambiguities? It is that ambiguity is
pervasive; but the *conscious experience of ambiguity* is quite rare. We
generally gain information about a world that is locally ambiguous, yet we
usually experience a stable, coherent world. This suggests that *before
input becomes conscious, it interacts with numerous unconscious contextual influences to produce a single, coherent, conscious experience.*
Consciousness and context are twin issues, inseparable in the nature of
things.

As we pointed out in Chapter 2, the global workspace architecture was
originally developed to deal precisely with the problem of unifying many
ambiguous or partial sources of information into a single, unified solution
(2.3.1).

The next section considers another source of evidence on contexts.

4.1.4 Decontextualization: Strong violations of context can become consciously accessible

Unconscious contextual assumptions can become consciously accessible.
Every statement we hear or read has presupposed (contextual) information that must be understood before it can make sense. The "washing
machine" paragraph shown just above is an example. But these contextual presuppositions remain unconscious *unless* they are violated. If we
suddenly speak of putting a five-pound weight into the washing machine,
we tend to become conscious of one contextual assumption. We will call

this process decontextualization. It is a theoretically central phenomenon. Consider the following example, which is quite normal, so that presupposed ideas tend to remain unconscious:

1   It was a hot day. Johnny walked to the store and bought some ice cream to eat. Then he brought home a snow cone for his mother.

But now consider the following version. (It will be helpful to read it slowly):

2   a It was a hot day in December.
    b Johnny walked three hours to the town store.
    c He was completely broke but not very hungry.
    d He bought a gallon of ice cream and ate to his heart's content.
    e He also brought a snow cone home to his mother.

The second story makes implausible a number of conditions in the presupposed context of the event "buying ice cream," so that we find this normally unconscious knowledge becoming conscious (see Figure 4.2). Story (1) left unconscious the fact that "walking to the store to get ice cream" is assumed to take a matter of minutes (not three hours); that hot days are likely in summer (not in December); that buying involves money (thus being broke excludes buying anything); that one would certainly not eat a gallon of ice cream if one were not very hungry; and that walking home for three hours on a hot day, carrying a snow cone, would cause it to melt. When these implausible claims are presented, at least some of the contradicted context tends to come to mind spontaneously.

We can think of this presupposed context as a set of *stable, predictable constraints* on normal discourse (Clark & Carlson, 1981; Foss, 1982). As long as a piece of presupposed knowledge remains predictable it also tends to remain unconscious. But when it is strongly violated, its consequences tend to become conscious in some way. This is similar to the pattern we find with violated expectations in stimulus habituation, with obstacles created in automatic tasks, and with increases in task difficulty for habituated mental images (see 1.4.1; 5.1). In all these cases novel information is created by the violation of established, predictable properties of the situation. Of course, when we make parts of a conceptual context conscious, this places the newly conscious material in its *own* unconscious context. Becoming conscious of contextual knowledge while it is acting as context is like chasing one's tail; it is ultimately impossible.

4.1.5 A summary of the evidence for unconscious contexts

We have detailed several factors so far. First, conscious experiences change later, related experiences long after the earlier ones have become unconscious. Presumably, the first experience creates a context within which the later one is shaped and defined.

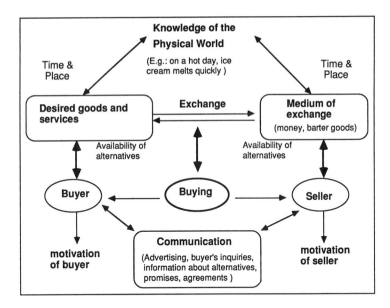

Figure 4.2. Presuppositions of the concept of "buying" that may become conscious upon violation. The knowledge necessary to understand an everyday concept like "buying" shown in the form of a semantic network. "Buying" presupposes other concepts, such as time, space, exchange, movement, transportation, communication, money or another valued medium of exchange, motivation, anticipated gain for both buyer and seller, and so on. It is incomprehensible, or something very different, without these concepts. But these presupposed concepts are not conscious in a routine act of buying. Some of the presupposed concepts may become consciously accessible when they are violated or when there is some uncertainty about them. Thus, the idea of carrying an ice cream cone for an hour on a hot day violates some presuppositions, which may then be broadcast via the global workspace. In GW theory, the presupposed network of concepts needed to understand a consciously accessed concept is called a conceptual context (4.4, Figure 4.5).

Second, the universal phenomenon of fixedness suggests that all conscious and deliberate processes are bounded by assumptions that are unconscious to the subject, though they may be obvious to outside observers. Selective attention and absorbed states may be variations on this theme of fixedness.

Third, there is extensive evidence for local ambiguity in all areas of life: the past, the future, other people's minds, our own feelings, visual and auditory perception, language understanding, and so forth. All these domains are rife with ambiguity; yet ambiguities are rarely experienced *as* ambiguities. Normally, many different contexts interact to create a single conscious interpretation of reality.

Fourth, strong violations of our contextual assumptions can become conceptually conscious – that is, we can refer to these surprises as objects of experience, and as they become conscious, we can sometimes change our previous contextual way of thinking about them.

We can assess contexts in two convenient ways. First, priming tasks can be designed to be sensitive to the information contained in a dominant context. Current cognitive psychology has dozens of examples of the use of such priming techniques (e.g., Baars, 1985; Swinney, 1979). Second, one can observe the occurrence of surprise in response to events that violate contextual expectations. Thus, changes in heart rate – a measure of surprise – have been used to assess the existence of phoneme boundaries in infants who could not possibly tell us about their experience. Measures of surprise could be used much more often with adults, because there is little reason to think that adult voluntary report of contextual structures is accurate; hence we may miss contextual violations in adults rather often because of our reliance on verbal report.

4.2   Several kinds of contexts

We can distinguish several kinds of contexts including, first, the Contexts of Perception and Imagery; the Context of Conceptual Thought; goal contexts, which evoke and shape actions; and finally, the context of communication that is shared by two people talking with each other, or by ourselves talking to ourselves. Notice that some of these contexts actually shape conscious experience as such, while others evoke conscious thoughts and images or help select conscious percepts. Perceptual–imaginal contexts clearly enter into the conscious qualitative experience. A goal context may simply serve to recall a word (6.0) or evoke a mental image. That is, not all contexts necessarily enter into the experience itself. However, these different kinds of contexts seem to interact with each other: Perceptual events and images have a lot of influence on conceptual thinking; concepts influence inner speech, images, and the selection of perceptual events; goals influence concepts, and vice versa. We will now examine the types of context in a little more detail.

4.2.1 The Contexts of Perception and Imagery

The Context of Perception

Imagine sitting in a tiny, well-lit movie theater looking at a metallic disk instead of a movie screen. The disk appears to be white. But now someone lights a cigarette, and as the smoke curls upward you see it floating through a slender but powerful light beam, coming from the rear of the theater, and aimed precisely at the metal disk. You look back at the disk, and suddenly notice that it isn't white at all, but black. This is the Gelb Effect (Gelb, 1932), and can be summarized by saying that the color of a surface is a function of the perceived incoming light. If we never become conscious of the incoming light, we will attribute the brightness of the disk to its surface color and not to the light. Once having seen the cigarette smoke intersecting the light beam, the disk is seen to be black. Similarly, if we turn a picture of the moon's craters upside down, the experience of depth is reversed, so that the craters are seen as hills. This is because scenes are interpreted under the assumption that light comes from above, as indeed it usually does. When the photo of the moon is turned upside-down, the light is still assumed to come from the top of the picture, and concavities are seen as convexities (Rock, 1983).

Perceptual research since the nineteenth century has uncovered hundreds of such phenomena. They can be summarized by saying that complex and subtle unconscious systems, which we call contexts, shape and define conscious perceptual experiences.

The Context of Imagery

Imagery has not been studied as extensively as perception, but over the past decade very interesting findings have emerged, suggesting constraints on visual imagery of which we are generally unconscious. These constraints tell us about both the *format* and the *content* of imagery (Kosslyn & Schwartz, 1981). The "field" of visual imagery has a close resemblance to vision: It has the same flat elliptical shape as the visual field, it presents us with one perspective on a potentially three-dimensional spatial domain, and the scanning time needed to move from one point to another in the Mind's Eye is a linear function of the distance between the two points, just as we might expect of the visual field.

Clearly as we learn more about mental imagery, we will continue to find more of these constraints, which are largely unconscious until they are brought to mind.

4.2.2 The Context of Conceptual Thought

Anyone who has tried to think very clearly about some topic must know from experience that our *stable presuppositions* tend to become unconscious. Whatever we believe with absolute certainty we tend to take for granted. Moreover, we lose sight of the fact that *alternatives to our stable presuppositions can be entertained.* Indeed, scientific-paradigm shifts generally take place when one group of scientists begins to challenge a presupposition that is held to be immutable (and hence is largely unconscious) in the thinking of an older scientific establishment. In his autobiography, Albert Einstein described this phenomenon in nineteenth-century physics (1949):

> All physicists of the last century saw in classical mechanics a firm and final foundation for all physics, yes, indeed, for all natural science. . . . Even Maxwell and H. Hertz, who in retrospect appear as those who demolished the faith in mechanics as the final basis of all physical thinking, *in their conscious thinking* adhered throughout to mechanics as the secured basis of physics. (p. 21; italics added)

Some pages later he recalls how he gained the insight that led to the Special Theory of Relativity:

> After ten years of reflection such a principle resulted from a paradox upon which I had already hit at the age of sixteen: If I pursue a beam of light with the velocity c (the velocity of light in a vacuum), I should observe such a beam of light as a spatially oscillatory electromagnetic field at rest. However, there seems to be no such thing. . . . One sees that in this paradox the germ of the special relativity theory is already contained. Today everyone knows, of course, that all attempts to clarify this paradox satisfactorily were condemned to failure as long as the axiom of the absolute character of time, viz., of simultaneity, *unrecognizedly was anchored in the unconscious.* (p. 53; italics added)

Kuhn (1970) quotes Charles Darwin to much the same effect:

> Darwin, in a particularly perceptive passage at the end of his *Origin of Species*, wrote, "Although I am fully convinced of the truth of the views given in this volume. . . . I by no means expect to convince experienced naturalists whose minds are stocked with a multitude of facts all viewed, during a long course of years, from a point of view directly opposite to mine. . . . [B]ut I look with confidence to the future – to young rising naturalists, *who will be able to view both sides of the question* with impartiality." (p. 151, italics added)

Darwin observed that many older naturalists were simply unable to consciously think consistently of the alternatives to their own, stable presuppositons. In psychology this phenomenon is easy to observe today, since the field has recently passed through something much like a paradigm shift (see Baars, 1986a). It is still remarkably easy to find psychologists who find it impossible to take the existence of consciousness seriously. For these people, the implications of consciousness as something scientifically real and important remain hidden and unconscious.

It would be interesting to find out why conceptual presuppositions tend to become conscious so readily in a simple example like the one cited above (4.1.4), compared to the case of scientific change, where Darwin, Einstein, and many others have complained so much about the inability of other scientists to entertain alternatives to their own presuppositions. Was it because these scientists were emotionally invested in their customary way of viewing the world? Or do more complex knowledge domains make it more difficult to see contextual alternatives and their consequences? Or both?

Perceptual versus conceptual contexts

There are some interesting differences between the perceptual and the conceptual context. In the case of perception, when the context is challenged we do not "perceive" the challenge directly, though we can conceptualize it. That is, in getting used to the swaying of a small sailing boat, we can think of the conceptual fact that the horizon is really not swaying, but the boat is. It is not clear whether this conceptual realization about the perceptual context helps the process of adaptation.

The Ames room provides another good example. As we noted above, a room with trapezoidal walls can appear normal so long as the observer is stationary and monocular. In that case, a person walking in the room will be seen to grow as he or she is approaching the low end of the trapezoidal wall, and to shrink while walking in the opposite direction. The visual system, forced to choose between revising its assumptions about the room or about the constant height of people, prefers to let human height change to keep the room the same. However, when the observer is allowed to bounce a few ping-pong balls against surfaces in the room, the challenge to contextual assumptions becomes overwhelming. The balls bounce off at odd angles for a normal room; they take longer to reach the opposite wall when it is farther away, even though it seems close by. Now the observer experiences a shift: The room is seen to be truly trapezoidal, and human height is experienced as constant. Previous unconscious assumptions are revised, and we now experience the room veridically.

Things are quite different in solving a conceptual problem. Einsteinian physicists who began to question the time axiom of Newtonian theory were able to change their presuppositions directly and voluntarily, even though their more traditional colleagues found this difficult or impossible. In conceptual contexts, we can at times make a piece of context consciously accessible, and in doing so change it. The new conceptual context then begins to shape the interpretation of scientific observations. Notice that once we question a presupposed idea, it is no longer presupposed, but focal and conscious. It is therefore interpreted in its own conceptual context. When we *talk* about our conceptual context we can make a piece of it conscious.

Scientific paradigms as largely unconscious contexts

Communication problems occur when people try to exchange ideas under different contextual assumptions. This is especially clear in the case of paradigmatic differences in a scientific community. One might expect science at least to be free of such communication problems, because scientists deal with a shared, observable empirical domain and because mature sciences make use of explicit formal theories. Not so. Historians have long remarked on the frequency of communication problems in science, but it is only with Thomas Kuhn's seminal monograph *The structure of scientific revolutions* (1970) that these communication problems have come to be widely acknowledged as part of the fundamental nature of science. Kuhn described two kinds of evolution in the history of science: Within a certain framework, or "paradigm," development is cumulative, since scientists share common tools, goals, typical problems, and assumptions about reality. Thus physics enjoyed a shared paradigm in the two centuries after Newton's *Principia Mathematica* until the late nineteenth century, when the paradigm began to develop difficult internal contradictions. Einstein's relativity theory solved some of those problems, giving rise to a new framework within which physicists could again communicate without serious problems for some time; but Einsteinian physicists had great difficulty communicating with those who continued to view the world in Newtonian terms. Kuhn (1970) calls this phenomenon "the *incommensurability* of competing paradigms":

Since new paradigms are born from old ones, they ordinarily incorporate much of the vocabulary and apparatus, both conceptual and manipulative, that the traditional paradigm had previously employed. But they seldom employ these borrowed elements in quite the traditional way. Within the new paradigm, old terms, concepts, and experiments fall into new relationships with the other. The inevitable result is what we must call, though the term is not quite right, a *misunderstanding* between the two competing schools. The laymen who scoffed at Einstein's general theory of relativity because space could not be "curved" – it was not that sort of thing – were not simply wrong or mistaken. Nor were the mathematicians, physicists, and philosophers who tried to develop a Euclidian version of Einstein's theory. What had previously been meant by space was necessarily flat, homogeneous, isotropic, and unaffected by the presence of matter. If it had not been, Newtonian physics would not have worked. To make the transition to Einstein's universe, the whole conceptual web whose strands are space, time, matter, force, and so on, had to be shifted and laid down again on nature whole. . . . *Communication across the revolutionary divide is inevitably partial.* Consider, for another example, the men who called Copernicus mad because he proclaimed that the earth moved. They were not either just wrong or quite wrong. Part of what they meant by "earth" was fixed position. *Their* earth, at least, could not be moved. Correspondingly, Copernicus's innovation was not simply to move the earth. Rather, it was a whole new way of regarding the problems of physics and astronomy, one that necessarily changed the meaning of both "earth" and "motion." Without those changes the concept of a moving earth *was* mad. . . .

These examples point to the . . . most fundamental aspect of the *incommensurability between competing paradigms.* In a sense that I am unable to explicate further, the proponents of competing paradigms practice their trades in different worlds. One contains constrained bodies that fall slowly, the other pendulums that repeat their motions again and again. In one, [chemical] solutions are compounds, in the other mixtures. One is embedded in a flat, the other in a curved, matrix of space. Practicing in different worlds, the two groups of scientists see different things when they look from the same point in the same direction. Again, that is not to say that they can see anything they please. Both are looking at the world, and what they look at has not changed. But in some areas they see different things, and they see them in different relations one to the other. That is why a law that cannot even be demonstrated to one group of scientists may occasionally seem intuitively obvious to another. Equally, it is why, *before they can hope to communicate fully, one group or the other must experience the conversion we have been calling a paradigm shift.* Just because it is a transition between incommensurables, the transition between competing paradigms cannot be made a step at a time, forced by logic and neutral experience. (pp. 149–51; italics added)

Why is it so difficult for committed scientists to change paradigms? From our model, it would seem that change is hard, at least in part because at any single moment the bulk of a paradigm is unconscious. In our terms, paradigms are conceptual contexts. If one tried to make a paradigm conscious, one could only make one aspect of it conscious at any one time because of the limited capacity of consciousness. But typically paradigm-differences between two groups of scientists involve not just one, but many different aspects of the mental framework simultaneously. This may also be why conversion phenomena in science (as elsewhere) tend to be relatively rapid, all-or-none events that seem to have a not quite rational component. In fact, Kuhn compares the experience of conversion to a "Gestalt switch" such as we observe with the Necker Cube (2.1, 4.1.1).

4.2.3 Intentions as goal contexts

Thus far we have talked about two kinds of contexts, the qualitative (perceptual–imaginal) context and the conceptual context. conscious experiences also interact with a third kind of unconscious context, which we will call the *goal context.* Goal contexts are useful in understanding problem solving, intentions, and voluntary control. We will postpone a detailed consideration of goal contexts until Chapters 6 and 7. However, it is important at this point to introduce the concept of an ordered *Goal Hierarchy* – simply, the idea that goals are ordered in significance at any point in time, and that higher (more significant) goals will tend to predominate over lower ones. This is by no means a new idea; it has been suggested by numerous motivational and cognitive psychologists (e.g., Maslow, 1970), and the computational implications of Goal Hierarchies

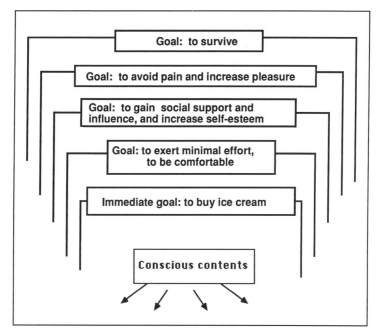

Figure 4.3. A significance hierarchy of goal contexts. A hypothetical set of
ordered goal contexts (a Goal Hierarchy) that together influence conscious
contents without themselves being entirely conscious when they do so. Notice
that higher-level goal contexts are more significant than lower-level ones. No
claim is made about the particular goals chosen: Under different conditions the
hierarchy might be somewhat different – surely, the goal of eating becomes more
significant after a long, involuntary fast. Such goals are largely contextual by
definition; they will tend to become conscious when violated in some way, but not
in the normal course of events (see Chapters 6 and 7).

have been worked out in some detail by artificial intelligence researchers.
Our emphasis at this point is on the control of conscious events by such
contextual Goal Hierarchies, which are diagrammed in Figure 4.3.

Note that Goal Hierarchies cannot be rigid over time. For instance, the
goal of eating must rise higher in the hierarchy after food deprivation. But
at any one moment the hierarchy is ordered; that is, at any particular time
we will prefer food over sex over watching TV. Some goals are more
stable over time: In general, survival has a higher priority than avoiding
boredom. We will not develop this notion here; we simply suggest that a
set of ordered goals can act as context for the flow of conscious
experience. The evidence for this claim is developed in Chapters 6 and 7.

4.2.4 Other types of context

Social and cultural contexts usually operate unconsciously. The sociologist Ervin Goffman (1974) writes,

> When the individual in our Western society recognizes a particular (social) event, he tends . . . [to] employ one or more frameworks or schemata of interpretation . . . to locate, perceive, identify, and label a seemingly infinite number of concrete occurrences defined in its terms. *He is likely to be unaware of such organized features as the framework has and unable to describe the framework with any completeness if asked,* yet these handicaps are no bar to his easily and fully applying it. (p. 21; italics added)

Anthropologists often encounter their own cultural presuppositions in a dramatic way when they enter a culture that violates those presuppositions; as usual, unconscious presuppositions can become conscious when they are severely violated. In conversation, a member of another culture may seem to thrust his face toward a Westerner an unacceptable six inches away. This may be experienced by a Westerner as shocking or offensive, but it makes conscious what is normally taken for granted: Namely, the fact that we, too, adopt a typical social distance. Thus unconscious customs and habits come to the foreground. Custom leads to adaptation and loss of consciousness; this is why children, novices, and strangers can guide us to become conscious again of things we have lost touch with in the process of becoming adults, experts, and members of various in-groups. These properties of context have major implications for sociology and anthropology. For instance, all cultures have periodic ceremonies, festivals, and initiation rites using dramatic or even traumatic symbolism; a major function of these events may be to create and renew memorable conscious experiences that invoke and reinforce the unconscious contextual assumptions of the society.

Much the same sort of thing is true for motivation and personality research. The genius of Freud has led us to believe that much of our lack of awareness of ourselves is due to repression. This may be true, but even without repression we should be ignorant of regularities in our own actions, beliefs, and experiences, simply because regularity by itself creates unconscious context (e.g., Nisbett & Wilson, 1977; see Chapter 9). It is possible that motivational mechanisms like repression and denial make use of contexts to ward off painful or confusing experiences (8.4).

Many kinds of knowledge can be profitably viewed in these terms. One of the most important is the *context of communication.* Indeed, we need some sort of shared context to conduct any social relations. To communicate we must share with each other unconscious assumptions about ourselves, our audience, our conceptual framework, and the perceptual world. The communicative context is a close relative of the conceptual context, but it is not identical. Here we can follow Clark and Carlson (1981), who define "the intrinsic context for understanding what a speaker means" as "the common ground that the *listener* believes holds at that moment between the speaker and the listeners" (italics added). Clearly the speaker's and the listener's context need not be identical, though they should overlap considerably if communication is to succeed. We would emphasize that this shared set of beliefs is probably unconscious at the time the participants hold it, although they will consciously recognize violations of the implicit context. Clark and Carlson cite formal demonstrations that common ground is necessary in social conventions, in speech acts, and in definite reference. Much the same can be argued for the "given-new contract," the agreement between two speakers to focus on new material, and to take shared givens for granted (e.g., Chafe, 1970; Clark & Clark, 1977).

When two people know each other very well they can often communicate with remarkable brevity. A word, a glance, an unexpected silence – these can often say volumes. The reason for this economy of expression is clear: People who talk together for many years share so much context that very little needs to be made explicit.

An elegant experiment by David R. Olson (1970) serves as a prototype for the communicative context. Olson asked one child to tell another child, hidden behind a screen, where to find a gold star located beneath a white, round block. What the first child said depended not just on the block referred to, but also on the other blocks that were present. If the other blocks were also white but had different shapes, the child would refer to the *disambiguating shape* by saying, "It's under the round one." If, on the contrary, the colors were different but the shapes were all the same, the child would say, "It's under the white one" – referring to the *disambiguating color*. Thus the description of the object differed according to the *context of alternatives which were assumed to exist in the mind of the listener*. This is apparently a general property of communication, one that applies to adults and to very different semantic domains as well.

Most listeners and speakers already share a tremendous amount of context: The children in Olson's experiment shared a great deal of knowledge about the world of objects, about the size, shape, color, weight, and playability of blocks, about gold stars, about language, and even about each other's knowledge about these things. Most of this context can be taken for granted; it does not need to be mentioned, nor does it need to be made conscious for communication to work. Only the information needed to disambiguate *relevant choices* in the shared context needs to be specified. This is why people who share a great deal of context seldom need to make it explicit.

Contexts in communicating with ourselves

The more context we share with other people, the less we must make conscious and explicit. This observation suggests something about our *inner* dialogue as well. Having lived with ourselves for so long, it seems likely that we can communicate to ourselves with minimal conscious inner speech; and each conscious thought can have reference to voluminous amounts of knowledge. We can hypothesize that what needs to be made explicit in communication is closely analogous to what needs to be made conscious in the mind of the speaker and listener (Chafe, 1980). That is, in general it may be true that we need to become conscious only of information that disambiguates some relevant context of alternatives, even in our own minds – everything else can remain unconscious. This view is closely related to the notion that conscious events are *informative,* that is, that they select one interpretation from a larger context of alternative interpretations (see Chapter 5).

4.2.5 The different kinds of contexts interact

Perception and imagery are key ingredients in the conceptual and goal contexts. In particular, conceptual thinking is affected by inner speech and by visual images – both of which are controlled by the Context of Imagery. Indeed, as Rosch and her associates have shown, much of our abstract thinking is heavily swayed by imageable "prototypes" (Rosch, Mervis, Gray, Johnson, & Boyes-Bream, 1975). The class of birds is represented not so much by an abstract description of birds as a biological genus, but rather by some particular imageable bird, like a robin, that stands for the abstract class. Similarly, the class of chairs is often mentally represented by the classical kitchen chair, made of wood, with a square back and seat, and with the natural wood grain showing through the lacquer. This prototypical chair is neither the average chair we encounter, nor is it an adequate abstract description of all chairs. Rather, it is something we can conveniently imagine consciously. Prototypical images serve to index abstract descriptions that cannot be visualized.

Similarly, we know that abstract thinking is heavily influenced by metaphors, which can usually be imaged, but which stand for more abstract things. Lakoff and Johnson (1980) discuss a number of such common metaphors, such as "memory is like a container," "love is like a journey," "electricity is like a stream," and "the atom is like a solar system." These metaphors influence thinking, sometimes far more than they should – a useful caution in this book!

Thus the conceptual context is heavily influenced by the contexts of perception and imagery. But influence runs the other way as well. Perception is relatively impervious to conceptual thought – try as we might, we cannot change the visual world by thinking about it – but conceptual thinking can evoke different visual images and inner speech. Conceptual processes may also influence the process of selecting perceptual events to pay attention to. In Chapters 6 and 7 we argue that imagery and perception have great influence on action goals as well.

In sum, different kinds of contexts interact. Especially significant is the way in which conceptual thinking and goals interact with the Context of Imagery. In Chapters 6 and 7 this point will suggest an answer to the question we asked in Chapter 1: What is the relationship between qualitative conscious contents, like percepts and mental images, and nonqualitative "conscious" beliefs, concepts, expectations, and intentions?

4.3   Modeling contextual knowledge

We can apply the familiar facts about cognitive representations to contexts. Piaget's description of schemata, cognitive views about scripts, semantic networks, organization in memory, story grammars, currently activated knowledge and the like – all these statements can be applied to contexts, as long as the knowledge structure in question is generally unconscious while influencing conscious contents (Anderson, 1983; Bransford, 1979; McClelland & Rumelhart, 1984; Norman, 1976; Piaget, 1952). This distinctive fact makes a great difference. We will use a notational convention (Figure 4.4b) in which contexts are shown as horizontal "frames," with horizontal length symbolizing duration in time, and vertical length representing cooperation or competition with respect to other contexts and with the global workspace. In general, "higher" contextual frames imply a more encompassing context that is presupposed by lower ones. Contextual frames are nested, and the higher ones "embrace" the lower contexts. Of course these diagrams are schematic only; details of contexts must be worked out in every domain. But here we are concerned mainly with the general properties of contexts. The following section aims to spell out the exact theoretical implications of the evidence we have been considering.

4.3.1 Contexts as stable coalitions of specialized processors

So far our models have had only two entities: specialized processors, which are believed to be unconscious, and a global workspace, whose

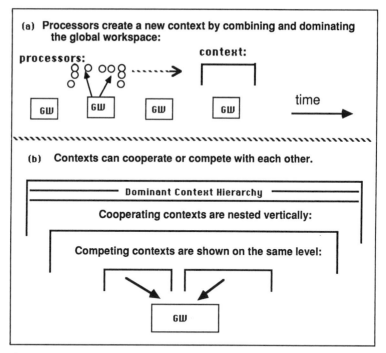

Figure 4.4. Modeling contextual knowledge. Some conventions for contexts in global workspace (GW) diagrams, designed to be as intuitively obvious as possible. A context (horizontal frame) is made up of a coalition of specialized processors (circles) that is fairly stable over time and can dominate the global workspace (rectangle). In diagram *a*, a context dominates the global workspace when it is positioned just above it so as to encompass its width. According to the theory, this is when the context can constrain conscious contents without itself being conscious. Notice that a global workspace can be repeated to symbolize the flow of conscious contents over time. In the lower drawing (*b*), two contexts on the same level are competing for domination of the global workspace. However, the competing contexts are themselves "nested" within a set of higher-level dominant contexts. Nested contexts are considered to be cooperating rather than competing with each other. The enduring set of dominant contexts is called the Dominant Context Hierarchy.

contents are conscious. We now add a third construct, a "context," a knowledge structure that is unconscious, but which constrains whatever becomes conscious.

How do contexts relate to the specialized processors discussed in previous chapters? After all, specialized processors are unconscious also. In fact, we can treat a context as a cooperating group of specialized processors with ready access to the global workspace. If contexts are to shape conscious experience they obviously must be able to interact with

GW messages quickly and easily. Some of this interaction may conceivably take place even before global messages reach the global workspace. But the arguments given in Chapter 2 about the ability for any ambiguity to be resolved by any other knowledge source, given enough time and learning, suggest that some contextual systems must interact with potentially conscious events through the global workspace (2.1). We will refer to the set of currently operative contexts as the Current Dominant Context Hierarchy, or Dominant Context for short (viz., Shallice, 1978). Any group of specialized processors that can cooperate to shape conscious experience, and that has a routine, committed way of processing information, will tend to behave like a context. Figure 4.4a makes this point simply by showing that unconscious processors together can look like a contextual frame. Another way of saying this is that contexts involve unconscious processors that are *already committed* to a certain stable way of processing, and that tend to shape global messages to their own committed organization. Contexts presumably develop over time, in a process of coalition-formation and competition, in roughly the same way that a majority party in a legislature evolves a working, stable coalition among its members.

4.3.2 The current Dominant Context imposes unconscious constraints on what can become conscious

Just by reading and understanding the foregoing sections, the reader will have gained a partial framework, or, well, . . . a *context* for the rest of this chapter. This suggests that you will experience the material that follows in a different way, *even when* you are not consciously recalling the earlier material. In this way do we humans continuously define and redefine reality.

Contexts are not conscious at the time they have their influence, though they might be conscious a second, an hour, or half a lifetime before the experience they help shape or evoke. The Dominant Context at any time is a coherent mix of perceptual–imaginal, conceptual, and goal contexts. Our experience at any time is controlled by numerous mutually consistent contexts. The reader's experience at this moment is likely to be controlled not only by his or her reading of the first part of this book, but also by much earlier decisions about the difficult issue of conscious experience, made perhaps many years ago. It is further controlled by an early life decision to learn to recognize the letter "d" and distinguish it from "b," "p," and "q," and by a later decision to learn a certain scientific prose style. When these contextual factors are mutually consistent, they can *cooperate* in gaining control of the global workspace. If they are mutually inconsistent – if, for example, the reader years ago decided that consciousness is utterly hopeless from a scientific point of view – the various contextual factors will compete.

4.3.3 Contexts do not completely predict conscious experiences

There is extensive evidence that completely predictable events fade from consciousness (5.0). We habituate to repeated sounds, we take for granted predictable thoughts, and we lose consciousness of routine skills. This implies that context, which constrains many potential degrees of freedom of a conscious content, does not constrain all of them. If some input were 100 percent predictable, we would be habituated to it, and it would be unconscious. The context of any experience must leave some degrees of freedom open. In the next chapter we review evidence for the loss of consciousness to redundant input and develop the argument that consciousness always involves *a reduction of uncertainty* within a stable dominant context. That is, the degrees of freedom left by the context are reduced by the conscious experience, until the input becomes entirely predictable and unconscious (5.1).

4.3.4 Internal consistency and the role of organization in contexts

Contexts are organized knowledge structures. This implies that they are internally consistent; they tend to resist changes that are inconsistent with them, and resist more strongly the greater the inconsistency; there is a tendency to complete partial input, and when one component changes, another one may have to compensate. All these phenomena are observable about contexts. For example, in the Ames room the height of the room is inconsistent with the person walking in the room – as he walks back and forth, his height is perceived to change. As observers we must revise our contextual assumptions either about human height or about the room. We first tend to give up our tendency to see human height as constant. Now we toss a ping-pong ball into the room, and that revision also fails; suddenly we perceive the room as trapezoidal, and human height become constant again. There is thus a trade-off between our perception of height and rectangularity; one or the other changes to maintain consistency.

The remarkable research tradition on perceptual adaptation goes back to the 1890s, using distorting goggles, mirrors, colored glasses, and the like to alter the visual world (Gregory, 1966). Thus the world may be viewed upside down, in mirror image, with different transformations in the two eyes or even in parts of each eye, and so on. The auditory realm can be transformed as well, for example by switching input between the two ears. The literature on perceptual transformations demonstrates a truly remarkable ability of the human nervous system to adapt within a few days to major changes in sensorimotor context.

Incompatible contexts compete; a scientist cannot simultaneously presuppose that time is constant and also that it changes, even when such presupposed knowledge is not currently conscious. A viewer of the Ames room cannot simultaneously assume that the visible surfaces are rectangular and that they are trapezoidal. If there is a conflict between two currently active contexts, it must give rise to conflicting conscious experience, given our previous assumptions. These conflicting conscious experiences presumably serve the cause of reconciliation between the two contexts. Take jokes as an example. A typical joke involves the creation of a misleading context, followed by a rapid restructuring of the information by a conflicting context. To cite a not very funny but classical music-hall joke: "Why did the chicken cross the street? To get to the other side." The question creates a context: We search for an answer that is not already obvious. The answer repeats something obvious, thus violating a contextual discourse constraint (4.1). The violated context may become briefly conscious – we may feel foolish not to have thought of this obvious answer – and becoming conscious of this old context may allow us to adapt to the conflict. The old context may thus become decontextualized, at least for a moment. Laughter may be one way to adapt to the conflict.

4.3.5 Cooperating and competing contexts: Model 2

Two conscious contents cannot be perceived at the same time. But two or more contextual constraints can dominate the global workspace. We previously listed the many simultaneous constraints that shape our perception of speech (4.3.1). Any conscious experience has many such contextual constraints: perceptual, conceptual, and goal-related. We can think of a compatible set of these contexts as cooperating with each other; incompatible contexts will compete. Figure 4.5 shows a convenient way to diagram both cooperation and competition. Cooperating contexts are shown in a hierarchy that dominates the global workspace. Competing contexts are shown at the same level as the dominant hierarchy, but not dominating the workspace.

In Chapter 6 we will develop these ideas to claim that intertwined contexts produce a flow of conscious events that looks very much like the famous stream of consciousness described by William James (1890).

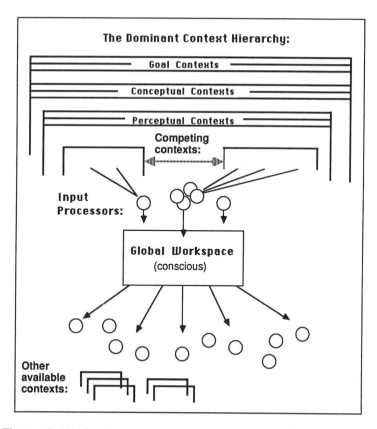

Figure 4.5. Model 2: Contexts compete and cooperate to influence conscious experience. The Dominant Context Hierarchy, showing nested goal, conceptual, and perceptual contexts. (Perceptual contexts are intended to include other qualitative contexts, such as the Contexts of Imagery, as well.) At the bottom of the hierarchy are two contexts competing to dominate the global workspace. Notice that potential contexts (the small frames at the bottom) are now shown among the specialized processors; they can be evoked by conscious contents and may then compete for dominance of the global workspace. Potential contexts that succeed in dominating the global workspace are added to the Context Hierarchy.

Now we can put all the elements together. Figure 4.5 shows GW Model 2, in which contexts have been added.

4.4   Some plausible properties of contexts

We can think of contexts as topics and themes in the ongoing conversation of the mind. Conversational topics have a beginning, a middle, and an end, suggesting that we should explore how mental topics may be evoked, how they are maintained, modified, and completed. We will describe the most plausible hypotheses, based on empirical findings and the logical implications of the theory so far. Needless to say, these hypotheses require much more testing.

4.4.1 Accessing and leaving contexts

The logic of our arguments suggests that to access a new context we need some distinctive conscious experience. A new context is by definition a not-completely-predictable event, and is therefore likely to require consciousness (5.0). A conscious experience that serves to install a new context may be as simple as walking into a room, reading a section heading in a book, or being introduced to a stranger. It may be quite momentary. Or it may be as complicated, confusing, and upsetting as learning to perceive a new art form, going through culture shock, or reluctantly learning some new insight into oneself. The common denominator is that a conscious experience gives us access to a new domain of knowledge that is itself largely unconscious, even though once accessed it will shape conscious experiences. To state it more formally:

A major function of conscious experience is to elicit, modify, and create new contexts – which in turn set the stage for later conscious experiences.

This point implies that *transitions* between contexts are psychologically crucial. In the first moments of a conversation, many unconscious constraints of the conversation are accessed. Thus if we were to probe for the parameters of a context, the ideal time to do so would be at its very beginning.

Contexts have a number of other implications, as we see next.

An uninterrupted dominant context creates an absorbed state

Occasionally people enter into states that are uninterrupted for a relatively long time: They may become absorbed in a fascinating book or creative project, in hypnosis (7.7), or in a demanding task, like shadowing speech in one ear. These absorbed states seem to be controlled uninterruptedly by a coherent context hierarchy. In absorbed states people resist distraction, lose track of time, and often report "losing themselves" as well, suggesting a drop in conscious self-monitoring (9.0.2, 9.2.2) (Tellegen & Atkinson, 1974). These are all important features of absorption, and we will discuss them in some detail later in this book (7.7; 8.5.1, 8.5.2).

Natural endings and forced exits

The experience of hearing a sentence in a conversation is constrained by a dominant context hierarchy, including syntactic, semantic, pragmatic, and discourse components. When the sentence ends, many of these contexts end as well: There are no further syntactic and lexical predictions after the end of a sentence; some semantic predictions may still be made about the next sentence; and some pragmatic purposes will still be unfulfilled. Thus at the end of a sentence, several contexts come to a natural ending. If the sentence is, "Nice speaking to you, goodbye," the semantic and discourse predictions also come to a natural end. Whenever one context ends, room is made for a previously competing context at the same level. Thus if we start a conversation to stop feeling bored, at the end of the conversation boredom may come back. This is implied by the notion of a context hierarchy, with potential competing contexts "lying in wait" for the end of the dominant context at the same level (4.3.5).

Natural endings in a context may be difficult to report, since the context itself is an unconscious structure. Metacognitive insight into contextual processes may be poor most of the time, unless the context is disrupted, so that it can become decontextualized and an object of consciousness in its own right. In an absorbed state we are generally unaware that we are absorbed. This state can come to a natural conclusion when its controlling contexts come to an end, and then we may not even notice that we were absorbed. But if the state is interrupted, we may well notice our absorption, apologize for daydreaming, etc. Metacognitive reports about our controlling contexts are more likely to be accurate in the second case.

Interruption stops a dominant context hierarchy before its natural ending. This issue of interruption and surprise is discussed next.

"Surprise" as a resetting of conscious contexts due to competition between incompatible contexts

Several psychologists have suggested that *surprise* may reset conscious contents (e.g., Baars, in press b; Grossberg, 1982; Izard, 1980; Tomkins, 1962; Underwood, 1982). It is a plausible idea, which can be readily interpreted in GW theory. In principle, surprise could occur with any new conscious content, but if the new content fits the current Dominant Context, it should not disrupt the context hierarchy. The next word in this sentence should not fundamentally jar the reader's conscious experience, because it fits all the levels of the current context. Truly surprising events violate deeper layers of context (Figure 4.6). In the first paragraph of this chapter we described the experience of going on a short sailing trip. On stepping back onto dry ground, the scene may seem to sway for a moment

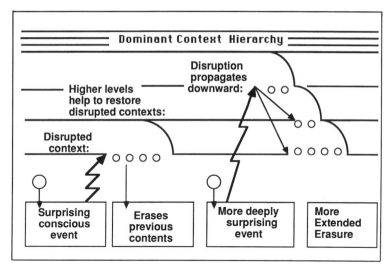

Figure 4.6. Surprise may erase conscious contents by disrupting dominant contexts; The disruption may propagate through the Context Hierarchy. Surprise tends to erase conscious contents because it disrupts the contextual framework needed to keep the old contents conscious. A disrupted context is presumably decomposed into specialized processors (circles), which made it up in the first place. Notice that the undisrupted higher-level context provides the knowledge and stability needed to repair the disrupted context. If surprise disrupts a high-level context, the disruptive effect will presumably propagate downward to other contexts that depend upon the higher levels.

because context predicts a certain motion in the surrounding world, and this prediction is violated. This kind of surprise is clearly due to competition between two incompatible contexts.

Similarly, a graduate student pursuing a Ph.D. may be surprised to find a book missing in the library. But most of his or her contextual assumptions and goals remain intact; it is easy to adapt to the surprising circumstance. On the other hand, if the student suddenly runs out of money needed to pursue the Ph.D., this change of context requires major changes throughout the system of life goals and local goals.

A violation of one level of context should "reset" the goal hierarchy, so that the violated context can fragment, but the higher (unviolated) level remains intact. If the book is not in the library, the goal of finding it may still remain intact, and one may simply try to find it some other way. If the book cannot be obtained, the required information may be found elsewhere. If the information cannot be obtained anywhere, the research project may have to be changed. If the research project fails, the student may have to go into selling life insurance – and so on. At each violation of goals the higher levels remain, and one can rebuild from there to reinstate a working goal context. Thus "surprise" does not usually imply a total overthrow of the context hierarchy, only its lower levels. That is, *one can think of the Dominant Context Hierarchy as a system that works to confine change to the lowest possible level.* High-level changes are costly, because they propagate throughout the context hierarchy and require widespread adaptation. Low-level changes are much to be preferred.

Competing contexts may be involved in episodes of momentary forgetting and "blanking out." Luborsky & Mintz (1974) have suggested that momentary forgetting may occur in psychotherapy when two themes conflict (Baars, in press, c), and Reason describes a number of cases of forgetfulness and action errors in these terms (Reason, 1983, 1984; Reason & Mycielska, 1982).

Surprise and interruption are central to the issue of emotion (Mandler, 1975a). Surprise creates an Orienting Response, with major activity in the sympathetic nervous system that closely resembles emotional upset. Surprise triggers changes in heart rate, in blood flow patterns, in the smooth musculature of the digestive tract, and in perspiration, just as emotional upset does. Personally significant information can be treated in GW theory as information that triggers deeper levels of the Dominant Goal Context; naturally this will disrupt lower levels as well, and it may trigger emotional experiences (Chapter 9). Deeper changes in the goal hierarchy may have consequences that propagate very widely throughout the context hierarchy.

4.4.2 Maintaining contexts with conscious reminders

It is simplistic to think that all contexts are entirely predictable over the long term. In any reasonably complex context there must be points of low predictability, where more conscious involvement is demanded. That implies that consciousness and mental effort are required, at least sometimes, to keep track of the current context or goal structure across the gaps in predictability. It seems that there are *underdetermined* choice-points in the control of action. If we fail to make these choice-points conscious, errors of action will occur. We can see this in absent-minded errors. Reason (1984) reports that errors like the following occur when people fail to pay attention to choice-points in the flow of action, even though most of the action is routine and can be considered to be controlled by a single dominant goal hierarchy. Following are some of Reason's examples of circumstances in which errors occur. (The examples are italicized.)

1   When a change of goal necessitates a departure from normal routine.
    (*I had decided to cut down on my sugar consumption and wanted to
    have my cornflakes without it. However, I sprinkled sugar on my cereal
    just as I had always done.*)
2   When changed circumstances demand some modification of a preestab-
    lished action pattern.
    (*We now have two fridges in our kitchen, and yesterday we moved our
    food from one to the other. This morning I repeatedly opened the fridge
    that used to contain our food.*)
3   When we wander into a familiar environment, associated with habitual
    activities, in a reduced state of intentionality [*sic*] (i.e., in a distracted
    state).
    (*I went into my room intending to fetch a book. I took off my rings,
    looked in the mirror and came out again, forgetting to pick up the book.*)
4   When features of our present environment contain elements similar to
    those in more familiar environments.
    (*As I approached the turnstile on my way out of the library, I pulled
    out my wallet as if to pay – although I knew no money was required.*)

All these examples seem to occur when automatic processes can handle
most, but not all, of the action, and the limited-capacity system is
occupied with other events. That is, consciousness is especially required
whenever there are underdetermined choice-points in the flow of events.
Presumably, making these choice-points conscious facilitates collabora-
tive processing that can resolve the ambiguities (2.3.2). Conversely, a loss
of conscious access to these uncertain choice-points threatens to "derail"
the action.

Reminding: Feedback between context and content
At the points of low predictability, unconscious contexts may need
conscious intervention to maintain their stability. It seems, for instance,
that in listening to speech, limited capacity is loaded most heavily
between sentences and even between the phrases of a single sentence
(Abrams & Bever, 1969). In speaking, peak load in limited capacity is just
before the onset of a sentence. These findings indicate that there may be
a continuous flow of feedback between conscious content and unconscious contexts, which over time helps to sustain the dominant context
hierarchy.

4.4.3 Modifying contexts: Coping with the unexpected

We have previously suggested that the context hierarchy may be disrupted by a surprising event, but that generally the disruption is kept as
low-level as possible. What happens with the disrupted context, however? How is it changed to deal with the new situation?

Surprise may cause the violated context to be decomposed into its
component specialized processors (Fig. 4.6). Some of these may become

consciously accessible, so that a group of specialists can now begin to work together on the job of fixing the fragmented context. That is consistent with the point made above (4.1.4, 4.4.3) that previously contextual material can become consciously accessible, at least in part, when the context is disrupted (decontextualized). Adaptation then becomes equivalent to cooperative processing between specialists, as discussed in Chapter 2. When the coalition of specialists from the fragmented context becomes practiced and proficient in its new configuration, it will presumably begin to act as a context again.

This may be the best way to solve the problem of fixedness in a single dominant context (4.1.2). When context controls conscious experience so much that a problem cannot be solved, it may be best to allow the context to be disrupted, so that its components can be reexamined. This is indeed the principle of "brainstorming" and other problem-solving techniques. However, decontextualization has costs in time and mental capacity. Fixedness may be especially problematic in panic situations, where one cannot afford to wait while the context is disrupted and reexamined (Norman, 1976).

The assimilation–accommodation dimension

Some challenges to a dominant context are more serious than others; a mild challenge may be ignored and assimilated, but a strong challenge must be treated more seriously (5.0). The following example is in the conceptual realm, but the same point applies to all kinds of contextual knowledge. Consider the following set of questions from Eriksen and Mattson (1981):

1   How many animals of each kind did Moses bring on the Ark?
2   In the Biblical story, what was Joshua swallowed by?
3   What was the nationality of Thomas Edison, inventor of the telephone?

Some readers no doubt noticed that each question contains a flaw, but most experimental subjects did not notice any problem. They simply answered "two" to question (1). But when they are asked "who built the Ark in the Bible?" they will correctly answer "Noah," showing that they do know the correct answer. Further, their immediate memory for the sentence is quite good, because they can repeat each question accurately, without spotting the incorrect name. But somehow they do not *bring their knowledge of the correct name to bear on the interpretation of the question*.

Now consider what happens when the flawed name is changed to one which violates context much more severely:

1   How many animals of each kind did Nixon bring on the Ark?
2   In the Biblical story, what was Jeffrey swallowed by?

3   What was the nationality of Benjamin Franklin, inventor of the telephone?

Now no one is fooled (Eriksen & Mattson, 1981). This "semantic illusion" illustrates our general claims about the context of experience very well. When the context is weakly violated, people usually do not even perceive the error; when it is strongly violated, they become conscious of it, so that what was previously context becomes conscious content (4.1.4).

We find similar phenomena in the well-known "proofreader effect," the general finding that spelling errors in page proofs are difficult to detect because the mind "fills in" the correct information. Here, too, we expect to find a difference depending upon the degree of error: Perhaps spelling errors that would change the pronunciation of a word are more egregious than those that do not, so that they are more likely to become conscious. Similarly, errors and dysfluencies in speech are surprisingly difficult for people to detect (MacKay, 1981). If we are listening for the intended meaning rather than for errors, as we normally do, minor errors are rarely noticed.

Input that violates context minimally is not consciously perceived; input that violates it moderately and that can be framed in another context is consciously perceived; and input that violates context totally and utterly is not consciously perceived in that particular framework. It may be dissociated – it is treated as something else; it may acquire its own context.

4.5   Implications for empirical testing

4.5.1 Related concepts

Context effects are so powerful and pervasive that every psychologist has surely observed them. But they are rarely stated in terms of the influence of unconscious events on conscious ones. Even current cognitive work on context tends to evade this issue, which is central in this volume. However, the existing research literature is easy to reinterpret in these terms. Perhaps the best worked-out theory of context is Adaptation Level (AL) Theory, originally developed by Helson (e.g., 1947, 1964). AL theory predicts that the perceived intensity of a perceptual or conceptual event depends on previous exposure to a range of similar events. Thus one's judgment of the severity of a criminal offense depends on previous exposures to a range of criminal offenses that differ in severity. After exposure to mass murder, mere assault seems less serious. The same pattern of adaptation by contextual manipulation applies to perceptual judgments and to such concepts as happiness, cost, and the like. There is also a considerable linguistic literature on such topics as focus and presupposition, given versus new information, topic versus comment, and so forth (Clark & Clark, 1977) – all of which correspond to context and content respectively. In the study of expert systems there is now an acute awareness of the presupposed and automatic nature of expert knowledge, compared to the same knowledge when it has been newly acquired (Anderson, 1983). On the theoretical side, Minsky's work on "frames" and Bransford's findings on "activated knowledge" seem closest to our claims about contexts (Bransford, 1979; Minsky, 1975).

4.5.2 Some testable predictions from Model 2

The evidence for contexts discussed above (4.1) can also be used to test our predictions. Priming effects, fixedness, top-down influences, and reports of violations of contexts may all be useful. There is currently a very interesting empirical literature on priming effects for assessing a variety of cognitive processes, which may be adapted to testing questions about context.

Contextual transitions as priming events

This chapter suggests that during contextual transitions things become momentarily conscious that are normally unconscious in the midst of a context. The example of gaining one's sea legs is illustrative. People should rate the swaying of a boat more highly if they have just stepped onto it, than later on. Similarly, we may quickly become conscious of our attitudes toward a friend at the very beginning of a meeting; a few minutes later those attitudes may have become inaccessible, at least until we take our leave. If we could probe someone at the beginning of a conversation, we should find that thoughts of friendship or hostility are more accessible than later on.

If a change in context becomes at least partly conscious, a switch in interpretation of an ambiguous stimulus should load limited capacity. If we measure limited capacity by a dual-task technique, for example (1.3.4), we should find that when we switch between two views of a Necker cube, two interpretations of a joke or an ambiguous sentence, or a change of mind about someone's motivation – all these contextual transitions should load limited capacity. Perhaps measures of surprise, like the Orienting Response, will also show measurable effects, though this may depend upon the depth of contextual violation involved (4.4.3; Figure 4.6).

Contexts may have many simultaneous levels

Context may be a many-leveled thing. If two contextual systems simultaneously constrain conscious experience and access, then a conscious experience that fits both of them should be favored. We have already described the experimental use of double entendres, linguistic ambiguities designed to fit two different contexts, and the fact that they are indeed chosen more often if both contexts are activated. Similarly, experimentally induced slips of the tongue, which tap into two simultaneous contexts, are more likely to occur than slips reflecting only one context (7.4). These are purely laboratory demonstrations, but Spence, Scarborough, & Ginsberg (1978) have shown that in spontaneous speech, terminal cancer patients produce more double entendres related to death and disease than controls. Similar studies could be carried out with any dominant mental set.

Blindness to conceptual presuppositions

Although there is considerable work on fixedness in problem solving, there is very little research exploring the apparent difficulty of accessing presupposed knowledge. Yet the naturalistic evidence in favor of "presuppositional blindness" is very strong – everyone must surely have encountered an inability to remember one's own basic beliefs, even when those beliefs continue to guide one's actions. Many people, especially scholars, routinely deal with students and skeptics who demand an explicit account of those beliefs, and naturally, if we are in the habit of doing this kind of "justificational" argument, accessing routine beliefs becomes easier. But this relative ease of access is misleading: It is not representative of the great bulk of mankind, which does not need to justify its presuppositions very often.

It seems that presuppositional blindness involves not just a problem in accessing overarching beliefs, but an inability to see and "hold on to" the negation of some belief. This is especially obvious in the cases of scientific change mentioned above (4.2.2), but it may also account for resistance to attitude change as described in numerous social psychological studies (Abelson, Aronson, McGuire, Newcomb, Rosenberg, & Tannenbaum, 1968).

4.5.3 Some questions Model 2 does not answer

So far, we have dealt with contexts without paying much attention to the ways in which they develop and are changed. We have not investigated them over time. In the next chapter, we will try to correct this deficiency. We will pursue the claim that conscious experiences, when they are adapted to, result in new contexts, which, in turn, serve to constrain later conscious experiences. Thus we are always defining and redefining our reality, by getting used to new experiences. The resulting perspective has strong implications for learning.

We have not yet addressed the issues of goals, intentions, and voluntary control. A complete theory must deal with these fundamental topics, and we develop an approach to them in Chapters 6 and 7.

4.6   Chapter summary

We have explored the pervasive influence of unconscious systems that act to evoke, select, and shape conscious experience. The evidence for such effects is very strong. Indeed, there is no conscious content without context. Psychologically we are always ensconced in the midst of a multitude of ongoing unconscious systems that shape and define our experience. Some of these unconscious systems have been with us from childhood, while others may have been evoked in the last few minutes.

In GW theory we can view contexts as collections of specialists that are committed to a certain way of processing input and that can come to dominate the global workspace, at least for some time. We can specify different contexts for perception and imagery (where they help shape qualitative experiences), and in conceptual thought, goal directed activities and the like (where contexts serve to access conscious experiences). The results can be modeled with little difficulty in an extended version of GW theory. It seems that one main function of consciousness is to evoke contexts that will then shape later conscious experiences.

Experimental psychologists often seem to feel that context effects are to be controlled and eliminated from an experiment if at all possible. This, we would argue, is a mistake. One can indeed suggest that some of the most serious conceptual errors in psychological history – errors that misled researchers for decades – began with naive attempts to remove phenomena from their natural contexts. We would argue rather that context effects are impossible to eliminate, and that we should not wish to eliminate them totally, but only to study them. There is no zero point in the flow of contexts. They are not incidental phenomena that confound our careful experiments: They are *quintessential* in psychology. There is no experience without context.

5   Model 3:
Conscious experience is informative –
it always demands some degree
of adaptation

> Into the awareness of the thunder itself the awareness of the previous
> silence creeps and continues; for what we hear when the thunder crashes
> is not thunder *pure*, but thunder-breaking-upon-silence-and-constrast-
> ing-with-it.

William James, 1890/1983 (p. 156)

5.0   Introduction: Information and adaptation

Has the "publicity metaphor" helped to clarify the issues so far?
Consider how the GW model resembles a publicity organ like a newspaper. First, a global workspace can distribute a message to a wide public of
specialized, relatively independent processors (2.2). Further, only one
consistent message can be broadcast at a time, so that the mental news
medium does not publish self-contradictory information at any one time
(2.1). And third, GW theory claims that there are contextual constraints
on the conscious interpretation of the world, comparable to the editorial
policies and practices of a newspaper that determine how it will select and
interpret the news (4.0). In these ways the publicity metaphor seems
helpful.

But we have not yet addressed some essential features of the publicity
metaphor. First: So far, we cannot tell old from new input; second: The
Model has no way to determine the *significance* of a piece of news; and
third: We have no way to keep the system from publishing the same old
message over and over again. In short, until now we seem to have a
newspaper that has no preference for news.

Yet the nervous system does have a great preference for news. There
is ample evidence from a great variety of sources that people and animals
actively seek novelty and informative stimulation, and that they have an
enormous selective preference for significant input (see 5.1.3). Repetitive,
"old" stimuli tend to fade from consciousness regardless of their sensory
modality, degree of abstractness, or physical intensity (short of the pain

177

threshold) (5.1, 5.2). Even a single neuron habituates to repetitive input, and becomes active again only when the input is changed (Kaidel, Kaidel, & Weigand, 1960). The GW system is designed especially to cope with novelty and informative stimulation, because it allows many knowledge sources to work together on a single, novel source of information. The premier function of consciousness, we will argue, is to facilitate this cooperative integration of novel information (10.0). The more informative an event is, the more adaptation is required, and the longer the event must be in consciousness to achieve adaptation (5.5).

Defining "information"

In this chapter we will use the word *information* in its conventional sense as a *reduction of uncertainty* in a set of choices defined within a stable context (Miller, 1953; Shannon & Weaver, 1949). The context of information must define at least two options: for example, 0 or 1 in the case of a computer, or "war" and "peace" in the case of a diplomatic code. Any arbitrary amount of information can be coded as a combination of binary codes. This is of course the well-established mathematical definition that has been so influential in communication engineering and computer science, except that we will be using it qualitatively and in a somewhat broader sense. Over the past few decades, the mathematical definition has also found increasing application in psychology. It has been found useful in modeling fundamental findings about reaction time (Hick, 1952; Hyman, 1953), classical conditioning (Rescorla & Wagner, 1972), basic level categories (Gluck & Corter, 1985), perceptual complexity (Garner, 1974), and so forth. Thus the mathematical notion of information seems to have some psychological reality.

How is information in this sense related to consciousness? There is good evidence (presented below) that we are conscious of an event only when it exists in a stable context, but not when it is so predictable that there are no conceivable alternatives to it. Conscious experience seems to exist only when there are some degrees of freedom within a stable context. Thus the notion of reduction of uncertainty in a stable context seems appropriate. Information is inherently context-dependent, and we have already presented a set of arguments that conscious experience is also highly context-dependent (2.1, 4.2).

Conscious experience of the world is not a direct function of physical stimulation. The same physical stimulus repeated over and over again will soon become less informative – and also less conscious. But a highly significant or variable stimulus habituates more slowly. We therefore need to make a distinction between *physical stimulation* and real *information*. On the other side of that coin, this is the difference between *repetition* and *redundancy*. The same physical energy impinging on the same sensory receptors may be either informative or not, depending upon the reduction of uncertainty in the relevant context. Sometimes the physical *absence* of an expected stimulus can provide information, just as its presence may be redundant. In this sentence, we need only omit one . . . to show that the absence of a stimulus can draw our attention – and the missing item may well become conscious for the reader. Thus information and stimulation are not the same; they can vary independently. In general, the probability of being conscious of any event increases with its information value and decreases with redundancy.

Finally, a single stimulus can carry different amounts of information when it suggests something beyond itself. In Pavlov's conditioning experiments, when the sound of the bell signaled that food was coming (a significance beyond itself), the hungry dog was much more likely to prick up its ears, the Orienting Response to the bell took longer to habituate, and learning occurred more quickly. One way to think about significance is in terms of purposes the hungry dog is likely to have, which create goal contexts for its perceptual systems to explore (4.2.3). Significant information can then be seen as a reduction of uncertainty within a goal context (5.2.3). Thus, the concept of information can be related naturally to the things that matter most to animals or humans. We can think of information as existing at different levels, just as we have previously suggested that contexts exist at different levels (4.2).

The strongest evidence for the close relationship between information and consciousness is the existence of what we call Redundancy Effects. Redundancy, the absence of information, is defined in information theory as the physical transmission of a signal after the uncertainty at the receiver is already zero. The choice between "peace" and "war" had great information value in 1945 for most of the Western world, but repeating "peace at home" over and over again after that point became increasingly less informative, *even though the context* of subsequent events in the Western world is accurately described by that word. Thus the word "peace" became increasingly redundant to describe local conditions in Europe and the United States, but not false. Note well that "peace at home" has become redundant precisely because it was understood and learned when it was still news. Further, it provides an ongoing context for interpreting more recent news. This knowledge does not disappear, but it does tend to become unconscious even while it helps to shape current conscious experiences.

There are many well-known cases in which conscious input fades with repetition – cases like stimulus habituation, automatization of skills and mental images, perceptual adaptation, shifts in the Adaptation Level of

Table 5.1. *Contrasts between informative and redundant phenomena**

Conscious phenomena	Comparable unconscious phenomena
Novel stimuli or concepts	Predictable repetitions of habituated stimuli or concepts
Changes in habituated stimuli or concepts	
Novel actions	Automatized actions
De-automatized actions	

* The specific phenomena include: stimulus habituation with repetition, stopped retinal images, automatization of practiced skills, automatic visual images, semantic satiation, inacessability of stable conceptual presuppositions, habituation of the Orienting Response, and lack of conscious access to routine contextual systems.

perceptual and judgment categories, "blank-outs" in the *Ganzfeld*, semantic satiation, loss of access to stable conceptual knowledge, and so on. These phenomena allow us to do a contrastive analysis, showing a direct relationship between conscious experience and the informativeness of an event (see Table 5.1).

Habituation of awareness to a repeated stimulus is the most obvious example of a Redundancy Effect. At this moment the reader is likely to be habituated to the feeling of the chair, the color and intensity of the ambient light and background sounds, the language of this book, and many other predictable features of the inner and outer world. Section 1.4.1 detailed Sokolov's arguments for the continued existence of *un*conscious representations of habituated stimuli. Sokolov argued that a mismatch in any parameter of a habituated stimulus will elicit a new Orienting Response. To detect such mismatches, we must maintain some sort of representation of the expected input. But this representation does not elicit an Orienting Response, or – in the terms used in this book – it is not normally conscious. Thus there must be an unconscious representation of a habituated stimulus that is similar in many respects to the conscious perceptual representation of the same stimulus when it first occurs. The Sokolov argument therefore allows us to contrast two stimulus representations under identical physical conditions; the conscious representation that occurs when we first take in a stimulus, and the representation that continues to exist after habituation (Table 5.1).

Information versus novelty (mismatch)
What can be the difference between the conscious and unconscious representations of the same stimulus? Several writers have suggested that

novelty or mismatch with expectations is involved in conscious perception. That is, that there must be a mismatch between input and expectations for a stimulus to be conscious. This is certainly true in the case of
surprise, as discussed above. But it cannot be true without qualification
(Berlyne, 1960). Any stimulus that violates previous expectation can only
do so in a context that is itself not violated – if input were to violate every
expectation, if it were *totally* new, it could not be experienced at all.
Therefore all understandable novelty exists within a relatively stable
context that is not novel.

The opposite argument has also been offered. Marcel (1983b) suggests
that a match between input and memory is required for perceptual input
to be conscious. But this cannot be completely true either: If there is a
perfect match between input and expectation, we have the case of
habituation and loss of consciousness. Thus, we find ourselves in a
middling position with respect to both the match and the mismatch
hypothesis: Yes, there should be some sort of match, but not too much.
Both the mismatch and the match hypotheses capture some, but not all,
of the evidence.

We will develop the argument that the notion of *information* is more
attractive than either simple match or mismatch. Information involves
both a match of context *and* a mismatch of the stimulus details. It further
suggests that the input must be usable, in the sense that many systems can
reduce their uncertainty relative to it. It also allows us to include the
notion of significance as a reduction of uncertainty in a relevant goal
context; and finally it seems to explain the well-established Redundancy
Effects.

If the concept of information is indeed preferable, what about the case
of surprise, which is indeed a mismatch of input and expectations?
Surprising mismatch reduces to a special case of information: It is the
case where the context of the expected input is itself violated. This
context then becomes "decontextualized," and its components must be
reassembled within the framework of a higher-level context. We have
discussed this case in some detail in section 4.1.4. The point here is that
the notion of information seems well-suited to handle a number of
important properties of conscious input; it can also explain mismatch
phenomena such as surprise.

Some possible counterexamples
Much of the argument depends upon the Redundancy Effects, those cases
where repetition leads to a loss of conscious experience. There are some
apparent counterexamples to the Redundancy Effects: cases where
repeated events do not fade, or where they seem to become *more*

consciously available with practice (5.4). For instance, conscious access to highly significant or unpredictable events is lost only slowly. In the case of chronic pain people do not lose conscious access at all. We suggest that these facts reflect the special role of significant information. But as we have mentioned, significance can be treated as a reduction of uncertainty in a higher-level Goal Context (5.2.3).

Further, there are cases in which practice seems to *increase* access to conscious events. For instance, practicing recall will bring memorized material to mind more readily (Erdelyi, 1985), and practicing visual search will cause the search target to "pop" into consciousness quite involuntarily (Neisser, 1967; Shiffrin & Schneider, 1977). Notice however, that what is being practiced here is not the visual or memory target as such, but the *process of search and recall*. That is, in these cases we gain automaticity in the skill of controlling *access* to consciousness (see Chapter 8), but the input that will become conscious is not highly predictable, and may be quite novel and informative. Thus, these facts do not contradict the claim that consciousness requires informative input. Indeed, the process of recall or search itself does become automatic and unconscious with practice. Only its results remain informative and conscious.

There are also cases where repeated stimuli fade from consciousness, only to return in a new guise (Pritchard, Heron, & Hebb, 1960; Warren, 1961, 1968). As we shall see in section 5.4, these apparent counter-examples can be readily grasped with a deeper understanding of information and redundancy. Namely, these cases seem to reflect the fact that the same input can still be informative if the context of interpretation changes. There is indeed evidence for this suggestion from a variety of sources. From the viewpoint of information theory, a change in context does create new information, even with repetitive input.

We conclude that Redundancy Effects are both powerful and pervasive, while apparent counterexamples can be explained plausibly in an extended information-theoretic framework. All this supports the idea that informativeness may be a *necessary condition* for conscious experience of some event. This viewpoint also suggests a new perspective on context (4.0): In a sense, context consists of those things to which the nervous system has *already* adapted; it is the ground against which new information is defined.

A terminological note

Our use of the term "information" is similar to the classical mathematical definition developed by Shannon and others (Shannon & Weaver, 1949), but we should note some possible differences. Psychological contexts are highly complex knowledge structures that have many more dimensions than the simple, binary, one-dimensional message contexts of classical information theory. But of course, we know that knowledge structures of any dimensionality and complexity can be reduced in principle to binary choices (Shannon & Weaver, 1949). Further, the classical definition presumes that reduction of uncertainty takes place in a stable context of choices, but psychologically, we know that contexts are not totally stable, but adapt to informative input whenever possible. The nervous system learns about predictable inputs; it is not passive like the contexts of conventional information theory. We argue in section 5.1.1, that conscious experience is associated with a range of phenomena in which the context of informative choices is *relatively* stable. Within these relatively stable contexts, the classical definition is quite useful. Finally, the formal definition of information is quantitative, but we will not develop a quantitative approach here. Quantification at this stage can apply only to a small, experimentally defined subset of the full range of phenomena. Others have already done this (see references cited above). We will focus here on making a case for a special relationship between consciousness and information in general.

Adaptation

After information, the second major concept in this chapter is *adaptation*. Here we will use it in a narrow sense, as the process of learning to represent some input, to know it to the point of automatic predictability. Learning to represent something involves, of course, a reduction of uncertainty (i.e., information). When there is a perfect match between input and its representation, the input is *redundant* with respect to its representation. Thus redundancy is the end-product of successful adaptation.

We can borrow Piagetian terms here to represent different ends of the adaptation continuum (Piaget, 1952). When confronted with a situation that is new and strange, people need to find new contexts for experiencing the input; the result resembles Piagetian accomodation. In other words, accomodation has to do with the discovery of usable contexts. On the other end of the continuum, when the input is highly familiar and predictable, minimal adaptation is required to assimilate it into readily available contexts. In the extreme case of redundancy, context and input match exactly.

Conscious experience of an event seems to occur midway between the outer poles of assimilation and accomodation. If we can automatically predict something completely, we are not conscious of it. But if the input requires a deep revision of our current contexts, we do not experience it either – it is too confusing or disorganized to experience *as such,* though we may experience fragments and tentative interpretations of the input. Somewhere between these two extremes, between the assimilation and accomodation poles of the continuum, we may have an accurate conscious experience of the event. From the adaptation point of view, an informative conscious event translates into a demand for adaptation. This is of course the claim stated in the chapter title: that conscious experience is informative – it always demands some degree of adaptation.

In sum, there is a close web of connections between certain fundamental ideas: information, consciousness, reduction of uncertainty, a drop in contextually defined alternatives, a demand for adaptation and learning, a gain in predictability and redundancy, and the creation of new contexts.

Adaptation takes place over time, and we develop now the notion that conscious experience corresponds to a certain stage of the "adaptation cycle" namely, the stage where there is a relatively stable context for understanding the input, but there is still uncertainty to be reduced within that context. Many processors can cooperate in reducing the uncertainty. A fundamental point is that the nervous system is always in dynamic adaptive activity – it is always working to adapt to conscious input – even when we *seem* to be conscious of only a single thing. Conscious experience cannot be understood apart from this process of dynamic adaptation. We turn to this issue next.

5.1   The adaptation cycle: Any learnable task goes from *context-creation* to *conscious information* to *redundancy*

In learning about a new source of knowledge we often start with considerable uncertainty and confusion. By paying attention to the problem, a sense of clarity is often gained, as we become conscious of what is to be learned. Finally, with practice, the material becomes highly predictable and fades from consciousness. These three stages make up what we will call the *adaptation cycle*: Starting only with the knowledge that there is something to be learned, the first stage of *context creation* is resolved as the elements to be learned are defined; in the second stage we have a working context for understanding the new material, which is now *informative* – that is, input now serves to reduce uncertainty within the working context. In the third stage we have *adapted* completely, and lose conscious access to the learned material. Consciousness is primarily involved in the first two stages, but in the first, the input is so ill-defined that we are not even truly conscious of it as such. Consciousness of the input as such is confined to the second stage, which we call the stage of informativeness.

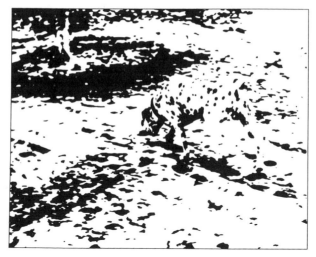

Figure 5.1. The Dalmation in the Park: Conscious experiences can help create context. This well-known camouflaged figure can be discovered using conscious hints that are typically not immediately conscious at the time they help to reveal the hidden figure. For example, one conscious hint indicates that the dark oval in the upper left quadrant is a planter, or a circular bush surrounding the base of a tree; another, that the very center of the picture contains the head of a dog sniffing the ground; another, that the two elongated clusters of black spots converging on the center represent two intersecting sidewalks. All these conscious hints may help reveal the hidden figure, but they are typically no longer immediately conscious when they influence the conscious experience of the hidden figure. Hence their effect is contextual, by the definition given in the text. (Photograph by R. C. James)

In the next sections we present a number of empirical findings that support these points.

5.1.1 Context-creation

Consider Figure 5.1, which looks at first to most people like a random collection of black and white spots. It is in fact a coherent picture of something, but in order to experience it consciously we need some context. Some may be provided by the picture's title, "Dalmatian in the Park"; some observers will find this hint helpful. (Note that if this helps, you may not be conscious of the title *as such* at the moment it seems to help – as in the case of other priming phenomena, the effect is contextual, since past experiences that are unconscious at this moment help shape current conscious experience.) Other observers find that it helps to notice that the diagonal black "lines" converging toward the center of the picture are the edges of a sidewalk in a park. Knowing this may help to reconstruct the three-dimensional properties of the picture. But, once again, depth information created by the converging sidewalks may be unconscious at the moment it constrains and helps reveal the conscious object. Other conscious hints that help to create context include the dog's nose sniffing the ground in the center of the picture, the tree above, the circular planter in which the tree stands, and the realization that a black-and-white photograph of a spotted Dalmatian in a shadow-flecked park can indeed look like this.

A good deal of learning begins in confusion. Until the confusion is dispelled, until guidance is provided either by the material itself, by a parent, guide or teacher, or by the use of knowledge and strategies from the past, we do not fully experience what is to be learned. This point is not limited to perception. At the end of section 4.1.3 we presented a confusing paragraph about washing clothes, but without mentioning the topic. Providing a title ("washing clothes") creates enough context for the paragraph that we can become conscious of its meaning as a whole, rather than as a fragmented and incoherent set of words and sentences.

Often in confronting new material we have only a goal context to work with. Someone tells us that here is something interesting or important – pay attention to it, and you will become aware of it. This is how the reader was guided in the Dalmatian demonstration above. It is how psychologists usually get people to do things in experiments. We tell subjects which goals to pursue, and observe how they perform: "Please pay attention to this, try to memorize that, tell us what you see there." Even just providing a goal context helps narrow down the possibilities.

Of course, the context of the experience is itself evoked by conscious events (4.4.1). Context-creation may involve tentative conscious inter-pretations of the input, or conscious fragments, or consciousness of a different level of analysis than the desired experience. In the Dalmatian demonstration, the reader was surely conscious of black and white spots even at the beginning. But in the stage of context-creation one is not conscious of the material to be learned *as such*. The Dalmatian becomes conscious only after context has been created for it.

5.1.2 Conscious experience corresponds to the information stage of adaptation

Harking back to the Dalmatian as a case in point (Figure 5.1), once we have the appropriate contextual constraints for a figure, we can evidently become conscious of it. But what does that mean?

Inherent in the notion of conscious experience is the existence of features of the conscious event. The Dalmatian has size, location in space, color, texture, and so on. But features involve discriminations of some sort: at the very least judgments of presence or absence, and implicit comparisons to contrasting features. The Psychophysical Law implies that perception of intensity always involves an implicit comparison to previous intensities (Stevens, 1966), and this point is not limited to intensity alone. Many aspects of a perceptual event, such as color, brightness, and pattern, are believed to involve implicit comparisons (e.g., Garner, 1974; Rock, 1983; Uznadze, 1966). Judgments of conceptual qualities are also thought to involve implicit comparisons (Helson, 1964). Research on person perception clearly shows that we perceive people in comparison to others (Levicki, 1986; Weiner, 1986). In sum, conscious experiences can often be shown to involve not one, but at least two alternative representations, one of which is implicit. Whenever we become conscious of something, internal processes are saying, in effect, "Aha! It's a dog with black and white spots, rather than a brown dog, or a cat, or some other object." Needless to say, this kind of implicit comparison must take place at many levels of analysis at the same time.

Another way of saying this is that conscious events are *objectlike;* they have many correlated features, which are implicitly differentiated from potential alternatives. This is quite different from habituated representations, which are not experienced as objectlike. Since habituated representations are highly predictable, we may presume that *their* potential alternatives are represented, if at all, as highly unlikely. In a later chapter, the objectlike nature of conscious experience will become very important (9.0).

A direct connection between conscious events and quantitative measures of information has been established in several cases. Take for example the notion of "basic level categories." In a number of studies Rosch and her colleagues have shown that people tend to think of the world in terms of prototypical members of categories. Thus we think of "furniture" not so much as an abstract class, but in terms of its typical members like chairs, tables, and beds; other members like ashtrays, drapes, and vases are much less likely to be thought of spontaneously (Rosch, 1975). Further, objects fit into a hierarchy of abstraction, with the most typical objects occupying a middle level in the hierarchy between great specificity and great generality. Thus a *Colonial kitchen chair* is quite specific; *kitchen chair* is more general, followed by *chair, furniture, artifact, inanimate object* and *physical object*. The word *chair* has been thought to be the most typical member of the hierarchy: It is easier to describe, recognize, draw, recall, and the like (Rosch et al., 1975). Typical objects are probably easiest to bring to consciousness.

However, there is now evidence that the level of an object hierarchy that is easiest to use at any given time depends upon the alternatives that are being entertained. If we are considering the esthetic pros and cons of man-made objects versus natural scenery, "chairs" are not necessarily the best example of man-made objects. Similarly, if we are debating the merits of Colonial versus modern kitchen chairs, very specific differentiating features are likely to come to mind. Depending on our purposes and implicit comparisons, different levels of the hierarchy of abstraction are likely to come to mind. Along these lines, Barsalou (1983) and Murphy & Medin (1985) have shown that conceptual structures are highly unstable and vary with the context of alternatives. Gluck and Corter (1985) have developed a set of quantitative predictions based on this reasoning. They have modified the well-known mathematical formula for information to measure *relative informativeness,* and find that the resulting model accurately predicts which level of a category hierarchy will be chosen under different circumstances. Gluck and Corter suggest that "the most useful categories are those that are, on the average, optimal for communicating information (hence reducing uncertainty) about the properties of instances."

There are other connections between likely conscious contents, implicit comparisons, and mathematical information theory. Garner (1974) has shown that people prefer to select stimuli that are neither very high nor very low in information content, suggesting that we tend to pay attention to events that do not require enormous adaptation, but that do require some. There is also good evidence that choice reaction time, the time needed to choose between explicit alternatives, is a function of the mathematical bit-rate, the quantitative measure of information (Hick, 1952; Hyman, 1953). Even classical conditioning is a function of the amount of information carried by the signalling stimulus (Rescorla & Wagner, 1972).

In communication, we select the most informative features to convey to the listener – that is, the features with the most valuable comparison. We have already mentioned Olson's revealing experiment in children's speech, in which the context of alternatives determines whether the child will say, "The gold star is under the *square* block" or "The gold star is under the *white* block" – even though the block in question is the same one (Olson, 1970). We can find this reasoning going back even to Aristotle, who defined a "definition" as a statement of a general category plus a differentiating feature within the category. "A mammal is an animal that suckles its young." "A chair is a piece of furniture for people to sit on." The general category provides a context of alternatives, and the differentiating feature reduces those alternatives to the correct subset.

This pattern is fundamental in linguistics. Conversations depend upon the "given–new" contract, the shared understanding that certain things are true, so that they do not need to be repeated, allowing new information to be brought to the fore (Clark & Carlson, 1981; Haviland & Clark, 1974). Similarly, individual sentences have a "focus" and a "presupposition": In the sentence, "It was the book that I lost yesterday," "the book" is brought forward in the sentence and made more focal. By comparison, "Yesterday I lost the book" does not have this special focus. There are numerous linguistic techniques for bringing some information to the fore and backgrounding other messages that are already shared. When hearing a sentence, people seem to pay attention primarily to whatever is new, focal, topical, and emphasized (Chafe, 1970; 1980). There is an implicit deemphasis of anything that is known, peripheral, and irrelevant at the moment.

If conscious events indeed exist in a context of implicit alternatives, how do we know that these alternatives are being reduced? After all, information is defined as a *reduction* of alternatives. Part of the answer depends, of course, on the Redundancy Effects discussed in section 5.1.3. But consider one of the most obvious aspects of conscious events: the fact that they are so fleeting. It is very difficult to keep a conscious image in mind for more than a moment. With rehearsal, we can refresh inner speech to an extent, but even rehearsed words tend to fade and satiate rather quickly (see 5.1.3). Perceptual events can be renewed in various ways, but we tend to stay with them only as long as needed to achieve some specific goal, and no longer. Conscious sensory memory, such as iconic or acoustical storage, lasts only a few hundred milliseconds. One explanation of the fleetingness of conscious events is that adaptive processes are continually learning from conscious events, reducing *their* alternatives, and nibbling away at the information provided. If that is true, then most conscious events lose most of their information value very quickly, as uncertainty is reduced by adaptive mechanisms. The evanescence of conscious contents is consistent with the notion of informativeness as a demand for adaptation.

Finally, notice that habituated or automatic events can become conscious again when their predictable conditions are violated. If they become unconscious due to redundancy, one way to make them conscious again is to violate the redundant pattern. And indeed, that is what happens when the foot pedal of a bicycle falls off, and we become conscious again of aspects of bicycle riding that were largely automatic before. Steering the bicycle, balancing it, and the like, now become informative again, as they become conscious. Again, consciousness is correlated with information content.

5.1.3 Redundancy Effects occur at all levels of processing

We are now ready to discuss the strongest source of evidence for the informativeness of conscious experience: the Redundancy Effects. If we were to ask the average student of psychology whether practice helps people deal with new material, the student would no doubt reply, "Yes, of course, repeating something helps you perceive and remember it." Rehearsing a telephone number helps us recall it, doesn't it? And if we do not understand a sentence, reading it over again surely gives us more time to think about it? There is, however, a fundamental class of cases in which repetition harms rather than helps conscious access. When we *already know* an event, repeating it further tends to harm our ability to consciously perceive, understand, recall, and monitor it. To say it slightly differently: Whether repetition helps conscious access or not depends upon the information value of the event in question. As long as information increases with each repetition, conscious availability will improve; but once the stimulus is known, repeating it only creates more redundancy, and a *loss* of conscious access. Table 5.1 presents this evidence in summary form.

Redundancy – the lack of information – is defined formally as the presence of a signal after the uncertainty at the receiver is already zero. Redundancy implies a perfect match of input with expectation. The context of alternatives described in the section 5.0 collapses to only a single representation, with one degree of freedom, and maximum certainty. In the Piagetian dimension of assimilation and accomodation, redundancy corresponds to the extreme pole of assimilation.

Of course, most of the time when we pay attention to something we do not wait for complete adaptation to occur. We are satisfied to understand an idea or clarify a perceptual event up to a point, and then go on to another. Redundancy Effects present the extreme case of absolute adaptation, but most of the time we are satisfied with *relative adaptation*. Once the conscious information is understood to some criterion, we go on.

We now turn to some specific examples.

Perceptual Redundancy Effects

Redundancy Effects for the different senses are quite clear in hearing, olfaction, taste, and touch; in all these sense modalities a repeated or lasting stimulus fades rapidly from consciousness. In the case of hearing, Miller (1955) was able to show a rapid decrement in the experienced intensity of even a single burst of white noise after several hundred milliseconds. In olfaction, we can observe every day how we lose track of an odor that may have been quite noticeable when we first encountered it. Most people are quite unaware of stable, surrounding odors, though these may be quite obvious to a newcomer. The act of sniffing, which changes the concentration of odor molecules over the smell and taste receptors, may serve to change the stimulus, to dishabituate previously adapted receptors. Similarly, it is a common experience that even the most delicious food becomes less noticeable after the first mouthful. Gourmet cooking often consists of selecting deliberate taste contrasts, to reawaken appreciation of otherwise habituated flavors. And the reader can probably verify that at this very moment a previously felt object – such as one's clothing – has now faded from consciousness.

One might object that vision seems different. Consciousness of visual stimuli does not seem to fade with repetitive stimulation, even when we stare fixedly at an object. But this argument neglects the existence of eye movements. Our eyes are in continual jumpy motion, both voluntary and involuntary, in addition to head and body motion. As long as the eye keeps scanning a differentiated visual field, new information will enter the retina. Therefore there may always be some element of uncertainty at the level of retinal receptors, as long as the eyes keep moving. It is difficult to completely stop even large eye movements, and there is a continual tiny eye tremor (*physiological nystagmus*) that cannot be stopped voluntarily at all. Thus, under normal conditions, light patterns coming into the eye are never wholly constant and predictable. However, one can artificially defeat physiological nystagmus, and then interesting things happen. For instance, Pritchard, Heron, & Hebb (1960) mounted a tiny projector on a contact lens that was firmly attached to the eye, so that the projected image moved along with all eye movements. Under these conditions, the visual image fades in a few seconds. The method of "stabilized retinal images" shows that even vision is subject to rapid habituation when it is not protected by constant eye movements. Similarly, when people look at a bright but featureless field (the *Ganzfeld*), they experience "blank-outs" – periods when visual perception seems to fade altogether (Natsoulas, 1982). The most extreme example along these lines is reported by Oswald (1960), who had a subject facing a bank of bright lights flashing on and off in rhythm to very loud rock music. He reports that the subject fell asleep, eyes open.

In nature, all the senses continually change their relationship to the input: The nose sniffs the air, changing the concentration of odors; the tongue tastes in an exploratory way, with the same effect; the hands and body explore by moving and touching (haptic touch); in most mammals the ears can be pricked up and oriented, and even humans tend to "cock" one ear to the source of sound when listening carefully; and of course the eyes are ceaselessly searching for significant information. Thus, the same physical event can enter a sensory system in many different ways, so that habituation can be avoided. But in the laboratory we can show that truly constant input fades rapidly from consciousness.

Note again that conscious fading does not mean that the event has disappeared from the nervous system. The Sokolov argument (1.4.1) shows that fading does not involve a fatiguing of receptors, or anything else that is dysfunctional. Rather, the fact that some stimulus fades from consciousness after repetition is highly functional; it is a sign that learning has occurred.

Conceptual Redundancy Effects

Habituation is not limited to perception: It may occur at all levels of analysis. Fading of conscious access to abstract concepts is shown by *semantic satiation*. A word repeated over and over again will soon seem different, somehow meaningless, estranged from its previous familiarity, as if it were being pronounced by some particularly impersonal robot (Amster, 1964). Semantic satiation is similar to stimulus habituation, but it seems to operate on the level of abstract meaning rather than sensation. It suggests, therefore, that the informativeness criterion does not only apply to perception and imagery, but to conceptual thought as well.

There has been some controversy about the empirical validity of semantic satiation (e.g., Esposito & Pelton, 1971), but the evidence for conceptual redundancy is actually quite pervasive. It is most common for experts in any discipline, who do not need to communicate their expertise to novices, to find it difficult to retrieve their knowledge explicitly (Anderson, 1983). This is likely to happen even though the inaccessible knowledge continues to inform their actions and experiences.

Research on Adaptation Level Theory indicates that conceptual events are evaluated in a context of alternatives that is shaped by previous experience with the same events (Helson, 1964). Thus, one's judged happiness is strongly affected by previous judgments of happiness. In general, when one achieves a new level of desired functioning – such as getting a higher level of income, a desired job, or a desired mate – people report high levels of happiness for some time. However, one rapidly becomes adapted to the new situation so that now events are evaluated *with respect* to the new Adaptation Level (AL). The reported level of happiness now tends to decline relative to one's expectations. In addition, people frequently raise their sights again, so that they actually become unhappy relative to their new desired state. Naturally, the Adaptation Level at any particular time – the level of one's successful predictions about the world – is not immediately consciously available, though it is established by conscious experiences, and it will become conscious again upon violation (5.3.4). In general, it may be said that those aspects of the world that we have learned *most completely* tend to be *the least* conscious.

Redundant goals also fade from consciousness, even though they continue to operate as goals

We can now make a direct connection between goals, information, and consciousness, because redundant goals are lost from consciousness as well (see 7.4.5). A graduate student may be very much aware at the beginning of graduate education of his or her goal of obtaining an advanced degree. But this goal tends to fade into the background as long as it remains highly predictable. Everyday concerns have more to do with the subgoals needed to carry out the goal of gaining an advanced degree than with this top-level goal. When the student goes to find a book in the library, it is not necessary to be reminded that this is done in pursuit of the ultimate goal. A subgoal can even fail without bringing to mind the high-level goal: One may fail to find the right book in the library; one may even fail to pass an examination. However, if all subgoals fail without alternatives, the top goal also comes into question and must become conscious again. If money for school runs out, if the student has a disabling accident, and so forth, the top-level goal of gaining an advanced degree comes into consciousness, as alternatives to it need to be examined. But as long as goals are predictable, they are as unconscious as any other potentially conscious content.

In actual fact, the goal of gaining a graduate degree may be a poor example, because it is a socially agreed-upon goal, one that can be communicated to others for whom it is not redundant but informative. Thus the goal of gaining a graduate degree is fairly easy to access, even when it becomes routine, because it often needs to be communicated. In the same way, teachers may be able to access information that *practitioners* with the same knowledge allow to become unconscious, because teachers must always be ready to communicate the presupposed information to students who do not share the presuppositions. From this point of view, it seems likely that constant private goals may be much more difficult to make conscious. Thus the goal of gaining the respect and affection of others may become presupposed and unconscious, even while we pursue its subgoals. Or the goal of advancing one's social control, or to outshine competitors, may become unconscious and still be pursued. From this point of view, adaptation to goals may behave much like repression (7.8.2) – that is to say, people will spontaneously disavow having such goals, even though the unconscious routine goals will continue to guide their actions.

Redundancy Effects are not limited to conscious processes: All
neural structures adapt to predictable input

Conscious experience is not the only thing that habituates. Selective habituation to repeated input seems to be a universal property of neural tissue (Kaidel, Kaidel, & Weigand, 1960). Even a single neuron will respond to electrical stimulation at a given frequency only for a while; after that, it will cease responding to the original frequency, but continue to respond to other frequencies. For example, a pulse train of 300 Hz will cause the neuron to fire – until it habituates. After that point, it will no longer fire to a 300-Hz stimulus, though it will continue to respond to stimuli less than 280 Hz or more than 320 Hz (Kaidel, Kaidel, & Weigand, 1960). Neuronal habituation is selective, just as habituation of the Orienting Response is selective (1.4.1). Further, Sokolov's arguments also seem to apply at this level: Fatigue cannot explain selective habituation, because the neuron continues to be responsive to nonhabituated frequencies.

This kind of selective habituation can be observed at many different levels of organization in the nervous system: in single cells, in small assemblies of neurons, in larger nuclei and pathways; in complete sensory and motor systems, and in the nervous system as a whole (Tighe & Leaton, 1976). This point is very important in our theoretical development because it suggests that *all* specialized processors attempt to adapt to (match) input, and become quiescent when they have done so. But what then is the difference between local neural habituation, and loss of conscious access to some experience? Below, we will propose that loss of conscious access is a global result of many cases of local habituation by specialized processors (5.3.1).

5.1.4 Adapted systems can provide new context for later conscious experiences

What happens after some conscious event is matched exactly? We have just stated that the input does not disappear; what does it do instead? Chapter 4 suggested that a major function of consciousness is to evoke the proper context for later conscious experience. We can now extend this point to the *creation* of new contexts. One interesting possibility is that systems that adapt to conscious input create new contexts, which then begin to shape future conscious events. Going back to the epigraph for this chapter, we can now begin to explain James's observation that "what we hear when thunder crashes is not thunder *pure*, but thunder-breaking-upon-silence-and-contrasting-with-it." Those systems that have adapted to the silence, and that therefore predict continuing silence, must make major changes as a result of the thunder clap. Further, they have become contextual with respect to the experience of thunder: They notify us not only that thunder has occurred, but that it was very different from the foregoing level of sound.

We will consider two examples in detail; first, the act of driving a car, and next, the case of scientific concept development.

A perceptual–motor example: Adapted conscious contents can create a new context

When we first learn to drive a car, we are very conscious of the steering wheel, the transmission lever, the foot pedals, and so on. But once having learned to drive, we minimize consciousness of these things and become mainly concerned with the road: with turns in the road, traffic to cope with, and pedestrians to evade. The mechanics of driving becomes part of the unconscious context within which we experience the road. But even the road can be learned to the point of minimal conscious involvement if it is predictable enough: then we devote most of our consciousness to thinking of different destinations, of long-term goals, and so forth. The road has itself now become contextual. The whole process is much like Alice moving through the Looking Glass, entering a new reality, and forgetting for the time being that it is not the only reality. Things that were previously conscious become presupposed in the new reality. In fact, tools and subgoals in general become contextual as they become predictable and automatic.

Before learning to drive there are many things we may consciously consider doing with a gear lever or a steering wheel. We do not know exactly how much force is needed to turn the wheel, or how to put the transmission lever in its various positions. We don't have the "feel" of these actions. These are all open choices – constrained, of course, by their own previous contexts. But there are many degrees of freedom in our representation of these factors.

Of course, even after adaptation the nervous system continues to represent and process the foot-pressure on the accelerator pedal and the force needed to turn the steering wheel. These factors do not disappear when they are lost from consciousness: They have simply become predictable through an adaptive learning process. Learning or adaptation may in fact be defined as a reduction of alternatives in a domain. When complexity has been maximally reduced, we have learned successfully. Our general claim in this chapter is that reducing alternatives to a single one leads to a loss of consciousness of the source of stimulation. Indeed, the loss of consciousness that occurs with habituation and automatization can be taken as a sign that learning is complete.

But why, when the act of driving becomes automatic, do we become conscious of the road? Presumably the road is much more *informative* within our purposes than driving has become. Dodging another car, turning a blind corner, braking for a pedestrian – these are much less predictable than the handling of the steering wheel. These are now the differences that make a difference. But once the road itself becomes routine and predictable, it too can become context for other events, and so on indefinitely.

Notice that *goals* provide some of the constraints for the conscious domain. Indeed, goals involve one kind of context of alternatives (4.0, 6.0). Paying attention to choices at street crossings determines whether we shall get to our destination (our immediate goal), and driving safely determines whether we shall survive (an enduring goal). Like other contexts, these goals are not usually conscious when they shape action and experience. In the act of dodging another car, we do not consciously remind ourselves that we want to survive. We can interpret purposeful actions as having a kind of informativeness, making a difference within a goal context of alternatives. Goal contexts specify a set of alternatives that our actions serve to select, so that our purposeful actions are also informative at various levels of significance. Not running over that pedestrian selects our goal of not harming people, of avoiding trouble with the law, and of getting where we are going with minimum effort. These are all significant goals – some are more significant than others, and some are subgoals for deeper goals. In all these cases we can think of conscious events and voluntary actions as being informative, in the sense of selecting alternatives within the contextual goal hierarchy (5.2.3; 7.0).

A contextual system does not have to remain unconscious for a lifetime. It can be *de*contextualized to become once again a domain of conscious experience. Suppose we are accustomed to driving a car with power steering, and one day the power steering fails. Suddenly the steering wheel becomes harder to turn, especially at slow driving speeds. Our contextualized predictions about the force needed to turn the wheel are violated; our strategy for driving the car must change. Now the act of moving the steering wheel becomes conscious again. Previously predictable events decompose into several different alternatives, as previously contextual processes become the objects of conscious experience. We notice that in order to turn the wheel with less effort we must keep the car moving. This was not a consideration before, but it has now become relevant. Presumably a global display of the newly conscious information helps to bring such new considerations to bear upon our overall goal of steering the car. This phenomenon of decontextualization of previously unconscious tools and effectors is very general. When we break an arm, this normally presupposed part of the bodily context becomes an object of experience, one that now involves conscious choices: The arm, too, has become decontextualized.

This view gives a new perspective on context (4.0): In a sense, context consists of those things to which the nervous system has *already* adapted; it is the ground against which new information is defined (see Figure 5.2). The same point can be made at the conceptual level, as we see next.

The case of conceptual presuppositions: Conscious contents can turn into new contexts

The development of conceptual presuppositions provides another example of context-creation of adaptation. We have previously presented the case that all consciously accessible concepts exist in a framework of prior unconscious presuppositions (4.2.2). Without such presuppositions, the concepts themselves are different. We now suggest that this presupposed knowledge is simply the result of previously conscious concepts. When we first encounter someone from a different culture, we become conscious of many things that are normally presupposed: The person may speak from an uncomfortably close distance, he or she will have different conceptual presuppositions, etc. If we live for some time in that culture, all these prominent features disappear, and we are shocked when we discover our old culture again. Previously presupposed ideas and actions now become conscious. As usual, it is contrasts and transitions that bring out these points. Experts have much less conscious access to such material than novices.

We can usefully refer to these phenomena in terms of *contextualization* and *decontextualization*. When we encounter some new assumptions about reality, we often need to make them explicit. That does not mean that we must define them verbally; it may be good enough to contrast two different points of view, a politically rightist versus leftist viewpoint, for example. Once we become familiar with the contrasts, they can become automatic and contextualized, so that they will shape subsequent thought without becoming conscious. If the new context is then violated, however, it must become decontextualized; some contrast between right-wing and left-wing politics, which was previously unconscious, becomes conscious again. (Decontextualization is really the same as objectification, mentioned above.)

Take the process of constructing scientific reality, as in the discovery of the atom. In modern times, the first serious proposals for the existence of atoms go back to George Dalton in the early nineteenth century, who discovered that an electrical current will decompose water into two parts hydrogen and one part oxygen. Dalton proposed that tiny *indivisible* (Greek: atomic) particles of hydrogen and oxygen must combine in a two-to-one ratio to form water. But this hypothesis did not establish the reality of atoms and molecules; it merely began a debate that continued for the rest of the nineteenth century, with many facts pro and con being

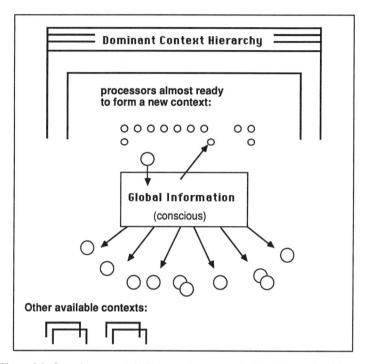

Figure 5.2. Conscious events help to create new contexts and to evoke old ones. Conscious events, when receiving systems adapt to them, can serve to create a new context. In the above diagram a coalition of processors is almost ready to form a new context, but requires some novel component that can only be provided consciously, by way of the global workspace. This component may fit into place either after habituation or, more quickly, after conscious perception or compre-hension—i.e., the case of priming (4.1.1). Once adaptation has occurred, the new context may help shape future conscious events without itself being conscious. Notice that existing contexts can also be evoked by a conscious content, without having to be recreated from scratch.

offered by both sides. Some scientists refused to believe in atoms, or only treated them as useful fictions, *façons de parler,* without any reality. They had many arguments in their favor: Not all substances fell apart into elements with simple ratios; the relationships between the supposed elements were confusing, and could not be organized coherently until quite late in the century. The reality of atoms was not universally recognized until the *various alternatives were shown to reduce to essen-tially one interpretation* (Figure 5.2). This reduction in alternatives culminated with Einstein's work early in this century (Kuhn, 1970). At that point, the reality of atoms became the conceptual framework of a new world view. No longer were atoms considered to be merely convenient fictions. They were "real" objects.

In general, it appears that scientific constructs are not considered "real" until other ways to interpret the evidence are lost from sight. At that point the community stops arguing about them, and begins to take the new construct for granted (Baars, 1986a). Indeed, the newly "real" objects can become the fulcrum of novel explorations that now *presuppose* the existence of the construct. Thus atoms have become part of the unquestioned context within which modern physicists are exploring subnuclear particles. For scientific constructs like atoms, it is not so much that they disappear from the consciousness of the scientists who accept this reality. Rather, the construct is accepted when alternatives are forgotten.

Thus in particle physics today no one challenges the reality of atoms; to do that would undermine the task of exploring subatomic and subnuclear particles. It would force researchers to challenge the context within which protons and quarks are defined. Challenging context is not impossible, of course. Einstein's relativity theory decontextualized Newtonian presuppositions about space and time, and quantum mechanics decontextualized Einstein's assumptions about determinism (Kuhn, 1962/1970). In both cases, physicists became conscious once more of the alternatives to their presupposed reality. But it is very difficult to decontextualize one's assumptions *and at the same time* engage topics *within* that set of assumptions. In driving a car, one cannot be absorbed in moving the steering wheel and successfully engage the road at the same time. In general, a context must remain stable, presupposed, and largely unconscious in order for us to engage the objects that are defined within it.

These parallels between a perceptual–motor task like driving a car and the pursuit of scientific reality are quite intriguing. They suggest that consciousness of the perceptual world and consciousness of a conceptual reality like science may follow similar laws. Notions such as predictability and uncertainty, informativeness and redundancy, context of alternatives, and decontextualization may have very wide application.

The thrust of this section has been that human beings *adapt* to information at all levels: perceptually, imaginatively, conceptually, motorically, and even motivationally. As they adapt, they lose conscious access to the learned material. The next section argues that people also *seek* informative input, so that there are actually two countervailing tendencies.

5.2 Human beings also *seek* information at many levels

So far we have discussed ways in which the nervous system adapts to some conscious event, thereby *reducing* conscious access to it. But the

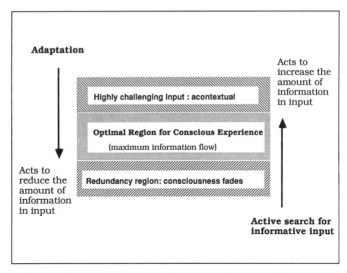

Figure 5.3. Adaptation versus the search for new information. Consciousness and information are closely related. The mind seems to preserve a balance tending toward optimal information flow. Informative input is defined as input that demands reduction of uncertainty, whether perceptually, conceptually, or in Goal Contexts. If there is extreme uncertainty, there is not enough context to constrain a conscious experience of an event. If there is too much certainty, on the other hand, the input is redundant and fades from consciousness. In general, extremes of uncertainty or redundancy are avoided if at all possible, and the system tends toward the middle of the range of novelty, where information content is greatest.

opposite process occurs as well: There is extensive evidence that people seek out novel and informative conscious contents. We do not wait for the perceptual world to fade. We always go on to seek new and interesting things. In sum, there seem to be two tendencies: one to reduce conscious access by adaptation, and a countervailing tendency to increase conscious access by searching for informative stimulation. These two tendencies may alternate, so that we seek conscious information, adapt to it, seek a new source of information, adapt to that, and so on (Figure 5.3). The process may approach a self-regulating homeostasis that tends toward optimal information flow. In this section we explore the *search* for information at different levels of conscious access: in perception, in conceptual processes, and in the domain of goals, where the search for information helps to define the significance of conscious input.

5.2.1 Perceptual systems aim for informative parts of the field

In nature, all of an animal's senses work together in active, coherent exploration. Upon hearing a surprising noise, a dog will prick up its ears;

it will look toward the sound; its pupils will dilate, lungs expand to help sniff the air, nostrils flare to allow better smelling; the animal will even taste the in-breathed air as it flows over the tongue. If the sound is interesting the dog will move toward it, constantly sniffing – looking, listening, and licking anything of interest. It is actively searching for information, for signals that make a difference in the search for food, for social and sexual partners, for dangers to avoid, and often for just plain novelty.

In the laboratory, by contrast, we usually examine only one perceptual system at a time; but the same overwhelming preference for information emerges there. There is extensive evidence that eye-movements focus on the most informative parts of a scene (Kahneman, 1973; Yarbus, 1967). Given a choice between predictable and unpredictable figures, people choose those that are moderately unpredictable: those with enough information to be interesting, but not so much as to be confusing or overwhelming with novelty (Garner, 1974). And it is well established that animals and people will work for informative stimulation without food or any other reward (e.g., Harlow, 1953).

As we see next, the same restless search for information characterizes conceptual processes, those that are abstract and not directly reducible to perception or imagery.

5.2.2   *Conceptual processes aim for informative points*

"Be informative" is a cardinal rule of normal discourse (Clark & Clark, 1977). In fact, violations of this rule are quite strange. When the same conceptual message is repeated over and over, we tend to turn away to other, more interesting and informative material. If we nevertheless *try* to pay attention to the same redundant material, we find that doing this is quite effortful, and ultimately impossible (Mackworth, 1970). People do not ask questions about the things they already know – we always speak with a point of information in mind, either for the speaker or the listener. All these facts suggest that people *seek* conceptual information in the sense described above.

But what about apparent exceptions, such as repeated insistent demands for help, or a child's pursuit of some desire? Surely messages like this can be repeated hundreds of times without adding new information. What about obsessive thoughts, which may recur thousands of times? All of these cases can be reconciled with the idea that people search for novel information, if we interpret them within a goal context. Goal contexts are much more lasting and invariant than perceptual contexts, and the same perceptual message – "Can I have that toy?" – may be repeated over and over again without losing its informativeness in the goal context (5.2.3).

We can again describe these phenomena in terms of Figure 5.3, with the difference that conceptual processes involve a more abstract level of representation. Clearly the search for information can operate at many levels of representation, just as adaptation to information occurs at all levels of representation.

5.2.3 Goal contexts define significant information to attend to

Much of normal conscious thought is devoted to goals and the means to achieve them. Thought-sampling studies show that college students devote about 40 percent of their time to clearly goal-related thoughts and images (Klinger, 1971; Singer, 1984). But even thoughts that *seem* purposeless may be driven by goals that are not currently conscious (Horowitz, 1975a,b; Pope & Singer, 1978; see Chapter 6). Even daydreaming may serve specific goals.

In this section we cite evidence that goal contexts define "significant" information; that is, that people are highly sensitive to signals that reduce uncertainty within goal-defined contexts. Those signals become the objects of attention: We seek to make them conscious. As in the example of a child demanding a new, fascinating toy, this point implies that input may be repetitive at other levels, but informative in a goal context. We are willing to seek out information that is redundant perceptually and conceptually, as long as it is significant within a Dominant Goal Context.

Goals are more important than arbitrary stimuli or concepts; indeed, psychological significance is defined by goals. They provide the higher-level context of information for any animal. Eating and drinking, avoiding danger and discomfort, competing and cooperating with other animals – all these activities are defined by goals. In that sense, goal-related input is inherently informative (6.0, 7.0). We can see this in the case of stimulus habituation: When a stimulus signals food to a hungry animal, it can be repeated many times before the Orienting Response habituates. But when the animal is sated, repetition of the same signal causes rapid habituation of orienting (Sokolov, 1963). Conditioning generally involves reinforcers that tap into biologically significant goals: food, drink, avoidance of pain, and the like. And classical conditioning is believed to depend heavily upon the amount of information given by the conditional stimulus about a significant (goal-related) unconditional stimulus (Rescorla & Wagner, 1972).

It is obvious that people scan the world for significant information, and make it conscious when possible. Attentional control to repetitive stimulation fades quite quickly in spite of our best efforts, but it can be revived by creating pay-offs for successes and failures; that is, when we create a direct connection between conscious vigilance and a currently significant goal (Mackworth, 1970). When there is a monetary reward or penalty, or when survival depends upon vigilance – as in the case of a war-time submarine sonar operator – then we can to some extent overcome the tendency of redundant stimuli to fade from consciousness. Thus the claim that goal contexts define significance, and that we actively search for such significance, seems well-supported. This connection is modeled here by showing that we can recruit a goal context to help maintain relevant information on the GW.

5.2.4 Section summary: Seeking versus adapting to information

This chapter has noted two countervailing tendencies: the search for information and adaptation to information. The first leads to more conscious access, and the second reduces conscious access: Obviously our model should reflect both of these countervailing tendencies, as they balance each other out (see Figure 5.2). So far, the picture seems quite consistent across the board. Perceptual systems are highly sensitive to information rather than physical energy. Conceptual and goal processes can similarly be viewed as sensitive to information – to distinctions that make a difference, that trigger adaptive processes. Further, there is a special relationship between information and consciousness, as shown by the fact that redundant stimuli fade from consciousness (the exceptions to this rule are discussed in section 5.4). Note again that in ordinary life, adaptation does not have to be complete: When routine events become partially redundant, other, more informative, events demand our attention.

5.3 Model 3: Interpreting informativeness in the theory

We can now begin to describe this pattern of evidence in terms of GW theory. Figure 5.4 describes the facts, showing how input can serve to select one of several alternatives that are defined within a stable context. As one choice is selected over and over again, the context begins to predict it routinely, until finally the presentation of the stimulus no longer requires conscious involvement. At this point a new unconscious connection may be established between the input and its mental representation, or there may be a momentary global display for shorter and shorter periods of time, until it becomes very difficult to report (2.4.2). The more predictable the input becomes, the more redundant it is with respect to its mental representation, and the less will it be conscious.

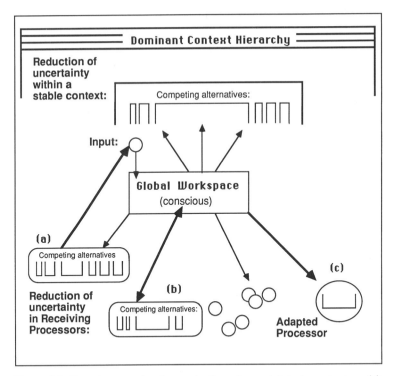

Figure 5.4. Consciousness involves reduction of uncertainty in contexts and in receiving processors. Consciousness seems to be a function of information, defined as a reduction of uncertainty within a stable context or receiving processor. Uncertainty is reduced by an adaptation (matching) process that continues until the number of active alternative interpretations is 1, as in (c). Processors feed back their "interest" in the conscious message as long as there is still uncertainty to be reduced, thereby helping to maintain this particular conscious content. (Notice that feedback is shown in two ways: as an arrow going from a receiving processor to the Input Processor (a), and as a two-way arrow, (b).)

This feedback loop helps explain the pervasive Redundancy Effects, which show that repeated input that is adapted to fades from consciousness. Presumably, adapted processors no longer feed back their interest, and hence fail to support the conscious message. The adapted processor on the right (c) has no feedback arrow, and its shape is represented as returning to the normal round shape of receiving processors.

5.3.1 *How does the system know what is informative?*

How does the GW system determine whether some input is informative? Sometimes we are simply told that some source of conscious information is important, that is, we accept the goal to pay attention to it (see Chapter

8). Indeed, that is what we did with the Dalmatian example: The reader was simply asked to pay attention to the demonstration (5.1.1). Thus sometimes what we make conscious is under the control of goals. However, even when we try to pay attention to a boring and repetitive stimulus, it becomes difficult to do so after a short while. Other, competing thoughts come to mind, and the stimulus fades in spite of our best efforts to pay attention to it. But surely some information is inherently interesting even if it does not serve a currently active goal (Harlow, 1953). Thus there must be some way in which the system can determine how informative the input is independent of goal-controlled attention.

The most plausible supposition is that the audience decides. Specialized processors that are interested in the global message may feed back their interest, and do so until all the usable information is absorbed, or until some other conscious content becomes more informative. We have previously called this the "Nielsen ratings of the mind," by analogy to the continuous assessment of the popularity of different television programs in the United States. In Model 3 we show this as a feedback loop coming from the Receiving Processors to the global message. Presumably we lose conscious access to a repeated stimulus if the Receiving Processors stop feeding back their interest. Figure 5.5 shows this kind of feedback loop.

Notice that Model 3 is quite consistent with the physiological evidence we discussed in Chapter 3 (Model 1A). There are indeed feedback loops coming from the cortex and elsewhere to the ERTAS. It is also consistent with the fact that all neural structures, down to single neurons, habituate in a stimulus-specific way. Specialized processors receive global information, and as they adapt to it, they no longer respond with feedback requesting more of the global message.

This is really a kind of coalition formation between the Receiving Processors and the processors that support the message. It is as if there were television sets with feedback monitors that let the broadcasting station know how many people are actively watching. When the program is popular, the audience supports the input processors – the actors, writers, and producers of the show. There is a coalition in support of the conscious content. But as the audience adapts to the broadcast, it becomes predictable and uninformative, so that fewer and fewer audience members continue to watch. The coalition breaks up, and may re-form around another global message.

In summary, conscious experience suggests that the Receiving Processors are feeding back their interest in adapting to the conscious global message (5.0). Another way of stating this is to say that any conscious message must be *globally informative*.

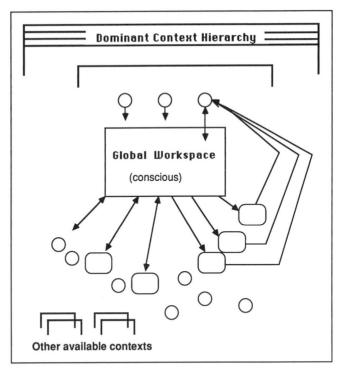

Figure 5.5. Model 3: Feedback from adapting processors. The Redundancy Effects can be explained in terms of feedback from adapting processors (symbolized as rectangles with rounded corners), which work to maintain global access for the conscious content they need to adapt to (see Figure 5.4). This is similar to Model 1A (Fig. 3.3), which suggested the existence of feedback loops based on neurophysiological evidence; the current model supports this suggestion based on functional, psychological considerations. (For the sake of simplicity, future models will not show the feedback loops but only two-way arrows to symbolize adaptation and feedback.)

5.3.2 It takes time for GW input to become conscious

Creating a coalition of global senders and receivers presumably takes time. A short tentative global message may first be broadcast. Some receivers may request more of it, resulting in a longer message, which gathers more support, and so on, in a "snowballing" fashion, until finally the global message becomes available long enough to report as a conscious event (3.2.1; 2.4.2). We have previously referred to this notion as the Momentary Access Hypothesis (2.4.3). It is consistent with Libet's (1978) finding that skin stimulation of moderate intensity may take as long as 0.5 seconds to become conscious, even though cortical activity from the stimulus can be recorded long before that time.

5.3.3 When one conscious event becomes redundant, the next most informative input becomes conscious

The model does not imply that all conscious events are completely adapted to until they are utterly redundant. Most of the time when we read or hear a sentence we do not wait for complete adaptation to take place – we only need to adapt to a single aspect of the input. The reader of this book is not going to repeat each word or sentence over and over again to the point of semantic satiation – it is enough to simply wait for the "click of comprehension." Instead, the model suggests there is *relative* adaptation: We adapt to a conscious event to some point, perhaps until we feel that we have comprehended it. After that, other potential conscious contents may be scanned, to see if there is one with greater significance or with greater ability to recruit a coalition of receivers to support its dominance.

5.3.4 Informativeness and objectification versus redundancy and contextualization

We have suggested that during the information stage of adaptation, there are choices in the stimulus, either implicit or explicit. To see even a simple black line on white paper means that there is an implicit figure–ground comparison; the brightness of the line and paper are implicitly compared to previous visual intensities, as well as to adjacent contrasting areas; and so on. There is no conscious content without implicit comparison.

This point has an interesting bearing on the general issue of contextualization versus objectification. Conscious contents seem always to be objectlike. Even abstract entities and processes tend to be reified and treated as objects – we speak of "mathematics," "democracy," and "process," as if they were objects like chairs, tables, and pencils. Of course when these ideas become thoroughly predictable, they become habituated and automatic and fade from consciousness, though even then they can constrain future conscious experience. That is to say, they have become context, by our definition of that term – they constrain conscious experience without being conscious. We can call this process *contextualization*. The reverse occurs in the case of violated presuppositions, discussed above. Presupposed contextual constraints can become conscious when they are violated, and hence they become objectlike (decontextualized). They change from the status of context and become objectified – turned into an object of experience and thought. The notions of contextualization and objectification have wide-ranging consequences (see Chapter 9).

5.4   When repeated experiences do not fade: Is informativeness a necessary condition for conscious experience?

The claim that informativeness is necessary for a conscious event depends heavily upon the Redundancy Effects discussed above – those cases where input is repeated over and over again and consequently disappears from consciousness. These effects are pervasive: They exist in all senses, in mental imagery, in motor skills, and apparently in conceptual processes as well. However, if there are clear exceptions to the Redundancy Effects, the hypothesis of a necessary connection between consciousness and information cannot be maintained. The existence of genuine counterexamples would destroy the "necesssary condition" claim. In this section I discuss some apparent counterexamples and show that these can generally be handled in a broad information-theoretic framework. The "necessary condition" claim, I conclude, seems quite defensible.

5.4.1   The apparent implausibility of Redundancy Effects in everyday life

On the face of it there is something implausible about the idea that *all* conscious experiences fade when they become automatically predictable. If that were true, how could we experience the same road to work every day of our lives? Or the same kitchen table, the same bedroom, the same faces of friends and family? Is there a *prima facie* absurdity in the informativeness claim? Some Redundancy Effects, like the stopped retinal images discussed above, occur only under laboratory conditions. Is it possible that the laboratory creates artificial circumstances that do not represent reality?

Some of the counterexamples pose genuine challenges, others do not. For instance, Neisser trained people to search for a single word in a list of words, or a face in a photograph of a crowd (see Neisser, 1967). People can learn to do this very well, so that the target face seems to "pop out" of the crowd quite automatically. In these experiments, automaticity in the task seems to *lead* to conscious access, rather than causing it to fade. But this is a false counterargument. If the task practiced involves conscious access, then of course practice in this task should lead to more efficient conscious access. What becomes automatic in the Neisser studies is the act of attending, the act of making things conscious, as opposed to the object that becomes conscious. The particular face in the crowd, or the fact that this face is to be found in this particular place, is quite new and informative (see 8.0). If this is true, the act of attending should fade from consciousness even if the target does not, and the Neisser studies do not provide a true counterargument to the claim that repeated conscious contents fade with redundancy.

Some other counterarguments are more difficult to handle. There are in fact clear cases where habituation of awareness does not hold, where we continue to be conscious of repeated experiences. Pavlov observed "spontaneous dishabituation" in dogs exposed to repeated sounds, and such things as chronic pain never permanently fade from the consciousness of its victims. Even stopped retinal images do not fade permanently; they tend to reappear in a transformed way, so that the word "BEER" will fade and reappear as "PEER," "PEEP," "REFP," and so forth. These cases may represent true counterexamples. I argue in section 5.4.2 that we can retain the informativeness hypothesis in spite of these counter-arguments if we take into account the fact that repeated material *can remain informative if its context of interpretation changes.* This is true of the formal definition of information (Shannon & Weaver, 1949), which permits a repeated message to continue to yield information if the context of choices within which the signal is received is altered. Information is a matter of the relationship of a message to its context, not of either message or context alone. Thus, in cases where a repeated event does not fade, we can ask whether its context of interpretation has changed.

We now explore these issues in some detail.

5.4.2 Some apparent counterexamples

Consciousness to repeated events is *not* lost in the following cases:

1   *Variability.* The same event seems to be repeated, but in fact there is variability in the input. Visual information provides a good example. We would expect that looking fixedly at a clock would cause it to fade from consciousness if the informativeness hypothesis is correct. In fact, the clock seems to stay in consciousness; but of course, this is only because we cannot control involuntary eye movements, especially physiological nystagmus. We only seem to be staring fixedly at the clock – in fact, the input is variable. Similarly, automaticity of skill learning does not occur if the skill is variable (Shiffrin & Schneider, 1977).

2   *Learning.* Fading does not occur if the repeated stimulus is incompletely learned, so that it is better understood with each repetition, and hence has not become truly redundant. This kind of repetition yields the classical learning curve, the relationship between practice and learning that is so much better known than the equally common Redundancy Effects.

3   *Relative adaptation.* Fading does not occur if we do not repeat the event to the point of complete adaptation. We stay conscious of an event if we move on to another one as soon as enough adaptation has occurred. We

try to listen to a repeating word, but in fact, a thought, a feeling, or an image begins to come to mind, even before the target stimulus fades. Most of the time we are satisfied with relative adaptation, as noted above.

4   *Ambiguity*. Redundancy does not occur as quickly if the stimulus is ambiguous and can be reinterpreted, so that it is consciously experienced as different.

We have already discussed the prevalence of local ambiguity in the world (2.3.2). Language is rife with ambiguity; the social world is profoundly ambiguous; the future is unknown and ambiguous; bodily arousal can often be interpreted in more than one way; and conceptual ambiguity is prevalent, even in science.

Good naturalistic examples of spontaneous reinterpretation of ambiguous events can be found in art, literature, music, mathematics, and science. Any piece of polyphonic music shows figure–ground ambiguity. If we pay attention to one melodic line, the others will fade into the "ground" of our perceptual experience. In this sense all polyphonic music can be experienced in many different ways. Further, even a single melodic line can be reinterpreted, because we are continually generating expectations about the next few notes before we hear them; if the composer is clever he or she will occasionally surprise us with an unexpected melodic turn. Truly great composers continually surprise and please us by the interplay of the predictable and unpredictable notes in the fate of an ongoing melody (Bernstein, 1976).

Musicians often find new and different sources of pleasure in the same composition, even when it is played hundreds of times over a period of years. Rather than fading from consciousness, the music is continually reinterpreted. This is true for other art forms as well. Serious works of art cannot be understood completely on first exposure. They require a many-leveled process of reinterpretation before we fully appreciate them. Reinterpretation can happen spontaneously, simply by allowing oneself to be conscious of the work, or under guided voluntary control.

5   *Significance and purpose*. Fading does not occur even with a repeated stimulus if it has significance beyond itself that has not been adapted to. Redundancy may be avoided if there is an ongoing *goal* in attending to the repeated stimulus, especially if the observer receives feedback on the success or failure of his goal. Presumably, the more important the goal, the more we resist redundancy, because the stimulus, which may be redundant perceptually, conveys continuing information in the observer's Dominant Goal Contexts.

Suppose two people are driving in a car to a new destination, but only the driver is involved in finding the way; the passenger is just enjoying the ride. When they go to the same place a week later, which one is likely to remember the way better? Common observation suggests that the driver will, even though the passenger has experienced the same physical flow of stimulation. The difference is that the driver engaged the world in a purposeful way, wondering whether to turn here or there, noting distinctive landmarks at critical choice-points, and the like. The driver's conscious experience was guided by a set of purposes, while the passenger's experience was relatively purposeless.

If people have different experiences of a single event when they are guided by different purposes, their memories should also be different. Thus Pichert and Anderson (1977) presented the same story about two boys playing in a house to two groups of subjects. The first group was told to take the perspective of a home buyer, while the second group assumed the viewpoint of a burglar casing the house. Different facts were recalled by the two groups. The "home buyers" were more likely to remember a leaking roof, while the "burglars" were more likely to remember the location of the color television (Bransford, 1979). This is consistent with the view that different purposes yield different experiences, or, as we will argue below, that inner contextual changes can create new experiences of the same event.

One effect of purpose is voluntary release from habituation – an aspect of voluntary attention (8.0). We can voluntarily make unconscious habituated stimuli conscious again. Simply by choosing to pay attention, the reader can again become conscious of the feeling of the chair, of the background noise, of the quality of the ambient light, and even of semantic presuppositions. I do not model this volitional phenomenon until Chapter 8, where I discuss voluntary attention. Note however that attempts at voluntary control shift the internal context of the signal. Thus this example seems to fit the claim (detailed below) that an internal shift of context can take place even if the physical input is repetitive, resulting in a new conscious experience.

6 *Contextual shifts*. Repetition sometimes leads to spontaneous perceptual transformations. When we listen passively to a repeated word, we soon begin hearing different words (Warren, 1961, 1968). Within a minute or so a repeated word like "break" will begin to be heard as "rake," "wake," "wait," "rape," "ape," "ate," "ache," and so forth. This remarkable Verbal Transformation Effect is different from semantic satiation (described in section 5.1.3) because here the subject is not saying the word, but merely listening to it.

A very similar phenomenon is observed with stopped retinal images. In this case, the transformations change according to the visual properties of letters rather than following phonemic or sound patterns (Pritchard, Heron, & Hebb, 1960). Thus "BEER" will turn to "BEEP," because the "P" and "R" are visually similar, while in the auditory case "break" may change to "wake" because the /r/ and /w/ are phonetically similar (Lackner & Goldstein, 1975).

Because our knowledge of the acoustic properties of speech has improved dramatically over the past twenty years, it has been possible to examine the Verbal Transformation process in detail. It is well established that sounds like /ba/ and /pa/ differ in only one articulatory property. In /ba/ the vocal chords begin to vibrate a few tens of milliseconds before the lips open, while in the case of /pa/ the lips open a short time before the start of voicing (Liberman, Cooper, Shankweiler, & Studdert-Kennedy, 1967). Using computer-generated speech one can systematically vary the "voice onset time" (the time difference between voicing and opening the lips) and locate the exact boundary between the perceived /pa/ and /ba/. Now we can examine the effects of selective habituation. If /pa/ is repeated over and over again, the boundary will shift in the direction of /b/; if /ba/ is repeated over and over again, the reverse occurs (Goldstein & Lackner, 1975; Lackner & Goldstein, 1975). This effect has been shown with natural as well as computer-generated speech. The implication is that if one day we heard all /p/'s and no /b/'s, our perception of these sounds would be grossly distorted, because the phonetic boundaries would shift. But the distortion would go in the right direction. If we heard all /p/'s, the /b/ category would expand, so that more and more cases would be interpreted as /b/'s. Thus the phonetic system acts to regulate itself, and to maintain a relatively constant number of /b/'s and /p/'s. In addition, the actual frequency of these "opponent" phonemes in the language is roughly the same – we normally hear roughly equal numbers of perceived /b/'s and /p/'s – so that the boundary stays at the same voice-onset time.

Thus the context of the information can vary, but the system is designed to keep it reasonably stable under most circumstances. This seems characteristic of all perceptual systems. Generally speaking, the stability of our perceptual contexts depends upon the existence of variation in the perceptual contents. The function of the distribution of /p/'s and /b/'s in a language may be to create enough variability to maintain the categorical boundary. This is similar to the case of physiological nystagmus, the function of which may be to avoid excessive redundancy of input. A similar argument also applies to opponent processes in other senses, such as color perception (Gregory, 1966). But context can change, especially if we are exposed to only one end of a continuum of variation.

This conclusion also comes from the Adaptation Level (AL) Theory of Helson (1964). Our ability to specify the expected stimulus value in perception or judgment depends largely on our experience of the extremes along the same dimension. We will judge criminality with less severity if we are routinely exposed to rapes and murders (even if only on television). As a result, our judgment of criminal severity changes. Political radicalization may work through the same mechanism: The more we are exposed to an extreme belief, the less extreme it seems, while the perceived norm will shift toward the extreme. Again, our experience of an event depends upon our previous related experiences, even when these are not conscious at the time. And again, the context changes when we are repeatedly exposed to one end of the continuum of variation.

Now we can go back to our original question. Why are there cases of repetition that result in conscious transformation rather than fading? One plausible suggestion is that in these cases the context has changed. As one extreme value of an opponent process is repeated over and over again, the context of interpretation may shift. This is clearly the case for Verbal Transformations, and it is at least plausible for stopped retinal images in the visual system. Of course mathematically, the same physical signal in a different context creates different information (Shannon & Weaver, 1949). In this way we can suggest a satisfying account for these interesting counterarguments to the informativeness hypothesis.

To summarize: Repeated signals may not fade from consciousness if they are incompletely known so that each repetition allows more information to be learned; if the signals are variable; if they are ambiguous, so that they can be re-interpreted; if they serve a larger purpose that is not redundant; or if the context drifts, so that the same input signal remains informative. It therefore seems that we can explain the apparent counterarguments to the "informativeness criterion" for conscious experience. Of course this question deserves much more testing.

5.4.3 Section summary

So far, we have suggested that all conscious experience must be informative – that true redundancy leads to a loss of consciousness of a message. The evidence for this is quite pervasive, ranging from repeated stimuli in all sensory modalities to repeated visual images, automatized skills, semantic satiation, and even stable conceptual presuppositions. There are counterarguments that seem compelling at first, but are less so upon further examination. Although more research is clearly needed on these questions, the position that informativeness is a *necessary condition* for conscious experience seems to be quite defensible.

5.5 Implications for learning

If consciousness always involves adaptation, there should be an intimate connection between conscious experience and all kinds of adaptive processes, including comprehension, learning, and problem-solving. We now explore these implications for learning.

5.5.1 Conscious experiences trigger widespread adaptation and learning

Learning of all kinds is surely the most obvious adaptive mental process in which people engage. To learn something deliberately, we typically act to become conscious of the material to be learned. But most details of the learning process are unconscious.

Information and learning are closely related. The most widely accepted model of classical conditioning is defined in terms of informative features of the conditioned stimulus (Rescorla & Wagner, 1972). Recent "connectionist" models of human learning also rely on mathematical rules that maximize the amount of information given by one event about another (Gluck & Bower, 1986; Sutton & Barto, 1981). These models do not have an explicit role for conscious experience. However, they may be moving in that direction.

From a theoretical point of view, we expect consciousness to be involved in learning of novel events, or novel connections between known events. The rationale is that novel connections require unpredictable interactions between specialized processors. Hence global communication from "any" specialist to "any other" is necessary (2.5). Widespread broadcasting serves to make this any–any connection.

What is the evidence for this claim? Perhaps the most obvious is the radical simplicity of the act of learning. To learn *anything* new we merely pay attention to it. Learning occurs "magically" – we merely allow ourselves to interact consciously with algebra, with language, or with a perceptual puzzle like the Dalmatian (5.1.1), and somehow, without detailed conscious intervention, we acquire the relevant knowledge and skill. But we know that learning cannot be a simple, unitary process in its details. The Dalmatian puzzle requires subtle and sophisticated visual and spatial analysis; language requires highly specialized analysis of sound and syntax – indeed all forms of learning involve specialized components, sources of knowledge, and acquisition strategies. These specifics of learning are generally unconscious when they operate most effectively.

The key step in deliberate learning is to become conscious of precisely what is to be learned. Doing this is sufficient for learning to take place, as shown by many studies of recognition memory. In general, if people are just made to pay attention to some material as an "incidental" task, recognition memory for the material will be quite good even a week later, provided that the material is distinctive enough not to be confused with very similar material (Bransford, 1979). Thus consciousness seems to facilitate learning. Whether consciousness is a *necessary condition* for learning is a more difficult question, discussed in section 5.5.3.

Finally, we are driven by our theory to a rather radical position about most learning. Very often conscious involvement in learning leads to adaptation, which alters *the context of experience*; but we know that a change in context in its turn alters subsequent experience. It follows that learning alters the conscious experience of the learned material. Evidence for this position seems strong for perceptual learning, knowledge acquisition, skill learning, immediate memory, episodic memory, and rule learning. It may be more debatable for associative learning. We explore this claim in the next section.

5.5.2 Learning alters the experience of the material learned

If it is true that learning involves the generation of new contexts, and if contexts shape and bound new conscious experiences, it follows that *we experience the same materials in a different way after learning.* Is there evidence for this implication? Certainly we talk about algebra as "the same thing" before and after learning it, just as we talk about the Dalmatian demonstration (5.1.1) as the same "thing" before and after comprehension. But both algebra and the Dalmatian are experienced differently after learning. Perceptual learning certainly changes the experience of the stimulus. Children are thought to experience the perceptual world differently after acquiring object permanence, for example (Piaget, 1952). Native speakers of a language can often discriminate phonetic distinctions foreigners cannot hear: Most English speakers simply cannot hear the Chinese tonal system. Even in learning to comprehend a puzzling sentence, there is a change in experience (4.1.2; Milne, 1982). In the "I scream/ice cream" example of Chapter 2 (2.3.2), the perceived word boundaries switch back and forth; and indeed, one of the great difficulties in learning foreign language is in learning to perceive word boundaries. Similarly, conceptual learning – of the sort that a student of science does in learning physics – clearly involves a change in perspective and insight into the field. The announcement of a new subnuclear particle must lead to a different experience of comprehension for an advanced physicist than for a novice.

What about associative learning? When we need to discover the connection between two known stimuli, or between a known stimulus and a known response, is there a change in conscious experience? This is not so clear. Perhaps the strongest evidence in favor of a change in experience comes from a series of brilliant studies by Dawson and Furedy (1976). These researchers showed that human Galvanic Skin Response (GSR) conditioning did not occur if subjects misinterpreted the relationship between the conditioning stimuli. In standard GSR conditioning a stimulus is given, such as a tone, followed by a shock which elicits a change in skin conductivity (GSR). Dawson and Furedy provided this stimulus situation, and normal conditioning occurred. But then they changed the subject's mental set about the stimulus sequence. Subjects were told that the task was to detect a tone in noise, and that the function of the shock was to mark the boundaries of the trials. (Experimental subjects will believe almost anything.) That is, they took the stimulus conditions (tone–shock, tone–shock, tone–shock) and made the subjects think of them in the reverse order (shock–tone, shock–tone, shock–tone). Under these circumstances, the tone no longer served as a signal for the shock. And indeed, though the stimulus conditions were unchanged, conditioning failed to take place.

What does this mean for the question of changing experience? We still do not know whether associative learning changes the experience of the learned connection. However, the Dawson and Furedy (1976) studies show that *if* we experience stimuli such that the tone does not seem to signal the shock, learning will not occur. It may therefore be that the distinction between "associative learning" and "knowledge acquisition" is a false distinction: All learning takes place within a knowledge context that defines the relationships between the stimuli. If that is true, it seems that learning changes this knowledge context even in the case of associative learning.

This somewhat radical hypothesis about learning has a perplexing implication. Namely, if we experience an event differently after learning, why do we still think of it as the same event? That is, how do we maintain *event identity* before and after learning? This is a profound and difficult question, which was raised by William James (of course) (1890/1983). It was also raised by Kuhn (1970) about scientific constructs after a paradigm shift. Indeed, scientific constructs like gravity and light are quite different in Relativity Theory as compared to Newtonian physics; yet they are called by the same names, and they are often naively believed to be the same things. Many physical observations relevant to light and gravity are unchanged, of course, but not all (Kuhn, 1970), and some new relationships are added with the coming of Relativity Theory: the bending of light by gravity, for example. Nonetheless, "construct identity" is maintained, at least in the sense that many physicists *believe* that in the Einsteinian framework they are simply understanding "the same thing" in a deeper way. The general implication is that *event identity is a function not only of the observations in question, but of the entire knowledge context in which it is defined.* This is *not* just true in physics, but in perception, in conceptual learning, and probably in learning in general.

The developmental role of forgotten conscious choice-points
There is another interesting implication of the hypothesis that learning changes the experience of the material learned. Any developmental process must involve choice-points between different potential paths. We may choose to learn to play the piano at the age of six; if not, we are

unlikely to become concert pianists. We may choose to distrust certain people at an early age as a result of traumatic experiences, and thus avoid finding out that our distrust is unjustified, and so on. At the moment of choice, we may be quite conscious of the alternatives; once having chosen, we enter a new context that is created by the choice, and within which the original choice is often not even defined. Once having learned algebra, it is extremely difficult to reexperience the confusion that was once so common about meaningless algebraic squiggles on a page. Thus we often cannot make previous choice-points conscious once we have entered the new context created by those choice-points. We may be utterly at the mercy of our previous choices, so that we cannot undo them. This suggests that some learning, and its consequent alteration in experience, may never be fully reversible. This is a point with major consequences for developmental psychology.

5.5.3 Is consciousness necessary for learning?

The fact that much effective learning begins with a conscious experience is known to every parent and teacher who has ever tried to teach distractable children. In daily life this is what the term "attention" means: It involves an attempt to control what shall become conscious (see Chapter 8). In the psychology laboratory we always call the attention of subjects to whatever is to be learned. Yet somehow the salience of this plain everyday fact has escaped the notice of many researchers, in part because it has been superseded by a controversy: that is, the question whether consciousness is a *necessary condition* for learning (e.g., Dixon, 1971, 1981; Eriksen, 1960; Holender, 1986; Marcel, 1983a,b). This controversy has been difficult to resolve conclusively, in good part because it raises the difficult question of defining empirically the "zero point" of consciousness. We have previously remarked on this difficulty, and on the importance of developing a theoretical approach that does not require a solution to this extremely problematic question (1.5.5). Unfortunately in the case of learning, most discussion of the role of consciousness seems to be assimilated to the "necessary condition" question. But even if conscious experience were not a necessary condition but only a helpful adjunct to the learning process, it would be difficult to doubt that in the real world consciousness and learning are very close companions. Thus the controversy about the *necessity* of consciousness tends to interfere with a more subtle question about the role consciousness plays in *most* cases of learning. We will not review the learning controversy here; we raise it merely to point out that, whatever the answer may be to that question, it does not negate the plain fact that most of the time when we

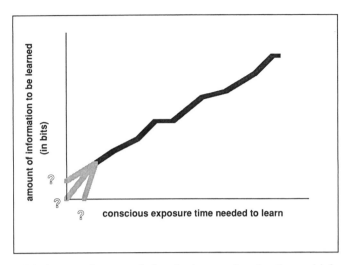

Figure 5.6. An upward monotonic function between learning time and information. A hypothetical curve showing the relationship between the amount of information to be learned and the duration of conscious exposure needed to learn it. Some monotonically upward function is generally found, under a number of different conditions. However, the zero point of the curve is heavily disputed – that is, it is not clear whether conscious exposure is a *necessary* condition of learning. But controversy over the zero point should not be allowed to obscure the wide consensus on the general shape of the curve.

want to learn something we make ourselves conscious of the material to be learned.

In order to avoid the unresolvable "zero-point" question, we suggest a more answerable one: Do we need *more* conscious involvement to learn *more* information? It seems likely that relatively routine and predictable information may be learned with minimal conscious involvement. The more novelty we must absorb, the more conscious experience we need. The evidence for this claim seems to be widespread and noncontroversial: The more words that need to be memorized, the longer we must pay attention. The more difficult and novel some material is, the more time we must spend being conscious of all its details and implications; and so on. Figure 5.6 presents a theoretical curve describing this situation. It shows an upward monotonic function between the amount of information that is to be learned and the amount of conscious involvement needed to learn it. Notice that the zero point of the curve is undefined, reflecting the difficulty of deciding whether consciousness is a *sine qua non* of learning. The figure suggests that we do not need to solve this problem in order to make interesting claims about the relationship between learning and consciousness.

5.6 Some experimental predictions

The key to theoretical success, of course, is making novel predictions that work. The following section presents some possibilities.

5.6.1 The "cold dog" experiment

There is evidence that unconscious (or at least, unreportable) words may prime subsequent conscious processes. Marcel (1983a,b) and others have shown that backward-masked printed words, which are not reportable, still improve lexical decision time for related words (i.e., the time that is needed to decide whether some string of letters is a word or not). While these results are apparently reliable, they have given rise to great controversy (Cheesman & Merikle, 1984; Holender, 1986). The debate is mainly about whether the unreportable words are truly unconscious or not. That is, it is about the "zero point" of consciousness, precisely the issue that is most difficult to decide. We do not take a position on this issue, of course, but GW theory does suggest an experimental prediction.

Briefly, when we have a very short unreportable exposure of a word compound like "hot dog," it should prime lexical decisions about related words, like "sausage." However, if the word compound is novel, like "cold dog," it should not prime a related term like "Huskie" or "frozen Fido." New word compounds require conscious involvement to bring many different specialists to bear on the problem of creating a coherent interpretation. There is indeed one report in the literature supporting this hypothesis (Greenwald & Liu, 1985).

5.6.2 Other testable questions

We have made the claim above that semantic satiation is one source of evidence for the generality of redundancy phenomena. In fact, it is difficult to do clean experiments with semantic satiation (Amster, 1964; Esposito & Pelton, 1971). For example, we do not know for sure that semantic satiation is semantic rather than a perceptual event, because when we repeat a word over and over again, both the meaning and the perceptual stimulus are repeated. To prove that semantic satiation is indeed semantic we would have to repeat different synonyms or paraphrases with the same conceptual meaning but different perceptual form, and show that satiation occurs. Reddy and Newell (1974) cite more than 100 paraphrases of a single sentence about a chess move. If we repeat all 100 paraphrases, we should expect to find semantic satiation if this is a truly conceptual, as opposed to perceptual, phenomenon. Our prediction is of course that semantic satiation to different paraphrases would take place.

There appears to be almost no work on the issue of blindness to conceptual presuppositions, although everyone must encounter this phenomenon in everyday life. Measures of recall could be easily used to test it.

How is automatization of skills related to stimulus habituation? They seem to be so similar that it is intriguing to wonder about a connection. One possibility is that skilled actions are guided by conscious and quasi-conscious goal-images (7.0). If that is so, perhaps automatization of skills simply involves habituation of the relevant guiding goal-images. This hypothesis may deserve further study.

Finally, it will be worth investigating the relationship between information to be learned and the amount of conscious involvement, using carefully designed stimuli with known information content (e.g., Garner, 1974). This should cast light on the heated issue of the relationship between consciousness and learning without raising the inherent methodological difficulties involved in seeking the "zero point" of consciousness.

5.7   Other implications

5.7.1 Subliminal perception

There are two ways to model subliminal or unreportable input in the GW model. First, if the input is routine, a perceptual system may analyze it without recourse to the global workspace. The second possibility is that the GW may be used for very rapid exchanges of information, and that linguistic and recall systems that can report conscious experiences simply do not have time to register this rapid global information. This is similar to the Sperling (1960) phenomenon, where stimuli are conscious briefly but cannot be recalled afterwards (1.1.2). In the second case, a limited amount of novel processing could be done, provided that other specialists in the system can react to the global information more quickly than the linguistic and recall specialists. Again, these alternatives may be difficult to test with our present methodology, but they are worth pointing out.

5.7.2 Phenomena involving more than one conscious experience

We have now finished considering the meaning of a single conscious experience. The following chapters focus on the relationships between multiple conscious events, allowing us to deal with issues like problem incubation, voluntary control, and conscious access to abstractions that are not experienced qualitatively.

5.8 Chapter summary

This chapter has explored the fundamental phenomena of habituation and automatization. We have argued that all conscious contents must be informative in that they trigger widespread adaptive processes. Receiving specialists must feed back their interest in the conscious content, so that they join the coalition of systems that support it. This is Model 3. It serves to put a conscious experience in a temporal context, described as the "adaptation cycle." All conscious experiences, it is argued, involve a stage of adaptation in which a defining context has been accessed, so that the conscious information can be understood; but not all degrees of freedom have been determined. Consciousness occurs during the stage where the remaining uncertainty in the defining context is being reduced. After that point, adaptation has taken place, and repetition of the same input will not result in a conscious experience. There is thus an intimate connection between consciousness, adaptation, information, reduction of uncertainty, redundancy, and context.

Information that fades from consciousness does not disappear; rather, it serves to constrain later conscious experiences. It may become part of a *new unconscious context, within which later experiences are defined.* One implication is that every event is experienced with respect to prior conscious events: "Into the awareness of the thunder itself the awareness of the previous silence creeps and continues . . ." as James says so eloquently in our epigraph.

The more information we must adapt to, the longer we need to be conscious of the material in order to create new contexts for dealing with it; and the more new contexts we create, the more our subsequent experiences will be reshaped. This suggests an unconventional view of learning and development. Namely, learning becomes a matter of developing contexts that cause us to experience the same reality in new and different ways. We have explored the evidence for this somewhat radical proposal.

In the upshot, this chapter suggests a third determining condition for conscious experience, on a par with *global broadcasting* and *internal consistency* (Chapter 2). To be conscious, a potential experience must be *informative*. Even the biological and personal significance of an event can be treated as its informativeness in a goal context. This point allows GW theory to deal with the issue of significance, a point that is often neglected in the current cognitive literature.

Thus we are compelled to view even a single conscious experience as part of a dynamic, developmental process of learning and adaptation. Increasingly it seems that the system underlying conscious experience is our primary organ of adaptation.

In the following chapter, we will explore the ways in which contexts help to achieve goals. Much of our stream of consciousness involves thoughts about goals, ways of achieving goals, failures to achieve them, and the like (Pope & Singer, 1978). In ordinary life, as in the psychological laboratory, we are always asking people to do some tasks by giving them a goal. "I would like you to listen for a tone [goal], and to press this button [subgoal] with your right hand [subgoal] as quickly as you can [subgoal] when you hear one." But people are never conscious at any one time of *all* the details of motivation, levels of planning and motor control, timing, testing of plans, and the like, that are needed to reach even a simple goal. The bulk of our goal-related processes are unconscious at any one time, even though they shape our action and experience; that is to say, they are mostly contextual. In the next chapter we show that some simple assumptions about goal contexts and conscious events lead to an understanding of the stream of consciousness – the "flights" and "perches" of the mind from one apparently unrelated experience to another.

Part IV

Goals and voluntary control

So far, we have considered what it means for something to be conscious. In this section, we place these considerations in a larger framework, exploring the uses of consciousness. Thus we move away from a consideration of separate conscious experiences to a concern with conscious *access*, *problem-solving*, and *control*.

Chapter 6 describes the commonly observed "triad" – conscious problem assignment, unconscious computation of routine components, and conscious display of solutions and subgoals. This triadic pattern is observable in many psychological tasks, including creative processes, mental arithmetic, language comprehension, recall, and voluntary control. It suggests that conscious contents often serve to assign problems to unconscious processors, which work out routine details, constrained by a goal context.

Intentions can be treated as largely unconscious goal structures that make use of conscious goal images to recruit the effectors and subgoals needed to reach their goals. This suggests ways in which conscious experience helps to solve problems in learning, perception, thinking, and action. The interplay between conscious contents and goal contexts also provides a plausible account of the "stream of consciousness."

In Chapter 7, a contrastive analysis of voluntary versus involuntary actions leads to a modern version of William James's ideomotor theory, suggesting that voluntary actions are also recruited by conscious goal images. The ideomotor theory can handle a number of puzzling questions about voluntary control; it implies that volition always involves conscious goal images that are tacitly edited by multiple unconscious criteria. Abstract concepts may be controlled by similar goal images, which may be conscious only fleetingly.

6   Model 4:

Goal contexts, spontaneous problem solving, and the stream of consciousness

Every actually existing consciousness seems . . . to be a *fighter for ends*, of which many, but for its presence, would not be ends at all.

William James, 1890/1983 (p. 144)

6.0   Introduction

Consider the following questions:[1]

1   What are two names for the ancient flying reptiles?
2   What technology develops artificial limbs and organs?
3   What are three synonyms for "talkative"?

These questions evoke a mental search for words that are known but rare. The search may take longer than expected, tending to create what William James called a "tip-of-the-tongue" (TOT) state, in which we have an intense feeling of knowing the word in question, even though it does not come to mind immediately (Brown & McNeill, 1966). This chapter is about this state in all its variegated forms.

In the last two chapters we explored the *contexts* of experience, defined as those systems that shape and bound conscious experiences without being conscious themselves. In this chapter we show how the very general idea of a *goal context* or *intention* allows us to deal in a natural way with tasks that extend over more than a single conscious experience. In practice, of course, all psychological tasks involve more than a single conscious event. The notion of a goal context allows us to understand a very large set of phenomena as variants of a single pattern. Creative processes in art, science, and mathematics seem to be under the control of goal contexts – but so are short-term events like word-search, question-answering, the interpretation of ambiguous words and figures, control of action, and the like (6.2.4). The stream of consciousness can be considered as a flow of experiences created by the interplay of many goal contexts, each tending to make conscious whatever will promote progress toward its goal (6.4).

---

1   Answers: 1. pterosaurus, pterodactyl; 2. bionics, prosthetics; 3. loquacious, wordy, voluble, verbose, long-winded, etc.

Notice that goal contexts are not necessarily *labeled* as voluntary. The ability to label one's own goals and to guide one's own processes requires an additional layer of metacognitive organization, to be discussed in Chapters 7, 8, and 9.

We begin with William James's well-known description of the intention to remember a forgotten word – the tip-of-the-tongue (TOT) state – and conclude, in modern terms, that the TOT state is a complex representational state that takes up limited capacity, that guides word-search and evaluates candidate words, but that does *not* have experienced qualities like color, warmth, flavor, pitch, or a clearly bounded locus in time and space. This state differs therefore from mental images, inner speech, feelings, or percepts, which do have experienced qualities (cf. Natsoulas, 1982). James suggests that perhaps one-third of our psychic life may be spent in such states of specific expectation. We will pursue the argument that the TOT state represents "a goal context searching for a conscious content."

Such goal contexts are different from conscious events that function as goals; both are needed for the system to operate. Given a conscious event that can be interpreted as a goal, the system works to recruit a goal context and a set of processors that engage in spontaneous problem solving. The resulting solutions often become conscious. If the goal cannot be reached, obstacles and subgoals tend to become conscious and recruit their own resources, until finally an acceptable conscious solution emerges.

This kind of spontaneous problem solving is extremely general. It can cover life plans, fantasies for the future, control of one's own body, retrieval of the right word at the right time, sentence comprehension, attempts to achieve social influence, and an endless variety of other goals that people think of achieving at one time or another. Even operant and classical conditioning can be seen as types of goal-directed problem solving. The material in this chapter is therefore crucial to the claim that conscious processes are functional: that they help people achieve their goals in life.

6.1   The tip-of-the-tongue state as a *goal context* or *intention*

6.1.1   *William James on the tip-of-the-tongue experience*

We begin with the following observations from William James about the state of attempting to recall a forgotten word (1890). Is such a state truly conscious or not? asks James.

Suppose we try to recall a forgotten name. The state of our consciousness is peculiar. There is a gap therein; but no mere gap. It is a gap that is intensely active. A sort of a wraith of the name is in it, beckoning us in a given direction, making us at moments tingle with the sense of our closeness, and then letting us sink back without the longed-for term. If wrong names are proposed to us, this singularly definite gap acts immediately so as to negate them. They do not fit into its mould.

Thus clearly something is going on – we are conscious of some sort of *definite* state, because if someone suggests the wrong word to us, we know immediately that this *is* the wrong word. And we also immediately recognize the right word when it comes to mind. In modern terms, we can successfully recognize *matches and mismatches* of the state of looking for a forgotten word – and the ability to accurately detect matches and mismatches implies that this state involves a *representation* of a target word. Since words can vary along many dimensions, it must be a *complex* representational state, much like a mental image or a percept.

Furthermore, this "tip-of-the-tongue" state resembles a mental image or a percept, because having it excludes other conscious contents. We cannot search for a forgotten word and at the same time contemplate a picture, think of yesterday's breakfast, or do anything else that involves conscious experience or mental effort. The TOT state occupies our central limited capacity.

But in one respect the TOT state differs from mental images, feelings, inner speech, and perceptual experiences. All these conscious events have experienced qualitative properties – qualities like size, color, warmth, or location. But the TOT state does not have experienced qualities (viz. Natsoulas, 1982). Two different TOT states are *not experienced* as sounding different, even though the words they stand for sound different. In some ways, therefore, the TOT state is like other conscious states such as percepts and images; in other ways, it is not like those conscious experiences at all, but much more like the contexts discussed in Chapter 4.

The same may be said whenever we intend to speak a thought that is not yet clothed in words:

And has the reader never asked himself what kind of a mental fact is his *intention of saying a thing* before he has said it? It is an entirely definite intention, distinct from all other intentions, an absolutely distinct state of consciousness, therefore; and yet how much of it consists of definite sensorial images, either of words or things? Hardly anything! Linger, and the words and things come into the mind; the anticipatory intention, the divination is there no more. But as the words that replace it arrive, it welcomes them successively and calls them right if they agree with it, it rejects them and calls them wrong if they do not. It has therefore a nature of its own of the most positive sort, and yet what can we say about it without using words that belong to the later mental facts that replace it? The intention *to-say-so-and-so* is the only name it can receive (italics in original).

James suggests that perhaps one-third of our psychic life consists of states like this; further, he seems to say that this state itself triggers off retrieval processes, which produce the words that will clothe the intention (James, 1890/1983). In other words, the TOT state is active; it initiates a conscious display of a series of candidate words, and "it welcomes them . . . and calls them right if they agree with it, it rejects them and calls them wrong if they do not."

6.1.2 Theoretical implications of James's observations

We can summarize in modern terms the theoretical claims made by James about the tip-of-the-tongue state:

1 The TOT state involves a complex representation of the missing word (as shown by the fact that it accurately matches and mismatches candidate words).
2 The TOT state occupies central limited capacity, like other conscious states. (Witness the fact that the TOT state is interrupted by incompatible conscious events.)
3 The TOT state helps trigger off word-retrieval processes, so that candidate words come to consciousness as long as this state dominates our limited capacity.
4 The TOT state only stops dominating our central limited capacity when the right word is found.
5 And yet in spite of all these properties the TOT state does *not* have experiential qualities like color, warmth, flavor, location, intensity, etc. It is therefore radically different from other conscious experiences like mental images, feelings, inner speech, and percepts.

These observations apply generally to intentions and expectations. To create experiences like this for *any* action, we need only ask someone to perform the action and then delay the moment of execution. To have a runner experience a "tip-of-the-foot" experience, we need only say "GET READY," "GET SET," and then delay "GO." At that point the runner is poised to go, the "intention" is at its highest pitch, and yet the action is not executed. There may be no sensory experience of the "intention to run," but the runner's concentration will still be impaired by interfering conscious events. The "intention to run" takes up limited capacity just as the tip-of-the-tongue state does.

Given these implications, let us sketch out a way in which the global workspace theory can model the TOT state, its antecedents, and its consequences.

6.1.3 Intentions in GW theory

GW theory treats the TOT state as a *current goal context*, an unconscious structure that dominates our limited capacity for some time – witness the fact that it competes with any conscious content. But the current goal context naturally operates in its own higher-order, more permanent context of preexisting goals (4.3.5). At this moment the reader's conscious experience is presumably shaped by the goal of reading this sentence. But as soon as the sentence ends, or the book is closed, it becomes clear that this local goal context exists always in its own complex hierarchy of goals, in which reading the sentence is merely a local subgoal.

The claim made here is that goal contexts are the same as the *intentions* of common sense psychology. We will use these expressions interchangeably. The term "goal context" emphasizes the contextual and nonqualitative nature of intentions and their similarity to other contexts, especially conceptual contexts (4.2.2). Indeed, we can say that conceptual contexts are equivalent to expectations, and goal contexts are equivalent to intentions. But intentions and expectations are very similar: Indeed, one can argue that they are basically the same. We speak of expectations when we have a future-directed mental representation that is dependent on external events for its satisfaction. An intention is the same, except that it depends on self-generated events. An intention, then, is an expectation about oneself.

A goal context does not have to be evoked by verbal questions. Any conscious stimulus that is incomplete, that invites further processing, seems to initiate a context that guides further unconscious work. This has been widely noted, for example by Gestalt psychologists, by the Würzburg school, by Zeigarnik, and by Ach (Murray, 1983; Rapaport, 1951). It is most widely known as the "Zeigarnik phenomenon," the tendency to complete incomplete mental contents. There has been some controversy about the evidence for it recently, which we will discuss below (6.2.2) (Holmes, 1967, 1968).

If it is generally true that intentions do not have qualitative conscious contents, then a current controversy about the ability to report intentions begins to make more sense. Nisbett and Wilson (1977) cite a number of social psychological studies showing that the intentions people attribute to themselves can often be quite incorrect. For example, in a department store display of socks or perfume, people will tend statistically to choose the right-most item; yet if asked why they chose the item, they will produce all sorts of reasons other than the one that seems to be operative. This is only one of dozens of demonstrations showing that people have poor access to their own reasons for doing things, even leaving out those cases where the rationalization is self-serving or defensive. But we also know that under optimal conditions people can report other mental processes quite accurately (e.g., in mental imagery, explicit verbal problem solving, rehearsal in short-term memory, etc.; see Ericsson & Simon, 1980). What is the difference then between reporting intentions and reporting mental images? Why are intentions so difficult to report?

One possible explanation is that intentions are complex, *nonqualitative*, but capacity-limiting events, which are not experienced in detail. To become reportable, intentions must be converted into an introspectible code, such as inner speech, visual images, or perhaps bodily feelings. These conscious contents may be easier to report accurately. This is not to say that intentions have no conscious correlates: There may be qualitative images, inner speech, and so forth, associated with the intention. Further, when the intention runs into difficulties there is a consciously expressible sense of surprise. But such conscious contents are *not the same as the intention itself.*

Below we will attempt to specify the role of consciously experienced goals as important parts of any intention (6.2.2; see also Chapter 7). But first, let us specify the notion of intention or goal context in more detail.

Intentions as multileveled goal structures

Intentions or goal contexts represent future states of the system, serving to constrain processes that can help reach those future states. But intentions are not simple goals. They must be multileveled goal *structures*, consisting of numerous nested goals and subgoals. Even a single spoken sentence is constrained by many simultaneous goals and criteria, including those that specify the desired loudness and rate of speech; voice quality; choice of words; intonation; dialect; morphology; syntax; choice of rhetorical style; semantics; discourse relations; conversational norms; and communicative effectiveness (Clark & Clark, 1977). Each of these levels of organization can be described in terms of general goals, which the action can match or mismatch. Each of these levels can go astray, and errors at each level of control can be detected and corrected immediately.

On top of these linguistic criteria we use language to gain a multitude of pragmatic ends, many of which combine to constrain any single speech act. Thus we may routinely want to appear educated in our speech, but not stuffy; tolerant, but not undiscriminating; we may want to capture the listener's attention, but not to the point of screaming for it. All such pragmatic goals simultaneously constrain any speech act.

Notice, again, that contexts can compete for limited capacity just as conscious contents can. But there is this difference, that we can only be aware of one chair (one conscious content), but that many goal contexts can simultaneously constrain limited capacity as long as they are mutually compatible (see Figure 6.2).

Once established, linguistic and pragmatic goal systems do not become

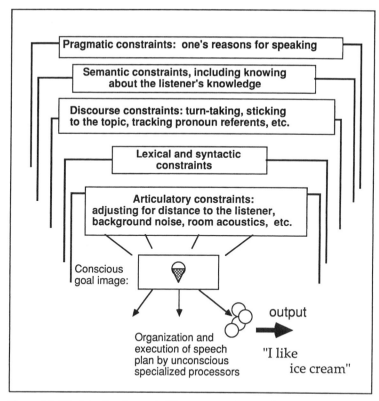

Figure 6.1. The intention to speak: Many unconscious goal contexts cooperate to constrain a single sentence. Any single conscious event is influenced by multiple unconscious goal systems, which together make up one kind of Context Hierarchy. Thus the conscious goal-image of the sentence to be spoken is constrained by all the goal contexts shown, which are not normally conscious. The conscious goal-image serves to recruit and organize the novel components of a set of specialized speech processors that actually control articulation of the sentence.

conscious as a whole. Thus, at the minimum, an "intention to say something" must involve a many-leveled goal structure, in which each major goal can activate numerous subgoals to accomplish its ends. At any one time, most components of such goal structures are not qualitatively conscious. Figures 6.1 and 6.2 represent such goal structures as graphic horizontal "frames," which together constrain any action.

The key observation is that goal contexts are apparently triggered by conscious events, and that they result in other conscious events. This *triadic pattern* appears to be of very great generality. We explore it next, and then modify our model to accommodate it.

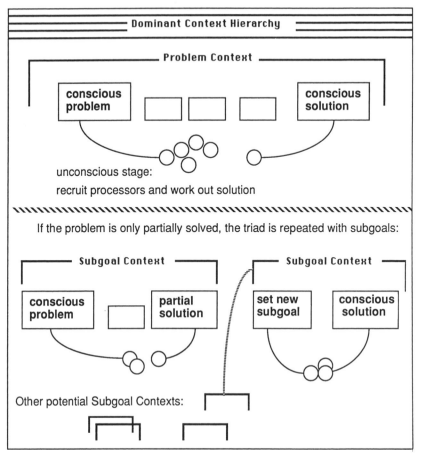

Figure 6.2. Model 4: The triadic pattern of spontaneous problem solving. Spontaneous problem solving is marked by gaps in conscious processing during which solutions to routine problems seem to be prepared. These become conscious after some time – seconds, days, or even longer. Shown above is a GW view of this triadic pattern of (1) conscious problem assignment, (2) unconscious recruitment and computation of a solution, and (3) conscious display of the solution. Note that unconscious problem solving requires both a largely unconscious Problem Context and unconscious Specialized Processors, which do the work of problem solving. Note also that the whole process occurs under the general purview of the Dominant Context Hierarchy, as shown by the fact that solutions that violate this larger context tend to be excluded. Most problem solving involves not one but a series of such conscious–unconscious–conscious triads before all subgoals are satisfied and the whole problem is solved.

6.2 The conscious–unconscious–conscious (CUC) triad

The common pattern here is:

1 a conscious *stage of problem-assignment*;
2 an unconscious *stage of processing* guided by an unconscious, limited-capacity-loading goal context;
3 a conscious *display of the solution.*

In the case of complex problems, these three stages can contain subgoals with their own triads (see Figure 6.2). For example, mental arithmetic might work roughly as follows:

1 Conscious goal-assignment: "multiply 12 × 24."
2 Unconscious search for subgoals.
3 Conscious subgoal assignment: "first multiply unit values by 24."
4 Conscious subgoal assignment: "multiply 2 × 24."
5 Unconscious search for answer.
6 Conscious report of subgoal: ". . . = 48."
7 Conscious subgoal assignment: "now multiply 10 × 24."
8 Unconscious processing: ("add a zero to multiply by 10").
9 Conscious display of subgoals: "48, 240."
10 Conscious subgoal assignment: "now add the two outcomes."
11 Unconscious addition process: ("48 + 240").
12 Conscious display of solution: ". . . = 288."

This example is only illustrative. There must be much individual variation. A very skilled mental calculator might only be conscious of steps (1) and (10), all others being automatic and unconscious. A novice might need more conscious intermediate steps than are shown here. The point is that a triad with this CUC pattern can be expanded into a series of triadic cycles, with as many cycles as there are subgoals to be satisfied. Table 6.1 shows this as a contrastive pattern.

6.2.1 Model 4: CUC triads in the model

It is easy to incorporate these ideas into our theoretical diagrams (Figure 6.2). We need only show the global workspace over time, and indicate that global messages broadcast both to potential goal contexts and to unconscious processors able to carry out the goals. Thus goal contexts can be recruited, and when they are, they compete for access to the global workspace. Once a given goal context becomes dominant, it begins to limit the conscious events that are likely to gain GW access. Thus an intention to retrieve the name of the ancient flying reptiles will restrict conscious contents until the right word comes to mind (6.0). However, as pointed out above, this intention must itself exist in a hierarchy of other intentions, so that, if the word remains out of reach, at some point a higher-level goal structure may decide that the game is not worth the

Table 6.1. *The triadic pattern in problem solving*

	Conscious		Unconscious	
Simple case	1a.	Conscious problem as-signment		
			b.	Unconscious processing and problem context
	c.	Conscious solution ap-pears		
More general case	1a.	Conscious problem as-signment		
			b.	Unconscious processing and problem context
	c.	Conscious subgoal solu-tion		
	2a.	Conscious assignment of further subgoals		
			b.	Add goal context
			c.	More unconscious prob-lem solving
	(Repetition of 1 and 2 until)			
	d.	Conscious solution ap-pears		

candle, and that one had better give up, wait, or look at a dictionary. Alternatively, other local goals can start competing against the intention to retrieve the word. In any case, local intentions are not absolutely dominant.

The triadic pattern results naturally from this model. Conscious events, themselves constrained by higher-level goal contexts, can recruit a local intention. In its turn, the local intention allows a mental image represent-ing a problem to become conscious. This serves to recruit processors and subgoals able to solve the problem. If these can operate automatically, they simply compute a solution to the problem. If they reach a dead end, they may be able to recruit their own conscious subgoal image to broadcast the obstacle, thereby mobilizing additional processors able to solve the resistant subproblem, and so on, and so on, until finally the original goal is solved. Alternatively, the original goal context may be competed out of dominance of the global workspace – in that case, we simply give up on the problem for the time being.

Notice that there is no *self-conscious* problem solving in this model. That is, the system does not know metacognitively that it is solving a problem. It simply does what it does, "spontaneously." We will deal with self-conscious metacognition in Chapters 8 and 9.

6.2.2 Conscious contents can trigger new goal contexts

In language, beginning a new topic or asking a question serves to access a goal context. Asking a question creates a set of constraints on subsequent conscious events: For at least a few seconds, conscious thoughts are constrained to be responsive to the question (Miyake & Norman, 1978). This is indeed how Brown and McNeill (1966) elicited TOT experiences experimentally: by asking subjects to find a fairly rare word corresponding to a definition (see 6.0). Again, the question is conscious, the constraints on answering are not conscious in detail, nor are the routine details of searching for the answer; but the answer, when it comes, is conscious.

Conscious events that are experienced as *incomplete* seem to set up very active goal contexts. They may vary from incomplete sentences or visual figures, to social or emotional issues, to unanswered mathematical or scientific problems. In each case, the conscious experience seems to set up unconscious constraints on future conscious events. This effect was demonstrated directly by Klos and Singer (1981) in the case of unresolved emotional conflicts in adolescents. College students with persistent parental conflicts were presented a conflict situation enacted dramatically; for example, an argument about borrowing the keys to the parents' car. The students were then asked to lie down in a quiet room and report their spontaneous thoughts. When the dramatic reenactment was unresolved, there were significantly more thoughts about it than when it was resolved (viz. Singer, 1984). The great advantage of this study is its human relevance; such findings may be more difficult to obtain in laboratory tasks that are perceived to be irrelevant to the subjects' everyday lives, but this should not be surprising (Holmes, 1968). In our theoretical vocabulary, irrelevant experimental tasks contexts are quickly dropped from the goal hierarchy, because they are inconsistent with higher-level goal contexts. In any study of goal contexts, personal relevance must be a critical variable.

6.2.3 Goal contexts can also evoke new conscious contents

If the TOT state is indeed "a goal context looking for the right content," it already provides us with one example of a dominant context triggering new conscious contents. The "Aha!" experience in problem solving is another example, as is the conscious popping up of answers to questions, the emergence of thoughts in free association, and the like. Thus it works both ways; conscious events can evoke goal contexts, and these can in turn evoke new conscious thoughts and images. This completes the conscious–unconscious–conscious triad.

6.2.4 *The great generality of triadic problem solving*

The triadic pattern is extremely common. We find it not only in explicit problem solving, but also in daydreaming (Klinger, 1971; Singer, 1984); it is the common pattern in controlling even simple actions, but it can also be found in long-term planning; it appears in perception – for example, in the well-known bi-stable figures such as the Necker cube and figure–ground illusions – as well as in memory retrieval, as shown by the tip-of-the-tongue phenomenon. Finally, and most widely recognized, it appears in high-level creative work. Let us examine a sampling of this general phenomenon, starting with examples from art, science, and mathematics – the highest levels of human creativity (Ghiselin, 1952; Hadamard, 1945; John-Steiner, 1985).

1 High-level creativity

The role of unconscious problem solving in high-level creativity was described early on by the mathematician Henri Poincaré, who devoted much thought to the psychology of mathematical creation. He wrote,

> Most striking at first is this appearance of sudden illumination, a manifest sign of long, unconscious prior work. The role of this unconscious work in mathematical invention appears to me incontestable, and traces of it would be found in other cases where it is less evident. Often when one works at a hard question, nothing good is accomplished at the first attack. Then one takes a rest, longer or shorter, and sits down anew to the work. During the first half-hour, as before, nothing is found, and then all of a sudden the decisive idea presents itself to the mind. . . . There is another remark to be made about the conditions of this unconscious work: it is possible, and of a certainty it is only fruitful, if it is on the one hand preceded and on the other hand followed by a period of conscious work. (Ghiselin, 1952, p. 38)

This last remark can be seen to describe what we have called the conscious–unconscious–conscious triad. This is also emphasized in the following quote from the poet Amy Lowell:

> How carefully and precisely the subconscious mind functions, I have often been a witness to in my own work. An idea will come into my head for no apparent reason; "The Bronze Horses," for instance. I registered horses as a good subject for a poem; and, having so registered them, I consciously thought no more about the matter. But what I had really done was to drop my subject into the subconscious, much as one drops a letter into the mailbox. Six months later, the words of the poem began to come into my head, the poem – to use my private vocabulary – was "there." (Ghiselin, 1952, p. 110)

Of course, creative people are often conscious of intermediate events in this process, which we would interpret as subgoal processing (6.2.1). And of course not all creative work is experienced as spontaneous – some of it is effortful and deliberate. This mixture of ingredients goes to make up a completed work. Listen to Mozart:

> When I am, as it were, completely myself, entirely alone, and of good cheer . . .
> my ideas flow best and most abundantly. *Whence* and *how* they come, I know not;
> nor can I force them. Those ideas that please me I retain in memory. . . . If I
> continue in this way, it soon occurs to me how I may turn this or that morsel to
> account, so as to make a good dish of it, that is to say, agreeably to the rules of
> counterpoint, to the peculiarities of the various instruments, etc.

> All this fires my soul, and provided I am not disturbed, my subject enlarges
> itself, becomes methodised and defined, and the whole, though it be long, stands
> almost complete and finished in my mind, so that I can survey it, like a fine picture
> or a beautiful statue, at a glance. Nor do I hear in my imagination the parts
> *successively*, but I hear them, as it were, all at once (*gleich alles zusammen*).
> What a delight this is I cannot tell! . . . When I proceed to write down my ideas,
> I take out of the bag of my memory, if I may use that phrase, what has been
> previously collected into it in the way I have mentioned. (Ghiselin, 1952; p. 44;
> italics in original)

It is clear that a major work is not accomplished in a single conscious–unconscious–conscious leap. In fact, Poincaré may simply have forgotten some intermediate events between the first effortful period of conscious problem assignment and the *Aha!* experience. Most problem solving requires a string of CUC triads.

So much for truly great creativity; we move now from the sublime – not to the ridiculous – but to the commonplace, and we find the same triadic pattern in such "simple" events as answering questions, retrieving memories, generating images, switching between the two interpretations of an ambiguous event, understanding analogies, generating free associations, and the like.

2   *Daydreaming involves spontaneous problem solving*

Thought-sampling studies indicate that, for most people, a substantial percentage of conscious activity does not serve a self-conscious purpose. Several studies by Singer and his colleagues and by Klinger (1971) suggest that these "daydreaming" activities may be quite goal-directed, even though people may not be able to state their purposes. According to Singer,

> "current concerns" – unfulfilled intentions, hierarchically organized in terms
> of closeness to fulfillment or personal value . . . – make up a goodly share of the
> conscious content derived from thought sampling. Our basic "rules" for admis-
> sion of material to consciousness seem to involve a screening strategy that is
> especially sensitive to our current concerns even in dichotic listening experiments
> or during sleep. . . . As we gain more information of this kind, it is my personal
> guess that we will find that a great deal of respondent (spontaneous) or playful
> fantasy has long-term planning, decision-making, and self-schema formation
> functions. (Singer, 1984; p. 25)

3 Analogy tasks

The following "remote associates" test devised by Mednick (1962) is a good example of a large class of analogy tasks. The task is to find the missing word. For our purposes it is useful to allow the answer to come by itself, without deliberate effort. For example, the following three words suggest a fourth:

    1 cookies   sixteen   heart   _____

The answer "sweet" fits with cookies, with phrase "sweet sixteen," and with the word "sweetheart." Here are some more examples.[2]

2	poke	go	molasses	_____
3	surprise	line	birthday	_____
4	base	snow	dance	_____
5	elephant	lapse	vivid	_____
6	lick	sprinkle	mines	_____
7	stalk	trainer	king	_____

On at least one of these items the reader should have a genuine *Aha!* experience. Note that we sometimes feel great certainty about the answer without knowing why it is right.

4 The "magical" quality of learning and retrieval

In Chapter 5, we maintained that most learning has this same "magical" character. We simply pay attention to some material for any reason at all, and learning seems to take place with no detailed self-conscious guidance. Most people do not have a set of recallable rules by which they learn.

Similarly, memory retrieval is typically unselfconscious. In memory tasks we often ask people to recall material deliberately. But in speaking, in walking about the world, and in performing a skilled action like driving a car, we retrieve information from memory with little self-conscious recall. Most retrieval is "magical" in the same sense that learning is.

5 Bi-stable figures in perception

We can find the conscious–unconscious–conscious triad in bi-stable perceptual figures as well. We are conscious of only one interpretation of the Necker cube until it changes unconsciously, and then we become conscious of the alternative interpretation. The intermediate stage is unconscious. Much the same is true of ambiguous words and sentences (Chapter 4), and the same pattern may be found in "hidden figures" like the Dalmatian in the park (5.1.1), which are bi-stable but not reversible. In the Dalmatian picture, we are conscious initially of the black-and-white blotches, and we are conscious of the final stage, in which we can perceive the dog, the tree, and the sidewalk. But we are not conscious of

---

2   Answers: 1. sweet; 2. slow; 3. party; 4. ball; 5. memory; 6. salt; 7. lion.

the details of the intervening stage in which the visual input is analyzed to arrive at the new conscious interpretation.

6 *Action control*

Action control has much the same CUC character, as we can see from the extreme case of biofeedback training. When people learn a biofeedback task such as controlling alpha waves in the cortical EEG, they are not conscious of the *way* in which they control the alpha waves. They are conscious, in some broad sense, of wishing to control a conscious feedback signal, but the intermediate steps are simply not available to awareness. However, the feedback signal itself is always conscious. Much the same is true for any motor task, such as wiggling one's finger. The intention to wiggle the finger has conscious or at least expressible aspects, and we are conscious of wiggling the finger; but the intermediate stage is unconscious. Most people do not realize that the muscles that move the finger are actually located not in the hand but in the forearm. But they do not need to know this – it is part of the automatic, unconscious problem-solving stage.

6.3 Empirical assessment of goal contexts

A goal is a representation of a future state that tends to remain constant as different means are explored for achieving it. Like any other context, a goal context serves to bias choice-points in processing. Perceptual contexts force the interpretation of the Necker Cube, or the moon's craters, in one direction rather than another (4.2.1). Conceptual contexts work to interpret the word "case" as "briefcase" rather than "sad case." Finally, goal contexts presumably cause different pragmatic interpretations of ambiguous information, as well as different choices in the control of action. These differences should then allow us to assess goal contexts by presenting subjects with the opportunity to interpret or act upon information that is ambiguous with respect to the goal (Baars, 1985).

Work done on experimentally elicited slips of the tongue provides a case in point (Baars, 1985; in press, c). A number of techniques are now available for eliciting predictable slips of the tongue. All these techniques create goal contexts in one way or another. For example, one can ask people to repeat the word "poke" over and over again. Since this is an action, it presumably involves a goal context. When the subjects are then asked, "What do you call the white of an egg?" they will tend to say "the yolk," even when they have the knowledge available that this is the wrong answer. Thus priming by repeating a similar-sounding word works to structure later motor control and memory retrieval, presumably by altering the goal context.

Slips may also reflect higher-level goal contexts. In *The Psychopathology of Everyday Life* (1901/1938, p. 81) Freud gives the example of "a young physician who timidly and reverently introduced himself to the celebrated Virchow with the following words: 'I am Dr. Virchow.' The surprised professor turned to him and asked, 'Is your name also Virchow?' " Slips like this are easy to produce in the laboratory; one only needs to create confusion between two alternative sentences, such as (1) 'Professor Virchow, I am Dr. X' and (2) 'I am Dr. X, Professor Virchow.' Competing sentences like these will result in inadvertent blends such as 'I am Dr. Virchow, Professor X.' (Baars, 1980; 1985; in press, c). Freud argues that the slip reveals the ambitious *purpose* of the person making it: The young physician wishes to be as famous as the great Virchow. In our theoretical terms, Freud believed that the slip reveals a goal context.

This hypothesis may be somewhat more difficult to test, but not impossible. It has been shown, for example, that male undergraduates confronted with an attractive female experimenter are more likely to make sexual slips of the tongue; when they are told that they may receive an electric shock during the experiment, they make more shock-related slips (Motley, Camden, & Baars, 1979). Thus slips seem to reflect important or immediate goals and preoccupations. It is difficult to separate goal contexts from related conceptual contexts that may be equally primed. Surely when we are confronted with an intensely desired object, our knowledge about it must also be activated. We should not expect to find evidence for goal contexts without related conceptual contexts. However, we would expect an increase in slips that actually express a wish when there is a goal versus merely a conceptual preoccupation. Thus when we are hungry and walk to the refrigerator, we should expect this to prime goal-related slips as opposed to the condition where we are not hungry and see someone else walk to the refrigerator. In both cases conceptual contexts should be primed; but in the first, specific actions related to the goals should be more likely as well.

6.4   Goal contexts and the stream of consciousness

The stream of consciousness can be seen as a complex interplay between conscious events and their goal contexts. Each conscious event can trigger a new goal context, which can, in its turn, evoke later conscious experiences (Figure 6.3). We introduce a graphic notation for contexts. Competition between incompatible contexts can cause a surprising "resetting" of conscious contents. As we have noted before (4.4.3), surprise may lead to momentary forgetting and a resetting of the global workspace due to competition between incompatible contexts (Baars, 1987). A TOT

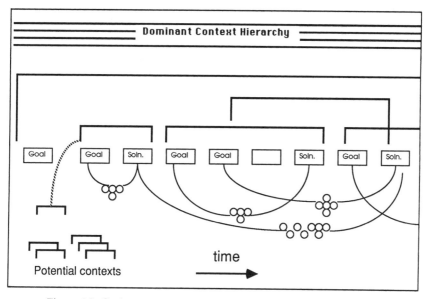

Figure 6.3. Goal contexts and the stream of consciousness. Putting a series of intertwined problem-solving triads together creates a "stream of consciousness." The solution (soln.) of one problem may pose a goal for another, so that goals in the above diagram may yield solutions that are also goals. From another point of view, it may be said that solutions tend to be conscious between the completion of one goal context and the beginning of the next: i.e., at points of indeterminancy, which are also those points in which reduction of uncertainty becomes possible. Thus we become conscious of the most informative points in the flow of processing. In the diagram, no new contexts are being created; new problem contexts are just selected from the potential contexts shown at the bottom. Note that spontaneous problem solving is not necessarily self-conscious; it may not be reported as problem solving. Metacognitive reports about one's own conscious processes require an added layer of organization (see Ch. 8). Note also that the local goals and solutions are constrained by the Dominant Context Hierarchy, which tends to rule out incompatible solutions.

state may result, which can be viewed as a new, dominant context looking for a new set of conscious contents.

6.4.1 Cooperating and competing goal contexts

Some goal contexts compete against each other for access to consciousness, but many goals must be compatible with each other (4.3.5). For instance, even a single sentence is constrained by many simultaneous goals and criteria: vocal, linguistic, semantic, and pragmatic. In Figure 6.3, nesting of contexts is intended to symbolize that the contexts involved are compatible, and indeed may be mutually supportive, while competing contexts are shown operating at the same horizontal level.

We have some direct evidence for the operation of compatible goal contexts from our experimental studies of unintended double entendres (Motley, Camden, & Baars, 1983a). Double entendres, of course, are compatible with two contexts of interpretation. Thus, if subjects are induced to feel angry by posthypnotic suggestion (context A), and if they are to select the best words to fill out non-emotional multiple-choice items (context B), they will tend to select items that are both angry and consistent with the overt context. Thus Baars, Cohen, and Bower (1986) presented sentences like:

1 I always lost at cards with him and wanted to _____ more often.
    a. beat him (*); b. win; c. succeed; d. come off well.
2 Toward the end of the day at the store, I still had a few customers to _____ .
    a. finish off (*); b. help; c. attend to; d. handle.

Angry subjects selected far more starred (*), ambiguously angry items than did happy subjects.

6.4.2 The goal hierarchy represents significance

One of the great gaps in current cognitive theory is the lack of a widely accepted account of significance or value. Some things are more important to people than others: more pleasurable, more painful, more valued, more likely to result in approach or avoidance. Contemporary cognitive theory thus far has not attempted to include this obvious and necessary dimension, but of course there is overwhelming evidence that significance matters. The great animal conditioning literature stands as a monument to this truism, as does the vast clinical and social psychological literature on emotion and motivation.

As pointed out in 4.2.3, the most obvious way to incorporate significance in GW theory is to use the hierarchy of goal contexts (see Figures 4.3 and 6.3). Some goals are more important than others, and some provide the contextual presuppositions within which other goals are defined. Thus the need to survive may be presupposed in the need to eat, to escape from danger, and so forth. The need to eat is presuppositional to the search for food. There is a partial ordering between different levels of the goal hierarchy, but it is not invariable. The primacy of food declines after eating and rises after food deprivation, so that the goal hierarchy is reordered.

Significant events usually drive less significant ones from consciousness. We will discuss these cases in Chapters 8 and 10 under the heading of *prioritizing* of conscious contents (8.2, 8.3.1, 10.5).

6.4.3 General-purpose goal contexts

Some goal contexts must be useful in many situations. All actions require control of timing, for example. Learning may require organizational skills that are useful across many different cases. It seems likely that there are *general-purpose goal contexts*, which can be called upon as subgoals in many different tasks. Presumably these can be recruited just like any other specialized processor. When a relevant message is broadcast, they can compete for GW access and, if they gain access, they can become part of the current goal hierarchy in the same way that any subgoal can (Figure 6.2). Chapter 8 will propose that there are special goal contexts in attentional control called options contexts (8.2.2). These are presumed to help select conscious contents according to their current significance.

6.5   Further implications

6.5.1 Why it is important for goals to compete for access to the global workspace

Several theories have been advanced with a similar notion of action systems competing for access to a limited-capacity channel (e.g., Norman & Shallice, 1980, and Shallice, 1978). However, these theories do not explain the advantage of doing so: Why would action control systems bother to compete for such access? GW theory gives one possible answer: If some goal context needs to recruit other processors and subgoals to carry out its goal, it must be able to dominate the global workspace long enough to broadcast a "recruiting message" for the appropriate specialists. In GW theory, access to the global workspace is the key element for the recruitment of any new configuration of systems. (This idea is further developed in Chapter 7.)

Further, competition for access to consciousness is one way in which dominant systems can also drive out or "repress" disturbing or erroneous goals. Thus GW theory very naturally allows us to model psychodynamic notions such as emotional conflict and repression in terms of competition between different goal systems for access to the global workspace. We have already noted the idea that *surprise* may involve a momentary erasure of the GW, allowing new information to gain access to consciousness (Baars, in press b; Grossberg, 1982; Luborsky, in press; Underwood, 1982).

6.5.2 *An answer to the problem of nonqualitative*
conscious events?

One of our running themes involves the relationship between conscious experience of qualitative events, such as perception and imagery, versus conscious access to nonqualitative events, such as currently conscious concepts and beliefs (1.5.4, 2.4.1). One interesting possibility is that all abstract concepts are accessed consciously by means of perceptual and imaginal events. That is to say, it is possible that even the most abstract concepts have qualitative mental symbols of some sort. This hypothesis was popular around the turn of the century among psychologists who were impressed by the fragmentary and fleeting mental images that often accompany abstract concepts (Woodworth, 1915). It has been advanced quite often by highly creative people like Einstein and Mozart in writing about their own creative processes (6.2.4; John-Steiner, 1985). We know, of course, that the "imageless thought controversy" that came along with this idea was apparently not very fruitful, but that does not mean it was wrong (Woodworth & Schlossberg, 1954). In Chapter 7 we will propose that many concepts may be triggered by fleeting conscious images. This *ideomotor theory* suggests a principled connection between abstract nonqualitative concepts and concrete, imageable conscious experiences.

It is attractive to simply suppose that nonqualitative concepts are part of the contextual structure developed above. Concepts can be evoked by qualitative events like percepts, inner speech, and mental images; and the conceptual contexts can, in return, trigger new qualitative contents. We can speculate that only qualitative events are broadcast globally. If this were true, the broadcasting arguments made before (2.5) would apply only to qualitative events and to the qualitative mental symbols for nonqualitative concepts, beliefs, intentions, and expectations.

This could explain many things: for example, the extraordinary power of imagery in memory and emotion (Horowitz, 1976; Paivio, 1971; Singer, 1984); or the great frequency of visualizable prototypes of abstract categories (Rosch, 1975). The power of prototypes, in turn, suggests the power of social stereotypes: Prejudice may consist of having standardized, uncomplimentary mental images of a despised group of people, and a failure to acknowledge that reality may be more complex than the mental image that symbolizes the group. In the realm of thinking, geometry has had great impact in mathematics, even though since Descartes all geometrical figures have been expressible algebraically. Geometry, however, can be visualized, whereas algebra cannot. All these qualitative conscious experiences may help to mainipulate more abstract nonqualitative entities.

6.6 Chapter summary

Starting from a consideration of William James's description of the tip-of-the-tongue state, we noted that there are complex representational states that dominate our central limited capacity, and which act as goals. These goal contexts or intentions are not conscious in the sense that they have no conscious qualities (Natsoulas, 1982); they are experienced differently from percepts, images, and the like. One can view such states as "goal contexts looking for conscious contents." We have discussed some ways to test these claims empirically, and explored their implications for spontaneous problem solving, the issue of significance, and the question of nonqualitative conscious events.

In the following chapter we see how these ideas can lead directly to a theory of voluntary control, a modern version of William James's ideomotor theory.

7 Model 5:
Volition as ideomotor control of thought and action

We know what it is to get out of bed on a freezing morning in a room without a fire, and how the very vital principle within us protests against the ordeal. Probably most persons have lain on certain mornings for an hour at a time unable to brace themselves to the resolve. We think how late we shall be, how the duties of the day will suffer; we say, "I *must* get up, this is ignominious," etc.; but still the warm couch feels too delicious, the cold outside too cruel, and resolution faints away and postpones itself again and again just as it seemed on the verge of bursting the resistance and passing over into the decisive act. . . .

Now how do we *ever* get up under such circumstances? If I may generalize from my own experience, we more often than not get up without any struggle at all. We suddenly find that we *have* got up. A fortunate lapse of consciousness occurs; we forget both the warmth and the cold; we fall into some revery connected with the day's life, in the course of which the idea flashes across us, "Hollo, I must lie here no longer" – an idea which at that lucky instant awakens no contradictory or paralyzing suggestions, and consequently produces immediately its appropriate motor effects. . . .

It was our acute consciousness of both the warmth and the cold during the period of struggle, which paralyzed our activity then and kept our idea of rising in the condition *wish* and not *will*. The moment these inhibitory ideas ceased, the original idea exerted its effects.

This case seems to me to contain in miniature form the data for an entire psychology of volition.

William James, 1890/1983 (Vol. II, p. 524–5; italics in original)

7.0 Introduction

We begin our chapter on volition with the image of William James on a cold winter morning, reluctantly trying to persuade himself to get out of bed. For James, this image goes to the very heart of the psychology of volition. He believed that a successful act of will does not typically emerge from some titanic inner struggle. Rather, he claims, we simply wait until the conscious image of the action can emerge for some time without competing images or intentions. At that moment the action occurs automatically, spontaneously, and without struggle.

246

We will first consider whether there is a problem of volition at all. To answer this question we seek contrasting pairs of actions that differ only in that one action is voluntary and the other involuntary. These empirical contrasts can constrain theory, just like the contrasts between conscious and unconscious events (1.2.2). The evidence indicates that the issue of volition is very real indeed. That is to say, the voluntary–involuntary contrasts highlight core psychological issues, such as automaticity due to practice, errors in speech and action, and psychopathology. Further, we can borrow James's solution to the problem of volitional control, and interpret it easily in terms of global workspace theory.

James explains conscious control of action by an *ideomotor theory* in which conscious goal images without effective competition serve to organize and trigger automatically controlled actions, which then run off without further conscious involvement. For James, conscious contents are inherently impulsive; everything else is automatic. The only conscious components of action are:

   a the "idea" or goal-image (really just an image of the outcome of the action);
   b perhaps some competing goal-image;
   c the "fiat" (the "go signal"); and finally,
   d sensory feedback from the action.

In this chapter we see how GW theory invites a natural interpretation of James's ideomotor theory. One use of the GW architecture is to have multiple unconscious systems inspect a single conscious goal and to compete against it if it is inadequate. That is to say, the architecture allows multiple unconscious criterion systems to *monitor* and *edit* any conscious goal or plan. This implies that any conscious goal-image that is conscious long enough to succeed in recruiting and executing an action has been tacitly edited by multiple criteria, and indeed I claim in this chapter that voluntary action *is* tacitly edited action. Conversely, involuntary actions, like slips of the tongue, are actions that *would have been* edited and changed, *if* there had been enough time and capacity for unconscious editing systems to be brought to bear upon the conscious action plans. This conclusion has a wealth of implications for the understanding of unintentional acts found in slips, automatisms, and psychopathology. It even suggests a theory of hypnosis and other "absorbed" states of mind, in which there is minimal editing of conscious events (Baars, in press a, c).

Of course William James himself could not speak in these terms, because of his resistance to the notion of unconscious mental processes (1.1.1). But his ideas make perfectly good sense in modern cognitive garb.

Before we proceed to develop these ideas, it is useful to be clear about the issue of volition itself. Many behaviorists and others have claimed that there is no problem of volition at all. What evidence do we have to the contrary, that "the will" matters?

7.1   Is there a problem of volition? Some contrasts between similar voluntary and involuntary actions

With the rise of physicalistic psychology at beginning of this century, many psychologists tried to make the case that there really is no question of volition, just as there was no true scientific issue of consciousness (e.g., Razran, 1961; Watson, 1925). Behaviorists and other physicalists at first believed that any apparently voluntary action can be reduced to a chain of conditioned, simple, *physical* reflexes. Later, when reflexes proved too simple and rigid, the unit of behavior was generalized to other stimulus–response relationships, but the goal still remained to reduce voluntary, goal-directed actions to simple, physical input–output relations (viz. Baars, 1986a; Kimble & Perlmutter, 1970). This was thought to eliminate any scientific question of volition once and for all. Was there any truth to this claim? Is there indeed a scientific question of volition?

For an answer we can look to pairs of actions that appear similar on the surface, but which differ in respect to volition. That is, we can carry out a contrastive analysis on the issue of volition, just as throughout this book we have contrasted comparable conscious and unconscious events (1.2.2). This is helpful not just to answer the questions about volition raised by Pavlov and Watson – it also defines major constraints to be satisfied by any theory of normal voluntary control. Any such theory should be able to explain why, of two similar-seeming actions, one seems to be voluntary and the other not.

There are some obvious examples of such contrastive pairs, as we see in Table 7.1.

7.1.1 Nonvoluntary versus counter-voluntary events

Notice first of all, that the "involuntary" events listed on the left side of Table 7.1 are of two kinds. First, automatic processes are part of every voluntary act, and while people cannot control them in detail, they are perceived to be consistent with our goals. We want them. A skilled typist does not control each finger movement in detail; a skilled reader does not perform letter identification consciously, and so forth. Yet because automatisms serve our voluntary goals, Table 7.1 calls these *nonvoluntary automatisms*. On the other hand there are clearly *countervoluntary actions* such as slips of the tongue. Here, too, there are automatisms at work, but they are perceived to be out of control, unwanted, against one's

Table 7.1. *Contrasts between voluntary and involuntary activities*

	Involuntary	Voluntary
Nonvoluntary automatisms: wanted, but not controllable in detail	Automatic components of normal actions	The same actions before automaticity
	Reflexes	Purposeful imitations of reflexes
	Actions controlled by brain stimulation of the motor cortex	The same actions before automaticity
	Autonomic functions (heart rate, peristalsis, skin conductivity, etc.)	Autonomic functions under temporary biofeedback control
	Spontaneous emotional facial expressions	"Social" expressions (Ekman, 1984)
	Automatic memory encoding (Hasher & Zacks, 1979)	Effortful memory encoding
Countervoluntary automatisms: unwanted	Slips of speech and action	Purposeful imitations of slips
	Pathological symptoms: out-of-control actions, images, inner speech, and feelings	Purposeful imitations of symptoms Regained voluntary control after "practicing the symptom"
	Voluntarily resisted automatisms (e.g., unwanted "bad" habits)	Voluntarily controlled automatisms

will. These two kinds of involuntary action may be closely related; for example, any automatic component can become countervoluntary simply by our resisting it. We can look at a word on this page, thereby triggering automatic reading processes that are not under detailed voluntary control. This wanted automatism can become countervoluntary simply by resisting it. Thus we can try to resist the act of reading while looking at a word, or a knee-jerk reflex after striking the patellar tendon. In this way any automatism can be made to be countervoluntary. This close relationship between nonvoluntary and countervoluntary actions makes it useful to consider both under the rubric of "involuntary" activities. Whenever there is a possibility of misunderstanding, we will choose an unambiguous term like "automatic" versus "countervoluntary" or "unwanted."

That being said, we can go on to discuss Table 7.1.

7.1.2 Slips of speech and action

Imagine repeating a slip of the tongue you have just made. The slip itself is experienced as involuntary; its imitation is voluntary. And yet the two isolated actions are much the same as far as an outside observer is concerned. Some famous slips by A. W. Spooner illustrate the point:

1 Instead of "our dear old Queen" – "our queer old Dean."
2 Instead of the hymn, "Conquering Kings their titles take" – "Kinquering Congs their titles take."
3 Upon dismissing a student, he intended to say "You have deliberately wasted two terms, and you will leave by the down train" – but actually said, "You have deliberately tasted two worms, and you will leave by the town drain."

Let us suppose Reverend Spooner actually made these slips (there is some doubt: see Fromkin, 1980). Now imagine that Spooner *repeated each slip* immediately after making it, as exactly as possible, so that it was said again by the same speaker, in the same tone of voice, at the same speaking rate, and so on. What is the difference between the slip and its voluntary repetition? Surely there is no basic *physical* difference, nor any real linguistic difference. The main difference is psychological. In the first case, the utterance was involuntary and unwanted; in the second, it was voluntary (Baars, 1985; in press, c).

But what a difference this invisible difference makes! In the first case, the speaker fails to execute his intention. If he becomes conscious of his error, he will experience *surprise* at his own utterance. Now we can observe the whole panoply of physiological reactions that make up the Orienting Response (1.4.1). He may be embarrassed and apologetic. Having failed to carry out his intention, he may try again. If, like Spooner, he is also head of one of the Cambridge colleges he may become a figure of fun in student folklore. If he makes involuntary errors so often that he can no longer function effectively, he may lose his position, be examined for neurological problems, and so on. None of these consequences follow from doing physically identical imitations of these slips, if they are voluntary. If Spooner were voluntarily making the slip to amuse his audience, or if someone were to quote a slip in a discussion of voluntary control, none of these consequences would follow; nor would the speaker be likely to be surprised by the "slip."

Thus two identical actions may be psychologically quite distinct, but not because of a difference in complexity, as the early behaviorists thought. Voluntary actions are not just complicated agglomerations of simple reflexes. Involuntary components added together do not result in a voluntary act. Something else is involved in volitional control. Let us consider two more contrasts of this kind.

7.1.3 The loss of voluntary control with practice

It is easy to see a voluntary act transformed into an involuntary one: We only need to practice it to the point where most of it fades from consciousness (5.1.1). We have previously pointed to experiments in which predictable skills that are highly overlearned that generally show a loss of voluntary control (LaBerge, 1980; Langer & Imber, 1979; Shiffrin & Schneider, 1977; Sternberg, 1966; see also Hasher & Zacks, 1979).

All actions have involuntary components. Most details of routine actions such as reading or writing must be automatic: We could never control their numerous details, given the limited capacity of the conscious and voluntary system. Usually only the novel features of an action are conscious and under voluntary control (7.2.2) (Reason, 1984). But non-voluntary automatisms can sometimes become unwanted or counter-voluntary.

This becomes clear when we try to control "bad habits" that have been practiced for years: Almost everyone seems to have at least one, whether it is overeating, smoking, making nervous gestures, and so on. These habits are characteristically difficult to control voluntarily; they especially escape control when conscious attention is directed elsewhere. No doubt unwanted habits have multiple causes, but it is easy to demonstrate that sheer automaticity makes it hard to stop an action once its normal triggering conditions are given. As we pointed out above, looking at a word *without* reading it seems to be quite impossible (viz., La Berge, 1980; Shiffrin & Schneider, 1977). The very act of looking at printed words seems to trigger automatisms; to block them we must look away, degrade the word visually, or perhaps focus on only a fraction of one letter. Sternberg's well-known experiment in automatic memory search makes the same point (Sternberg, 1966). The subject really cannot stop the search process once the target letter is found; it just runs on to the end of the memory set (see section 1.4.2). Reason (1983, 1984) has presented a detailed analysis of catastrophic accidents showing that many of them may be due to hard-to-control, highly practiced automatisms that were triggered out of context at some critical decision point just before the accident. Several of these accidents led to the death of the person making the error – about as strong an argument for the involuntary nature of automatisms as we might wish to have.

7.1.4 Involuntary automaticity involves a loss of conscious access

Loss of voluntary control over details of an action seems to follow a loss of conscious access to the details. Langer and her co-workers have conducted some elegant experiments to support this point (e.g., Langer & Imber, 1979). These investigators were pursuing the hypothesis that perceived competence affects one's performance: The more skilled we think we are, the better we perform – providing we cannot monitor our performance directly. One way in which we lose touch with our own competence is by automatization; when we become skilled readers, musicians, or truck drivers, we lose conscious access to many details of our own actions, and hence become more vulnerable to false attributions about our own performance. This line of reasoning led Langer and Imber to devise a simple coding task that people could learn to the point of automaticity in a matter of minutes. Letters of the alphabet were to be recoded into a two-symbol code; the letters A–I were "a triangle plus the nth letter after A"; letters J–R would be "circle plus the nth letter after J," and so on. Thus the letter "B" would be "triangle plus 2," "L" would be "circle plus 3," and so on. A preliminary group of subjects reported that they were still conscious of task details after recording two sentences; after six sentences, they were no longer conscious of the steps. The task had become automatic.

Langer and Imber now compared the effects of conscious access and automaticity. A Moderate Practice group recoded only two sentences, reported being conscious of details, and was able to specify more steps in the task than the High Practice group, which recoded six sentences and reported automaticity. Now Langer and Imber devised an arbitrary task in which some of the subjects were called "Bosses," others were called "Assistants," and a third group received no label. In fact, the three groups did the identical task; the assumption was that the labels would affect the self-confidence of the subjects. Afterward they were asked to do the coding task once again. Bosses performed much as before, no different from the no-label group; but Assistants now performed much worse *if* the coding task was automatic. Assistants who were highly automatic in the coding task made four times as many errors as before, and took 40 percent longer to finish. In the Moderate Practice condition, where the coding task was not automatic and was therefore consciously accessible, Assistants did as well as Bosses.

The simplicity and effectiveness of this study is quite remarkable, and the interpretation is quite clear: If we have no conscious access to our own performance, and if some reliable source of information *seems* to indicate that we are doing quite badly, we tend to accept misleading feedback because we cannot check our own performance. With direct conscious access to our performance we are much less influenced by misleading labels. These results suggest that three things go together: losing voluntary control over action details, losing consciousness of them, and losing the ability to *monitor and edit* the details. Indeed, the ability to monitor and edit a planned act may be the essence of voluntary control (see 7.3.2).

While we may speak of "conscious" monitoring and editing, the fact is, of course, that we are generally not conscious of the rules and criteria by which we do our monitoring. If we find a syntax error in inner speech, we do not consciously say, "Aha! lack of number agreement between noun and verb!" Not even linguists do that. Rather, we simply "know" immediately that the conscious plan is in error. The rule systems that spot the error are quite silent in their details. Thus it is not consciousness that *does* the monitoring and editing; rather, conscious experience of the event *facilitates* editing and monitoring by making some content available to many unconscious rule systems, just as the GW architecture facilitates the ability of many specialized processors to review a global message.

Thus any complete theory of voluntary control must explain the automaticity dimension: why, with practice, we lose both conscious access to and voluntary control over the details of an action.

7.1.5 Pathological loss of voluntary control

Psychopathology is the study of repeated, dysfunctional errors that are often *known to be* errors by the person who makes them – "slips" of action or experience that escape attempts to control them over and over again.   Most psychopathology in the neurotic range involves a loss of voluntary control over inner speech, feelings, mental images, or overt actions. Loss of control over *inner speech* is a factor in obsessive or delusional thinking and in some auditory hallucinations; out of control *bodily feelings* play a role in pathological anxiety, conversion hysteria, and depression; uncontrolled *mental images* are at the core of phobias; and when *actions* run out of control we find compulsive or impulse-control pathology.

We can illustrate all these points with a single patient who suffered from a variety of symptoms. Consider Anna O., the classical early patient of Breuer and Freud (1884/1950), who suffered from a very severe case of conversion hysteria. As Erdelyi describes the case,

Anna O. became Breuer's patient in 1880 at the age of 21 when, under the pressure of nursing her dying father, she suffered a nervous collapse. She developed a veritable museum of symptoms which included a labile [variable] pattern of incapacitating paralyses of the limbs; depression and listlessness; terrifying hallucinations of snakes, which transmogrified into death's heads and skeletons; painful coughing fits, especially in reaction to music; a period of severe hydrophobia, during which she could not bring herself to drink water; amnesias [blackouts] for recent events; a blinding squint; severe paraphasia [loss of language ability]; anorexia [unwillingness to take food]; and several other serious dysfunctions. (Erdelyi, 1985; p. 20)

It is the loss of desired control that makes these symptoms pathological. Not moving one's limbs is quite all right if one doesn't want to move them; depression and sadness due to a loss is quite normal; strong squinting is a good idea in the middle of a sun-drenched desert; even images of snakes and death's heads can be quite normal for a reader of Gothic fiction (after all, thousands of people voluntarily go to horror movies or read Gothic tales); even amnesias for recent events can be normal when we want to deliberately forget or ignore them. These events become pathological when people do not want them. Those who suffer from these symptoms try hard and often to master the involuntary feelings, thoughts, actions, or images, but they fail over and over again, in spite of often desperate efforts (e.g., Horowitz, 1975, a, b, 1976). It is not the *content* of the thoughts, feelings, and actions that is problematic: it is their occurrence out of an acceptable context, out of the perceived control of the sufferer. Thus the issue of voluntary control is at the very core of human psychopathology, and an understanding of psychopathology must be grounded in an adequate theory of volition (see 7.8).

There is a clinical intervention that is sometimes very effective that seems to act directly on the mechanism of voluntary control. This paradoxical technique is called "negative practice," or "practicing the symptom" (e.g., Azrin, Nunn, & Frantz, 1980; Dunlap, 1942). If a person has a specific phobia, he is told to voluntarily bring forth the fearful images and thoughts; if he is a stutterer, he is to try stuttering voluntarily whenever he stutters spontaneously; and so on. Although this technique has been known for decades, it has only recently begun to be systematically tested for a variety of problems. Some of the results are quite remarkable. Children who have stuttered for years are told to stutter deliberately for 30 seconds each time they do so involuntarily. As a result, they often stop stuttering in a day or two, with a 75 percent success rate (Levine, Ramirez, & Sandeen-Lee, 1982). There are many cases in which the paradoxical technique works remarkably quickly to stop anxiety attacks, compulsive actions, tics, involuntary phobic images, La Tourette symptoms, and the like. We see here a case in which countervoluntary automatisms are turned into wanted automatisms, just the opposite of the case of "bad" habits discussed above. Of course, practicing the symptom is not a cure-all; but it has been reliably observed to stop pathological symptoms with remarkable speed, often after years of helpless struggle.

Of theoretical interest here is the neat contrast between voluntary and involuntary control in the paradoxical technique. A habitual stutterer has typically struggled thousands of times against the tendency to stutter. This repeated attempt to exert voluntary control rarely works. The paradoxical intervention requires him to stutter deliberately, *to do voluntarily what normally happens involuntarily* – and rather magically, in many cases the problem disappears. One fascinating possibility is that practicing the symptom (which is, after all, only a switch in the direction of voluntary effort) operates through the voluntary control system. If this is true, then it may be that the symptom itself is an error in voluntary control. Much psychopathology may involve "errors of the will." These speculations pose some important questions. We will return to them when we attempt to model the voluntary–involuntary contrasts of Table 7.1 (see 7.5).

7.1.6 Voluntary action is consistent with one's dominant expectations

The cases discussed above – slips, automaticity, and psychopathology – suggest that *countervoluntary automatisms always surprise the actor*. This is also true for nonvoluntary automatisms such as reflexes when we resist them. Thus any nonvoluntary automatism can be made to be surprising by being resisted. Under these circumstances the automatism violates dominant expectations (the Dominant Context Hierarchy).[1] Conversely, voluntary action seems always to be consistent with one's dominant expectations.

There is direct evidence for this proposal from the study of slips in

1 The key role of surprise in the operational definition of voluntary control supports the previous point that expectations and intentions are quite similar. Surprise is a violation of expectations, and its existence may be used to infer the presence of an expectation.

speech and action (Baars, 1980, in press, c; Reason, 1984). First, of course, we know that people often express surprise when they make a slip. The Galvanic Skin Response (GSR) is a well-established measure of surprise. GSRs monitored immediately after experimentally elicited slips are quite large when a sexually explicit slip is made, much smaller when a neutral control slip occurs, and nonexistent when the subject makes a correct response (Motley, Camden, & Baars, 1983b). Thus the more surprising (dominant-context-violating) the slip, the larger the GSR. Further, many slips are spontaneously self-corrected immediately after they are made, again suggesting that they surprise the speaker (Baars & Mattson, 1981). This evidence supports the idea that *countervoluntary action violates the expectations of the actor,* even when an outsider might not notice anything unusual (Baars, in press, c).

7.1.7 Some neurophysiological observations

Neuroscientists have never stopped using words like "voluntary" and "involuntary" to describe some obvious phenomena. Reflexes are obvious examples of involuntary actions; so are autonomic functions like peristalsis, heart rate, sweat-gland activity, and the like, as opposed to the control of skeletal muscles, which is voluntary in the usual sense. We now know that autonomic functions can come under voluntary control at least temporarily when people are given conscious feedback signals activated by the autonomic functions (2.5). Biofeedback training seems to bring autonomic responses under the control of the conscious–voluntary system. All these cases present obvious contrasts between voluntary and involuntary control of the same physical functions.

Another remarkable example of a neurophysiological contrast between voluntary and involuntary control is cited by Penfield and Roberts (1959). These neurosurgeons used a low-voltage electrode to explore the exposed cerebral cortex of conscious patients in order to identify and avoid critical areas where surgery might cause serious damage. In one case, as the surgeon probed the motor cortex, the patient's hand moved, and the patient was asked, "Are you moving your hand?" – whereupon she replied, with perfect accuracy, "No, doctor, *you* are moving my hand." How could the patient possibly tell the difference between the brain mechanisms that were under "her own" versus the surgeon's control?

Surprise about one's own performance is similarly evidence for intentions (goal contexts), even if these intentions were previously not reportable as such. These points make sense if intentions are simply expectations about one's own performance. In GW vocabulary, they are just different kinds of contexts.

We do not know, but her ability to make this distinction suggests that there is a major difference between voluntary and nonvoluntary control.

In sum: Is volition really a psychologically significant issue? Our discussion indicates that, for *physically identical* events, voluntary control makes the difference between automatic actions and those that are conscious in detail; between reflexes, slips, and unwanted habits, compared to the same actions that are deliberately imitated; between "social" and spontaneous facial expressions; and, finally, between actions triggered by direct brain stimulation and those that are initiated in the normal way by the actor. Thus, volition is at the crux of many basic psychological issues. From here on, we will assume that common sense is well justified in giving volition a fundamental psychological role.

7.2   Voluntary action resembles spontaneous problem solving

In Chapter Six we worked out a way of understanding the conscious–unconscious–conscious (CUC) triad found in so many types of problem solving. Thus in answering a question we are conscious of the question in detail, but not of searching for the answer, though the answer is again conscious (6.2). In creative problem solving we are aware of the type of solution we need, but not of the incubation process that eventually brings it to awareness – and so on. Further, we have addressed the whole question of what is meant by an *intention* by considering the tip-of-the-tongue (TOT) state, concluding that even as we are searching for the right word, there is a dominant state of mind that guides the search that competes for limited capacity, but that does not have qualitative conscious contents like color, texture, or flavor. We have called this "intention to say so-and-so" a Dominant Goal Context (6.1).

Voluntary control resembles spontaneous problem solving in many ways. As James suggests, in voluntary action a conscious goal image may be carried out unconsciously, and the results of the action often become conscious again. To illustrate this, we will ask the reader to turn this book upside-down. (It is helpful to actually carry out this little experiment in self-observation.) Clearly the reader is conscious of the request to turn this book upside-down, and perhaps of some visual image of how this might be done. However, the request is ambiguous: Is the book to be turned in the horizontal or the vertical plane? This ambiguity may be conscious for some readers and unconscious for others. The mechanics of controlling hand and arm muscles are surely not conscious, although *choice points and obstacles* ("how do I turn the book upside-down without spilling my coffee?") may be conscious. And of course the results of the action will be conscious.

Further, there is a set of *constraints* on the action – represented in GW theory by the *Dominant Goal Context* – which is not likely to be conscious at any time during the action (see Figure 6.3). We probably turn the book over with maximum economy of movement, rather than sweeping through the air with graceful, elaborate gestures. Then there are constraints imposed by the need to maintain physical control of the book; we are not likely merely to flip it up into the air and let it fall helter-skelter. Even further, there are constraints of convenience, such as keeping track of one's place even while indulging in this little thought experiment. We must stop reading while the book is being moved, and we make automatic postural adjustments to balance the changing forces on the body. Finally, there may be social considerations: If we are in public, is anyone watching our peculiar behavior? Although some of these considerations may be momentarily conscious, many of them will be unconscious, but even these still serve to constrain the action.

In a real sense the action that results from this complex set of momentary conscious and unconscious constraints is a *solution* posed by *problems* triggered by the conscious goal, and bounded by numerous physical, kinetic, social, and other contextual considerations. It makes sense therefore to treat voluntary control as a kind of problem solving (6.0).

7.2.1 Cooperating automatic systems control most of a normal "voluntary" action

The bulk of spontaneous problem solving is unconscious (6.2). The same is surely true of voluntary actions. Much of our intention to perform a particular act must be formulated unconsciously, and the muscular effectors and subgoals needed to carry out the intention are also largely unconscious. Thus, many systems cooperate in creating a voluntary act. It is good to keep this great amount of cooperative processing in mind during the coming discussion, which will focus mostly on the *competitive* aspects of voluntary control.

Notice, by the way, that some sets of systems may cooperate most of the time, only to begin competing when the action runs into trouble. If many systems work together to structure normal speech, a slip of the tongue may violate some but not all of them. When Spooner slipped into "our queer old Dean," he violated no criteria in terms of English syntax, in vocabulary, pronunciation, or phonetics. The only systems able to detect the error are semantic and pragmatic: those that control meaning and communicative purpose. Those are the only levels of control violated by the slip. It would seem to follow that those systems may begin to compete against the error, while the others continue to cooperate. Thus, the coalition of automatic processors that controls the details of normal speech may decompose in the face of an error that violates some but not all levels of control.

7.2.2 We become conscious of underdetermined choice points in the flow of action

If we are unconscious of these routine, cooperating systems, what are we conscious of? Our previous discussion (5.2.3) suggests that the most informative aspects of action should be conscious: that is, those that are unpredictable and significant. It is the underdetermined choice points in the flow of action that should be conscious most often. In speech, hesitation pauses are known to occur at points of high uncertainty (Goldman-Eisler, 1972). Clearly, making people conscious of their routine speech will slow down or interrupt the flow of speech, because previously parallel automatisms are now monitored through the limited-capacity bottleneck; thus hesitation pauses may reflect high conscious involvement. There is considerable independent evidence for limited-capacity-loading events at junctures in the flow of speech, such as clause and sentence boundaries (Abrams & Bever, 1969). These junctures are likely to be points of high uncertainty. While this evidence does not prove that there is more conscious involvement at these points, it makes the hypothesis plausible.

Given these considerations, we can now explore the ideomotor approach to voluntary control.

7.3   Model 5: The ideomotor theory in modern garb

James's ideomotor theory fits neatly into the global-workspace framework. According to this view, a single conscious goal-image, if it does not meet with competition, may suffice to set off a complex, highly coordinated, largely unconscious action. For William James the ideomotor concept emerged from a puzzle in the experience of starting an action: Do we ever experience any command at all? Introspective reports on action commands were vague and contradictory, and this question became a major source of controversy between Wundt, James, and the Würzburg School (James, 1980/1983). James suggested that there is, in fact, no experience at all of commanding an action; rather, an action is organized and initiated unconsciously whenever a certain goal-image becomes conscious without effective competition.

We can partition the ideomotor theory into five interacting hypotheses:

1 The *Conscious Goal-Image Hypothesis* (as just stated) claims that all actions are initiated by relatively simple, momentary images of the goal. For many actions these images may be visual, because the visual system is very good in representing spatial properties of action. However, auditory, tactile, taste, or olfactory images are not ruled out. The act of walking to the kitchen to prepare lunch may be initiated by a taste-and-smell image of an attractive peanut-butter-and-jelly sandwich.

2 The *Competing Elements Hypothesis* is the notion that competing events may drive the goal-image from consciousness. Competing events include conscious goal-images as well as the nonqualitative intentions we have discussed previously (6.0). This idea has many important implications. It allows new conscious thoughts or images to interfere with the planning of an action, and it also permits editing of the goal by many different intentional goal systems.

3 The *Executive Ignorance Hypothesis* suggests that most detailed information processing is unconscious and that executive processes have no routine access to the details of effector control (Baars, 1980; Greene, 1972). Control of the muscles that are used to carry out an action is simply unconscious.

4 The *Action Fiat Hypothesis* claims that the moment of willingness to execute the action may be conscious, especially when the time to execute is nonroutine. (James calls this the "fiat," the mental permission to start the act).

5 Finally, the *Default Execution Hypothesis* is the tendency of the goal-image to execute in the absence of any effective competition "by default." This is really just another side of the Competing Elements Hypothesis, but it is useful to emphasize it with a special name.

In addition to these five points, we should be reminded that subgoals needed to accomplish the goal may become conscious if the goal cannot execute automatically (7.3.1). But let us suppose for now that all subgoals are automatic and unobstructed, so that they can execute without further conscious involvement.

To make these abstractions easier to imagine, take the example of retrieving a word, intending to say it, and then saying it. We have previously noted that complex activities like word retrieval and speaking involve many separable components. Because of the limited capacity of consciousness we cannot afford to think consciously about many details in the act of speaking; we want to access all components of speaking at once, so that "the speech system" behaves as a single processor. But when we change from speaking to listening, or from speaking to eating, we may want to *decompose* the unitary speech system, to reorganize its components into new configurations for listening, for chewing food, for inner speech, and the like.

The ideomotor theory suggests that the "speech processor" as a whole must be recruited, organized, and triggered by a single conscious goal image. This image is itself controlled by a higher-level goal structure – for example, the reader's general willingness to go along with demonstrations in this book. The following example explores ideomotor control in detail.

7.3.1   The fit with GW theory

1   Conscious Goal-Image Hypothesis: Conscious goal-images can activate unconscious goal structures.

If we ask the reader, "What are two names for the flying dinosaurs that lived millions of years ago?" the question is obviously conscious. Now, according to the ideomotor theory, this conscious experience initiates an intention to retrieve a word that matches the intention. Further, the conscious question triggers unconscious search processes that produce candidate words that may match or mismatch the intention (6.1). Because the words are rare, the momentary intention is likely to be prolonged into a tip-of-the-tongue state.

In GW theory, a "conscious goal-image" is of course a global, consistent representation that provides information to numerous specialized processors (2.2). It is not surprising that a conscious goal would trigger local processors that control the muscles that carry out the goal. Indeed, as we have argued early in this book (1.4.5), specialized processors are often goal-addressible: They are activated by goals. One nice feature of the GW system is that the goal-image can be quite arbitrary or fragmentary, since it is the specialized processors themselves that have the real "intelligence" of the system, and that interpret the implications of the goal-image in their own ways (Greene, 1972). Note that the goal-image can trigger both the subordinate specialists able to carry out the action *and* the intentional goal context that constrains planning and execution without itself becoming conscious (Figure 7.1).

In fact, the goal-image itself results from yet a higher-level goal context. Speaking is normally in the service of some other goal – communicating a thought, calling attention to oneself, gaining information – which is, in its turn, in the service of even higher-level goals.

2   The Competing Elements Hypothesis: Conscious contents can be edited by multiple unconscious goal systems.

Suppose the reader first retrieves "tyrannosaurus," instead of "pterosaurus"? Clearly we do not want to execute this incorrect goal-image. Various knowledge sources should interfere with its execution; Some may remind us that "tyrannosaurus" is too long, or that it has a different meaning. Such contradictory knowledge should have access to the global workspace so that it can compete against the incorrect conscious goal-image. GW theory thus suggests that editing of flawed conscious plans is

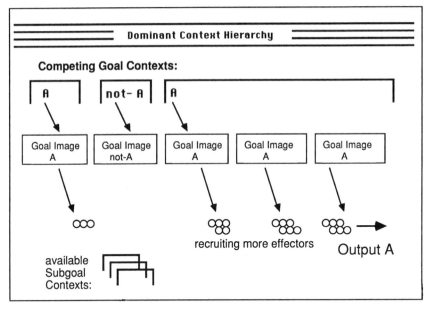

Figure 7.1. Model 5: A modern ideomotor theory of voluntary control. James's ideomotor theory suggests that conscious thoughts are inherently impulsive. If a conscious goal-image is not carried out, it is because contrary images or intentions blocked it. This is consistent with the view in GW theory that conscious events are globally broadcast, so that they can recruit and trigger the unconscious goal systems and effectors needed to carry out an action. In this diagram, goal-image *A* encounters brief competition from the countervailing image *not-A*, but over-comes this opposition and executes output *A*. One interesting feature of the GW model is that in principle any specialized processor can block execution of any conscious goal-image. The evidence for such "universal editing" is described in the text.

not some "added-on" capacity, but an integral aspect of the architecture of the cognitive system.

In GW terms, the goal-image may also set off processors that generate competing goal-images. Perhaps some of these contradict the first goal-image or present alternatives to it (see Figure 7.1). If some unconscious system detects a bad error in the goal-image, it may trigger competing images that act to destroy the flawed conscious goal – to edit and correct it. But once a single goal-image wins out long enough, it will be executed. Its details are obviously off the global workspace, and hence unconscious. Figure 7.1 presents this series of events in detail.

Global workspace architecture supports editing of a global plan by potentially *any* rule system. Take a single sentence spoken by a normal speaker. Errors at any level of control can be detected *if* the sentence become conscious (e.g., MacKay, 1981). There are many ways errors can creep into a sentence, and a correspondingly large number of unconscious rule systems that constrain successful sentences. There are many ways to be wrong and only a few ways to be right by all criteria. Thus, we can very quickly detect errors or anomalies in pronunciation, voice-quality, perceived location of the voice, acoustics, vocabulary, syllable stress, intonation, phonology, morphology, syntax, semantics, stylistics, discourse relations, conversational norms, communicative effectiveness, or pragmatic intentions of the speaker. Each of these aspects corresponds to very complex and highly developed rule systems, which we as skilled speakers of the language have developed to a high level of proficiency (e.g., Clark & Clark, 1977). Yet as long as we are conscious of the spoken sentence we bring all these rule systems to bear on the sentence – we can automatically detect violations of any of them, implying that the sentence is somehow available to all of them (2.5).

In principle, the set of "editing systems" is an open set. We can always add some new criteria for correct performance. This is one reason to suggest that conscious goals are universally edited. Obviously the most effective competition is from goal contexts in the Dominant Goal Hierarchy, since these already have GW access during preparation and execution of the action (4.2.3; 6.4.2; Figure 7.1). But entirely novel aspects of the action can in principle be monitored and edited by onlooking processors, providing they can compete for access to the global workspace. Thus if one prepares to say a sentence, and suddenly a buzzing fly darts into one's mouth, the action can be aborted even though this situation was not anticipated as part of the goal context. Novel considerations can compete against the global goal.

If all conscious goal-images are inherently edited by onlooking processors, it follows that conscious goals that are actually carried out *must have been tacitly edited* by relevant systems. Further, because *any* system can potentially compete against the goal-image, we can talk about this system as allowing *universal* editing. In section 7.3.2 we argue that this is indeed a criterial property of voluntary action: Voluntary action is action whose conscious components have been tacitly edited prior to execution.

> *3   Executive Ignorance Hypothesis: Conscious goal-images can recruit a coherent set of action schemata and effectors, even though we do not have conscious access to the details of those processors.*

Let us suppose that the reader has recalled the name "pterosaurus" (or "pterodactyl") as an answer to the question posed above. This is a conscious representation of the word. Now, how do we recruit the largely unconscious systems that control pronunciation of this difficult word? It is useful to recall here how complex and fast-moving the speech apparatus really is, and how little of it is accessible to awareness at any single time (Executive Ignorance). It seems plausible that the conscious word, in combination with a goal context, can recruit and organize the complex effector system needed to pronounce it.

Executive Ignorance of action details is already implicit in GW theory. As long as the details of action are unconscious, GW theory suggests that executive goal systems operating through the global workspace do not have direct access to such details.

4   The Action Fiat Hypothesis: The moment of execution may be under conscious and voluntary control.

We can wait to say "pterosaurus" until we get a conscious signal; by contrast, in speaking a stream of words, we rarely seem to control the onset of each individual word consciously. But with an isolated word or action, given enough lead time, we can report fairly accurately our intention to execute the action at some specific moment. One key difference is whether the moment of onset of the action is automatically predictable; if it is, it is rarely conscious; but if the moment of onset is unpredictable, conscious control becomes necessary.

How should we represent the Action Fiat Hypothesis in GW theory? If goal-images tend to execute automatically, it makes sense to suppose that timing an action involves *inhibiting execution* of a prepared action up to the right moment, and then releasing inhibition. Presumably, specialized processors sensitive to timing act to hold up execution of a goal-image until the right moment (see Figure 7.3).

5   Default Execution: Given a compatible dominant goal context, a conscious goal tends to execute automatically.

Once "pterosaurus" becomes conscious in the presence of an intention to say the matching word, something rather magical happens: We suddenly notice that our mouth has begun to pronounce the conscious word. The intervening steps of motor control are simply not conscious. In James's words, "consciousness is impulsive" – unless, of course, other goal systems begin to compete for access to consciousness.

The notion that specialized processors tend to execute automatically in the absence of contrary conscious messages is already implicit in basic GW theory. There is nothing to stop an unconscious processor from executing an action except contrary conscious images and intentions. If those are absent, we can expect actions to run off by themselves.

6   Mismatch, surprise, and corrective feedback

Conscious feedback resulting from an action can reveal success or failure to many unconscious goal systems, which may then develop corrective measures.

Imagine trying to say "pterosaurus" and actually saying, "ptero . . . ptero . . . pterosaurus" – a momentary stutter that is quite common in normal speech. Although we have no routine conscious access to the complex articulators and timing systems that control speech, it seems that those specialized systems *do* have access to conscious events. In general, when we allow errors to become conscious, chances are that we can learn to avoid them in the future. In GW theory, consciousness of feedback from the flawed action sets into motion unconscious specialists that attempt to repair the dysfluency.

When we notice a speech error consciously, we often "repair" it quickly (Clark & Clark, 1977; MacKay, 1981), but we are never conscious of details of the repair. Responding to overt errors is similar to anticipatory editing of covert errors, except that editing takes place before the action is executed (7.3.2). Correction of overt errors is useful in preparing for a more error-free performance next time around.

We have previously suggested that surprising events may involve disruptions of one level of context, even while higher levels are undisturbed (4.4.3). Thus repair of contextual violations may start at a higher level than the level that was violated. The same thing may be true of errors in action. If we stutter, the error is at the level of articulation, but higher levels of control – phonemic, lexical, syntactic, and so forth – are unaffected. Thus higher-level goal systems may seek another way to reach their goals. It is rarely the case that the entire Dominant Goal Hierarchy is disrupted, fortunately for us (9.3.4).

In sum, the Jamesian ideomotor theory can be incorporated straightforwardly into GW theory. In fact, it is difficult to see how one could believe that a conscious goal-image is executed unconsciously without the concept of a distributed system of intelligent processors, able to interpret and carry out the relatively crude conscious goal.

The tip-of-the-tongue experience for "pterosaurus" helped to illustrate the intuitive plausibility of the ideomotor theory, and its rather nice fit with GW theory. But it does not provide proof. In section 7.4 below we will discuss the evidence for or against each hypothesis, and its implications for a broad theory of voluntary control. But first, we are ready to make a basic theoretical claim about the nature of voluntary action.

7.3.2 *Voluntary action involves tacit editing of conscious goals*

If there is indeed universal editing of conscious goals, the conscious aspects of any action *must have been* tacitly edited for consistency with one's goal hierarchy before the action was performed. Take the example of premeditated murder. If a normal, rational person has thought for weeks about committing murder, and proceeds to do so, we immediately make the inference that contrary thoughts *must have been* entertained and rejected: The murderer must have anticipated the chances of being caught, the likely disapproval of others, and perhaps the suffering of the victim and his family. That is, we immediately infer that competing alternatives will have been evaluated for any conscious impulse to action that was considered for some time, especially if the action has heavy potential costs. If the action was taken in spite of these editing thoughts, we make appropriate inferences about the value system of the murderer, or about mitigating circumstances. The important point for us here is the idea that conscious impulses are presumed to have been edited before action, assuming there was enough time to do so.

What components of action are likely to be conscious, and therefore tacitly edited? The theoretical answer fits our previous supposition (7.2.2): We tend to be conscious of those aspects of action planning that are novel, informative, significant, or conflictful (see Chapters 4, 5, and 6). Those features that require the integrative capacities of a global workspace system are precisely those that are likely to be conscious – and those are of course exactly the ones that are likely to need editing.

A major claim in this chapter is that *voluntary action is, in its essence, action whose conscious components have been edited before being carried out*. In contrast, countervoluntary actions such as slips are editing failures: actions that *would have been edited and changed* had there been an opportunity to do so before execution. Of course, most components of a normal action are unconscious; these components cannot be globally edited before execution. However, even automatic components of action must have been conscious at some time in the past. Therefore they must have been implicitly edited at that time to make them consistent with the Dominant Goal Hierarchy – and, indeed, the close connection between editing of conscious components and voluntary control follows from our previous point that voluntary action is intrinsically consistent with the current Dominant Goal Hierarchy (7.1).

There is direct evidence for an editing capability of this kind, and when we turn to the voluntary–involuntary contrasts (7.5) we will find that the major difference between closely matched voluntary and countervoluntary actions is this ability to edit.

The five main parts of the ideomotor hypothesis seem to fit the GW framework remarkably well. The interpretation does not seem forced or awkward. Further, as we look at the world from the resulting point of view, many other pieces of the puzzle begin to fall into place (7.6, 7.7, 7.8). The payoffs of bringing the ideomotor concept into our model are therefore attractive, and the theoretical costs seem minimal. But what about empirical support? Do the facts justify our taking the ideomotor theory seriously? Let us see.

7.4 Evidence bearing on the ideomotor theory

A good deal of evidence is consistent with the ideomotor theory, though the case is not air-tight. Consider the following points:

7.4.1 Evidence for the impulsivity of conscious goal-images

The "Chevreul pendulum," a classic demonstration of the impulsive force of conscious goals, has been used since the nineteenth century to persuade hypnotic subjects of the power of their own unaided thoughts (James, 1890/1983). One simply takes a pendulum consisting of a string with a weighted bob at the end, and tries to hold it completely steady. Now, while trying to keep it steady, the subject begins to *think* of the pendulum as swinging away from and toward him, on a north–south axis. Without any perceived effort, the pendulum will begin to swing north and south. Again, making every effort not to move the pendulum, the subject begins to imagine it swinging right to left, in an east–west direction. The pendulum soon begins to follow the subject's thoughts, even though there is no noticeable effort or movement of the hand! It seems as if conscious images are more powerful than deliberate intentions.

It is not easy to adapt this classical demonstration to the rigors of modern investigation. The ideomotor theory needs a great deal more empirical support than is provided by demonstrations such as this. But it is difficult to doubt that there are conscious events related to goals: People can report their own conscious thoughts and images regarding a planned action, and usually predict their actions accurately in the short term. But do those conscious events actually trigger off actions? This is difficult to be sure about, especially in view of the fact that some fleeting conscious goals that are difficult to report may nevertheless evoke action (1.5.5).

We do know that there is a momentary increase in mental workload immediately before the onset of an action (Keele, 1973). This is consistent with the idea that there is at least a momentary conscious goal prior to action. Libet (1985) has presented arguments that we may become conscious of an action only *after* the brain events that immediately trigger it. But this cannot be true in every case: Surely there are many cases where people are conscious of what they are about to do seconds or hours before they do it, as shown by the fact that they can accurately predict their actions beforehand. The reader may make a conscious and reportable decision right now to turn the page, and actually do so: This is hardly surprising, but any theory that cannot handle this elementary fact is incomplete.

More evidence for the influence of conscious goals comes from the experimental literature on mental practice, showing that consciously imagining an action can sometimes improve performance as much as actual physical practice (Drowatsky, 1975; MacKay, 1981b). Conscious imaging of goals is used extensively in clinical practice and to improve athletic performance (Singer, 1984). There is no doubt that conscious images of goals can have powerful influence on effective action.

Further, we know that the opposite case also holds: *Loss* of conscious access to an action can lead to a loss of control. Langer and Imber (1979) showed that automatization of a coding task leads to a loss in ability to evaluate one's own performance, and Reason's analysis of errors and accidents also shows a plausible relationship between automaticity and loss of control (Reason, 1984). Automatization presumably means that goal-images become less and less available, and therefore the actions themselves become less and less modifiable.

Some of the most direct evidence for the role of conscious events in influencing action comes from conscious priming of experimentally evoked slips of speech and action. There are now several techniques for eliciting these slips in the laboratory (e.g., Baars, 1980, 1985, in press c; Motley, Camden, & Baars, 1983b). One of these techniques uses phonological priming – that is, conscious exposure to words that resemble the slip – to elicit spoonerisms. We have previously discussed how the reader can ask someone to repeat the word "poke" about half a dozen times, and then ask, "What do you call the white of an egg?" Most people will answer, "the yolk" even when they know better (6.3). They have evidently been primed by the conscious word "poke" to retrieve a similar-sounding word from memory (Kimble & Perlmuter, 1970). This technique may work because it duplicates the normal effect of conscious goal-images, which prime the action to be taken.

In general, spoonerisms can be elicited by consciously priming the speaker with word pairs that resemble the predicted error (Baars, 1980, in press c). Thus the slip *barn door–darn bore* can be elicited by showing a subject a series of word-pairs like *dart board, dark bowl, dot bone,* and so forth. Because subjects do not know ahead of time which word-pair they must say out loud, they must be prepared to say each one. This state of readiness apparently primes the system to make an error when the target *barn door* is presented.

There are several other techniques for eliciting errors. All of them seem to create competing speech plans that compel subjects to choose very quickly between the two alternatives (Baars, 1980). Sentence errors such as the following are triggered by creating uncertainty about the order of two phrases in a target sentence. If people are unsure about whether to say, "She touched her nose and picked a flower" or "She picked a flower and touched her nose," they are likely to say inadvertently, "She picked her nose . . ." There are several ways to create this uncertainty. The easiest is to present the stimulus sentences, and after each one simply signal the subject either to repeat the previous sentence in the order given, or to reverse the phrases of the sentence. This technique produces predictable word-exchange slips at an adequate rate. Materials can be designed so as to elicit almost any involuntary statement from the subjects (Baars, 1980; in press).

All slip techniques to date create a state of readiness in the speech system to act in a certain way – i.e., they create goal contexts. Once this is done, we can ask whether adding a conscious image related to the target slip will increase the chances of a certain slip. For example, if we gave people the conscious word pair "terrible error," would that increase the chances of the slip "bad goof"? Motley, Camden, and Baars (1979) showed that it does indeed. Further, if people are presented with a social situation such as the presence of an attractive member of the opposite sex, slips related to the situation are made much more often (see Baars, in press, c). In all these cases, a conscious prime coming just before a potential related slip will sharply increase the chances of making the slip. This suggests that conscious events can help recruit actions. While this evidence does not totally confirm the impulsive force of conscious goal-images, it does support this part of the ideomotor theory.

7.4.2 Evidence for editing by global competition

If a momentarily conscious goal-image is necessary to set up and trigger an action, competing conscious events should be able to delay or inhibit it. Everyday experience fits this pattern well. If we ask someone to recall a rare word, and then interrupt with any other demanding conscious task, the desired word will simply not come to mind long enough to allow the person to say it. This rather obvious observation cannot be ignored. It suggests that editing may simply take place by competition for access to the global workspace, presumably coming from processors that can spot errors in the conscious goal-image. This competition can then keep the error from dominating the global workspace long enough to recruit and trigger action. It is theoretically pleasing that we need add no new elements for editing to take place: It is simply another application of the general fact that the GW architecture permits local specialists to compete against global messages.

Other observations are consistent with this view. Meichenbaum and Goodman (1971) have shown that impulsive children can use inner speech to improve self-control. If impulsivity consists of having very powerful conscious goal-images that do not encounter immediate competition, then training children to use conscious inner speech may help them to compete against the undesirable goal-image. The impulsive goal-images may become less consciously available, and may thus have less time to organize and execute unwanted actions. On the other side of the editing coin, Langer & Imber's findings (1979, discussed above) indicate that practicing a task to the point of automaticity leads to a loss of ability to monitor the action. Apparently conscious goal-images are less and less easy to monitor as an action becomes more and more automatic (Pani, 1982; see 1.2.4).

Another source of evidence for anticipatory editing comes from experimentally elicited slips (Baars, in press c). One can get subjects to make slips of the tongue that violate the general rules of language or usage; these slips can then be compared to very similar slips that do fit the rules. Thus, in the laboratory, people will make slips like:

	1	darn bore – barn door (meaningful words)
(*)	2	dart board – bart doard (nonsense)
	3	nery vice – very nice (syntactically correct)
(*)	4	vice nery – nice very (wrong syntax)
	5	lice negs – nice legs (sexual comment that may be socially inappropriate)
	6	reel fejekted – feel rejected (depressed comment)

Likewise, we can elicit word-exchange slips like:

(*)	7	She touched her nose and picked a flower. – She picked her nose . . . (socially embarassing)
(*)	8	She hit the ball and saw her husband. – She hit her husband . . . (aggressive affect)
(*)	9	The teacher told the myths and dismissed the stories. – The teacher dismissed the myths . . . (hard to pronounce)
(*)	10	She looked at the boy and talked softly. – She talked at the boy and looked softly. (semantically anomalous)
(*)	11	Is the gray sea below the blue sky? – No, the blue sky is below the gray sea. (false)

By designing slips that violate some level of control, and comparing them to very similar rule-*governed* slips, we have found a number of cases where the rate of rule-violating slips drops precipitously, sometimes even to zero (e.g., Baars, 1980; Baars & Mattson, 1981; Baars,Motley, and MacKay, 1975; Motley, Baars & Camden, 1983). All starred (*) slips listed above violate generic rules, and these slips show lower rates than similar slips that obey the rules. If the drop in rule-violating error rates is due to some editing process, the fact that this occurs with so many different rule-systems – pronunciation, phonological, lexical, syntactic, social, and so forth – supports the idea of *universal editing*.

Ordinarily we think of "editing" as a review process in which a newspaper editor checks the output of a journalist against certain criteria – criteria like linguistic adequacy, fit with editorial policy, and the like. In general editing seems to involve two separate entities, one of which is able to detect errors in the output of the other.

To show that editing in that sense occurs in normal speech production, we need to demonstrate that people in the act of speaking can detect mismatches between a speech plan and their criteria. Motley, Camden, & Baars (1983b) report that for a task eliciting sexually expressive slips (*lake muv – make luv, bice noddy – nice body*), there is a large and rapid rise in the electrial skin conductivity on sexual slip trials *even if the slip is not actually made*. On neutral control items there is no such effect. Since the Electro-Dermal Response is one of the standard measures of the Orienting Response – a reliable physiological index of surprise – these results suggest that a mismatch was detected even when the slip was successfully avoided. Thus egregious errors can be detected even before they are made overtly, and suppressed. This is exactly the notion of editing suggested above.

We cannot be sure in these experiments that the edited speech plan was conscious, but we do know that conscious speech errors can be detected by many largely unconscious criteria. Not all errors in spontaneous speech are detected, not even all overt errors (MacKay, 1981a). But once speakers become conscious of an error they are likely to correct it. In fact, normal speech is marked by great numbers of overt self-corrections or "repairs" (Clark & Clark, 1977). In any case, only part of the process of error-detection and correction is conscious and reportable. Certainly the slip itself is so, often, but detailed mechanisms of detection and correction are not. Therefore, even though we do not know for sure that the edited slips in the above experiments were conscious, we can certainly suggest that unconscious editing of conscious errors occurs quite commonly.

7.4.3 Evidence for executive ignorance

Try wiggling a finger: Where are the muscles located that control the finger? Most people believe that they are located in the hand, but in fact they are in the forearm, as one can tell simply by feeling the forearm while moving the fingers. What is the difference between pronouncing /ba/ and /pa/? Most people simply don't know. In fact, the difference is a minute lag between the opening of the lips and the beginning of vocal cord vibration. These examples can be multiplied indefinitely. We simply have no conscious, reportable access to the details of action.

7.4.4 Evidence for the action fiat

We can prepare for an action and suspend execution until some "go" signal. The time of the "go" signal can be conscious: Witness the fact that people can tell us when they will execute the action. In that sense, people clearly have conscious access to, and control of, the "action fiat."

The separation between *preparation* and *execution* seems to exist even when execution is not delayed. All actions seem to have these two phases. For example, in the cat, where the neurophysiology of action control has been worked out to a considerable extent, there seems to be a natural division between preparation and execution. As Greene has written:

> When a cat turns its head to look at a mouse, the angles of tilting of its head and flexion and torsion of its neck will tune spinal motor centers in such a way that its brain has only to command "Jump!" and the jump will be in the right direction. . . . The tilt and neck flexion combine additively to determine the degrees of extension of the fore and hind limbs appropriate to each act of climbing up or down, jumping onto a platform, standing on an incline, or peering into a mousehole; the neck torsion regulates the relative extensions of left and right legs when preparing to jump to the side. These postures must be set as the act begins; for if they were entirely dependent upon corrective feedback, the cat would have stumbled or missed the platform before the feedback could work. A few of these reflex patterns of feedforward are adequate for the approximate regulation of all feline postures and movements required in normal environments for a cat. (1972, p. 308)

When is the action fiat conscious? We can suggest that this depends on predictability of the time of action, just as consciousness or automaticity in general depends upon the predictability of any action subsystem. The action fiat should be conscious when the time of execution is nonroutine.

7.4.5 Evidence for Default Execution

How do we know that conscious goals tend to be executed in the absence of contrary conscious or intentional events? Part of the reason comes from the kind of demonstration of automaticity we suggested before: Try looking at a word without reading it, or in the case of rapid memory scanning, try stopping automatic memory search before the end of the list. (Sternberg, 1966; 1.4.2)

Or consider once again the absent-minded errors collected by Reason and his colleagues. Reason reports that *strong habit intrusions* occur in the course of normal actions when the actor is absent-minded or distracted, hence unable to be conscious of the relevant aspect of the action. These cases argue for Default Execution. It seems as if a prepared action executes even when it should not, if contrary conscious events do not block the faulty action. This failure to block a faulty goal-image can have catastrophic consequences. Reason (1983) has analyzed a number of accidents such as airplane crashes and road accidents, and concludes that many of them may be caused by the intrusion of automatic processes, in combination with a low level of conscious monitoring.

A child of six knows how to keep such errors from happening: You have to *pay attention* to what you're doing. That is, be conscious of the novel circumstances and goals. When we pay attention, erroneous Default Executions do not occur. However, it seems likely that the same principle of Default Execution is used to execute *correct* actions most of the time. We seem to automatically carry out conscious goals, unless contrary images and intentions block the conscious goals.

7.5 Explaining the voluntary–involuntary contrasts

Earlier in this chapter we suggested that any complete theory of volitional control must explain the difference between the voluntary–involuntary contrasts: similar-seeming pairs of actions that differ only in that one is experienced as voluntary while the other is not (Table 7.1). Three categories of contrasting facts were explored in detail: the case of slips, of automaticity, and of psychopathology. Here we attempt to show how the theory we have developed so far can handle these facts.

An involuntary action tends to escape inspection, editing, and control. It is often known to be wrong at the very moment it is carried out. We may hit a tennis ball with the sinking feeling that it is going awry, and yet our own psychological momentum may be unstoppable. Or we may make a slip of the tongue that never would have been made if we had only had a little more time to think (Chen & Baars, in press; Dell, 1986). When we make an error out of ignorance or incapacity, we do not speak of involuntary errors, errors that we know are errors, and that would have been avoided *except for* – what? One plausible explanation is that involuntary errors involve a failure of anticipatory editing, as described above. Editing occurs when systems that have spotted a flaw in a conscious goal begin to compete for global access to keep the goal from executing; but this editing function fails to work in the case of slips, unwanted automaticity, and the persistent errors of psychopathology. How could this happen?

Let us consider how editing might fail in our three primary cases: slips, unwanted automaticity, and psychopathology.

7.5.1 Slips: A losing horse race between errors and editing

If conscious goal-images tend to be carried out by default when there are no competing elements, and if editing systems need time to compete effectively against faulty goal-images, there must be a "horse race" between execution time and editing time. ("Execution time" can be defined as the time from the onset of the conscious goal-image to the start of the action; "editing time" is the time from the start of the goal-image to the beginning of effective competition that stops execution of the act. See Figure 7.2.) In the case of slips, the editing systems lose the horse race, because execution time is faster than editing time. The faulty action executes before editorial systems have a chance to compete against its goal-image.

There is one obvious case where this may happen: We know that practiced images fade from consciousness or become very fleeting, and that highly practiced, predictable actions become more efficient and less conscious. Pani's (1982) study on the automatization of images show this pattern. As we have discussed before (1.2.4), Pani showed that conscious access to visual images used in solving a problem drops consistently with practice. In terms of our model, we can suppose that images become globally available for shorter and shorter periods of time, until finally they are globally available so briefly that they *can no longer be reported, even though they continue to trigger highly-prepared effector systems*. Highly prepared processors presumably can react very quickly, while the act of reporting goal-images may take more time. Alternatively, it is possible that goal-images are simply lost from the global workspace; that they are not even fleetingly available. In the remainder of this discussion I will assume that the first case is true – that with practice, goal-images are still broadcast globally, but more and more fleetingly. Naturally this hypothesis must be tested (see 7.9.1).

If goal-images become more and more briefly available with practice, the previously discussed studies by Langer and Imber (1979) begin to make sense. These authors found that more practiced subjects in a coding task were *more* willing to accept an incorrect assessment of their own performance than less practiced subjects. These authors argue that overlearning a task can reduce the knowledge the subject has about *how* the task is performed, and under these circumstances subjects should be more vulnerable to negative assessments of their own performance, because they can no longer evaluate their performance by themselves. This is exactly what we would expect, given the assumption that the goal-image becomes less and less available with practice. Automatic, highly prepared effector systems can continue to carry out the task (because they have become more well-prepared and efficient with practice, and therefore need less of a goal-image to be triggered). But asking someone to do something novel, such as evaluating their own performance, should become more difficult because the global goal-image to be evaluated is available only fleetingly.

Thus the goal-image controlling the countervoluntary act may be available long enough to trigger a *prepared* action, but not long enough to be vulnerable to interference from editing systems.

In Figure 7.1 we see our usual model, with the goal-image A able to trigger off processors that tend to carry out goal A, barring competing messages from other systems that may not approve of A, which we will call $\sim A$ ("*not-A*") messages. If A is globally available only very fleetingly, but long enough to trigger well-prepared processors, editing may fail because the effectors may be faster than the editing systems. Systems like $\sim A$ in Figure 7.2 find it difficult to interrupt and modify the goal-image A. In this way, an action may "slip out" in an uncontrolled way because competing processors could not catch it in time. Goal-image A can come and go very rapidly, because there are automatic systems able to execute it, and competing $\sim A$ messages are too slow to stop its execution.

Notice a very significant point here: There is a trade-off between *competing against A* and *repairing A*. In order to correct A, to modify it, to suggest alternatives, and the like, it is important for many processors to have global access to it. A must be available for a fairly long time if it is to be modified by other systems. This is of course the whole point of making something conscious – that many different unconscious experts can cooperatively work on it (2.3.2). But $\sim A$ systems compete against A in order to stop its execution, and therefore make it *less* consciously

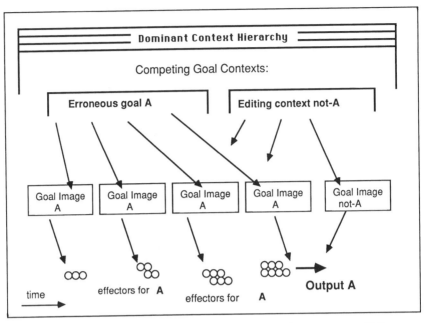

Figure 7.2. A slip of the tongue as a failure of competing systems to edit the error in time. The diagram shows a "horse-race" between an erroneous goal-image (*A*) and a conscious error-message (*not-A*) attempting to block *A*, but too late to prevent its execution. There is indeed evidence that erroneous goals like *A* may themselves result from competition between correct goals that fuse to create an erroneous one. Slips of the tongue, which are errors that are known to be errors at the time they are made, may be explained in this fashion. Very similar explanations may be offered for countervoluntary automaticity and even the involuntary aspects of psychopathology. In general, a well-learned automatic action can be carried out more quickly, and with less conscious involvement than the editing systems that try to catch up to the conscious component of the error.

available. If it is less available, there is less time to modify *A*, and to improve it. This trade-off will be very important in our discussion of psychopathology below.

Figure 7.2 tells why faulty goal-images may be carried out in spite of the fact that their faultiness is known; but it does not tell us why the inner error occurred in the first place. In the case of slips, I have argued in related work that competing goals are often the cause of errors (Baars, 1980, 1985). For example, there are often two different ways to express a single thought. The two alternative goal-images may compete for global access, they may fuse or alternate. When there is a limited time to resolve this goal competition, errors are likely to occur, especially if other events load limited capacity at the same time (Baars, in press, c; Chen & Baars, in press; Dell, 1986).

The horse race between execution time and editing time is key to the view of involuntary action we will maintain in this discussion. It has strong implications not only for understanding slips of the tongue, but also for unwanted automaticity and psychopathology.

7.5.2 Countervoluntary automaticity: The case of "structural" slips

Once the triggering conditions for any automatic process are provided it becomes difficult to stop voluntarily. Habitual cigarette smoking has an involuntary quality, as do compulsive eating, nervous movements, and the like. Once we simply look at a word, it is essentially impossible to stop reading it. The large experimental literature on these phenomena makes the same point (LaBerge, 1980; Shiffrin & Schneider, 1977). Habit is indeed the "great flywheel of society," to quote James's well-known phrase, and there are times when the flywheel runs out of control, resulting in fatal accidents (Reason, 1984). Whenever we try to resist an automatic habit, it will start to behave "erroneously" with respect to our purpose. Such errors have much in common with the slips discussed above. Just as in the case of slips, automatic execution time is plausibly faster than voluntary editing time. Thus we can apply the same "losing horse race" model in the case of unwanted automatisms. They seem to reflect the same mechanism.

Of course, automatisms are not immune to change. Changing them often requires repeated efforts. It may often be helpful to block or slow down the action to make it more conscious and easier to edit and modify. Further, we may need repeated trials to improve conscious access and reestablish voluntary control.

7.5.3 Psychopathology: The case of repeated editing failure, perhaps due to excessive control effort

If we are going in the right direction in this discussion, what can we say about repeated errors that are *known* to be errors – the case of psychopathology? The voluntary system we have explored so far aims above all to achieve goals and minimize errors. But in psychopathology we find a great range of behaviors that violate voluntary goals, repeating similar errors with remarkable persistence. Psychopathology seems to involve a repetitive failure of the entire voluntary control system. How could such persistent failures arise?

We have suggested that the lack of conscious availability might be responsible for a loss of editing ability. We can block and repair errors by making them consciously available longer. If there is a repeated editing failure in pathological symptoms, what could stand in the way of this normal editing process?

One answer may be that *the very attempt to block wrong goal-images may stand in the way of adaptation to the error*. We have referred to the trade-off between modifying a goal *A* and blocking its execution. That is, if we block a goal-image, we stop the goal from executing, but we also lose the opportunity to modify and improve it. In order to repair a faulty goal-image, we must allow it to be conscious for some time. But in the case of pathological errors, editing systems may attempt to wipe the goal-image from consciousness as quickly as possible. In psychopathology we may be trying to block the faulty goal-image so quickly and completely that we have no time to fix the problem.

Take the example of a fearful image of an airplane crash. Every time we think about taking an airplane trip, we may have a vivid fearful image of the plane going down in flames. If we allow ourselves to contemplate the image for a while, we may notice that we can also mentally reverse the plane crash – its flaming wreckage may turn imaginatively into a whole new airplane, and leap back into the sky to continue its journey. Just by allowing the image to remain conscious, many unconscious processors will have access to it. These unconscious processors may be able to modify the conscious image in various ways, thus creating a greater sense of control (Singer, 1984). The problem may come when we do not allow ourselves to contemplate the fearful image at leisure. Rather, we edit it quickly so as not to deal with its awfulness (Beck, 1976; Ellis, 1962). In that case, we do not provide the time needed to change the image, to create alternatives, and the like. Then the fearful mental image may become a rapid, frightening, and uncontrollable phobic thought. It is this trade-off between "editing by competition" and "repairing by conscious exposure" that may cause phobic images to take on a life of their own.

If that is true, then allowing the phobic image to become fully conscious, changing it to a safer image, and in general gaining more voluntary control over it, all should work in the control of phobias. And indeed, these techniques are the essence of phobic control: systematic desensitization, imagery techniques, flooding, and practicing the symptom may all work by allowing the phobic image to remain conscious long enough to notice that the reality is not as awful as the anticipation.

From this point of view the "paradoxical" techniques that are sometimes so effective take on great importance. Asking children to stutter voluntarily apparently solves the problem of stuttering in a number of cases; asking phobics to practice fearful imagery may help that problem, and so on. These results make perfect sense from our perspective: Voluntary stuttering presumably causes a goal-image to remain conscious for a longer time, without destructive competition to reduce its duration. And if it is available longer, other systems can act upon the goal-image to modify it, so that it comes under the control of systems that failed to control it before. Paradoxical practice of the to-be-avoided action increases our ability to avoid the action.

It would be foolhardy to claim that this is the only mechanism of psychopathology. But voluntary efforts to resist the unwanted symptom may be one central factor that sustains and aggravates a variety of repetitive dysfunctional behaviors. This hypothesis has great simplicity, there is some good evidence for it, it is quite testable, and it flows naturally from our entire discussion in this chapter.

In summary, we have explained the contrastive facts shown in Table 7.1 by means of a modern ideomotor theory. It seems likely that voluntary control is guided by momentary goal-images, even though those images are difficult to assess directly. The five major points of the ideomotor theory seem to have some empirical support, although more is needed. There is a satisfying fit between the ideomotor theory and the theoretical approach to consciousness we have pursued throughout this book. As we see next, the ideomotor theory seems to generate fruitful hypotheses about a number of other problems, including the nature of decision making, perceived effort and control, the nature of nonqualitative conscious contents, and even the understanding of absorbed states of mind and hypnosis.

7.6 Wider implications

7.6.1 What does it mean to make a decision?

Most of our actions are bound by past decisions that are not currently conscious. As children we learned to pronounce the difficult phoneme cluster /ask/ as "ask" rather than "aks," with a lot of conscious concern for the different sounds. Once learned, the difficulty of such a task fades into the background, and we need not make the same decision again. All actions contain the residue of commitments made at previous conscious choice-points, decisions that are no longer conscious. If the goal hierarchy has an established commitment to a certain option, there is no need to become conscious of the excluded alternatives. On those potential choices we now have established policies.

But perhaps some aspect of almost any action is consciously decided at the time it is performed – its timing, its propriety in a particular situation, etc. Much of the time people can make voluntary decisions about consciously entertained choices. We can decide to read a chapter in this book, to adopt certain life-choices in adolescence, and occasionally we can even make clear and effective decisions to stop or start long-term habits. These are all choices with conscious alternatives. If consciousness is the domain of competition between such alternative goals, our model should be able to show how we make decisions that stick, as well as those that do not last.

The simplest approach is to say that one can broadcast alternative goals, such as "Should I *A* . . .?" followed by "Or shouldn't I *A* . . .?" and allow a coalition of systems to build up in support of either alternative, as if they were voting one way or another (Figure 7.3). The stronger coalition presumably supports a goal-image that excludes effective competition, and which therefore gains ideomotor control over the action (7.0). Thus voluntary actions may be preceded by a long set of problem-solving triads, as described in Chapter 6.

But where does the conscious goal-image come from in the first place? If the Dominant Goal Hierarchy is not strongly violated, it presumably does not generate conscious goals (4.0). In that case, it may still constrain conscious images without itself becoming conscious. But where do conscious goal-images come from then? There are some obvious possibilities. Sometimes the Dominant Goal Hierarchy is challenged by internal or external events, and the conflict serves to make conscious elements that would otherwise be contextual (4.4.3). Further, some conscious choices are presented by the outside world, as when someone offers us a tempting dessert, an attractive item on sale, or a career opportunity. Other conscious choices are surely created by internal changes, such as the beginning of hunger or the onset of puberty. Some may be created by continuing unresolved conflicts between deep goal structures, such as the need to control others *versus* a desire to be liked by them. And some conscious choices may be generated by an ongoing process of entertaining long-term dilemmas that have no simple solutions (e.g., Luborsky, 1977).

All these points raise the possibility of *indecisiveness*. As James knew so well, the question of getting out of bed on a cold morning appears as a struggle between conscious alternatives. Perhaps most of our ordinary decisions have some of this quality, but some extended struggles may be won by patience rather than force. As James notes in the epigraph to this chapter, one can simply wait until the cold of the morning fades from consciousness; if a fortuitous thought about getting up then emerges, it may be able to dominate consciousness without competition. Thus the

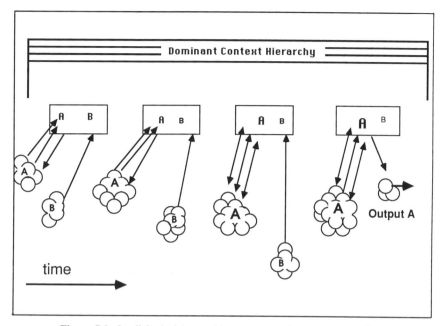

Figure 7.3. Implicit decision making as a vote between competing groups of processors. Implicit decisions about conscious events may occur as a voting process between coalitions supporting *A* vs. *B*. Contents *A* and *B* may be broadcast simultaneously or alternately, providing they alternate quickly enough to recruit coalitions in favor of each. The double-headed arrows indicate that support may flow back to the voting coalitions of processors in a self-supporting feedback cycle in which "the rich get richer and the poor get poorer" (McClelland & Rumelhart, 1981). Ultimately *A* is broadcast long enough, to the exclusion of *B*, that effectors can be recruited to carry out *A*. This diagram does not portray conscious, explicit decision making in which we experience a flow of conscious thoughts about the right course of action or about explicit problems in algebra or chemistry (e.g., Newell & Simon, 1972). That would involve metacognitive, conscious comments on other conscious events and voluntary control of future conscious contents, whereas the present diagram describes intuitive, spontaneous, inexplicit decisions about conscious alternatives.

persistently recurring thought ultimately wins out. The idea that important goal systems may "win out" by sheer persistence, by returning to consciousness again and again, is consistent with evidence from thought monitoring showing that unresolved personally important issues tend to recur spontaneously (Klinger, 1971; Pope and Singer, 1978).

Indecisiveness may be the case where neither of the two contending goals ever completely fades away. Young children often seem indecisive compared to adults. They may be quite impulse-driven, sometimes hesitating back and forth, back and forth, between two attractive goals.

Young children may not yet have a consistent Dominant Goal Hierarchy. Over time, many repeated cases of effective coalition-building between the most successful goal contexts may result in the relatively stable adult Goal Hierarchy, so that consistent goal contexts become dominant and automatized like any other skill.

We have noted that conscious goals that are consistent with the Dominant Goal Hierarchy will last longer than those that violate it (7.8.3). It also follows from our current model that some conscious goal images may fit the deeper levels of the Goal Hierarchy better than the more superficial levels. In that case the more deeply-driven goal-images may last longer, or they may return more often until they lead to effective action. One way to make new goals effective is to tie them in with existing deep goals. Thus one may have a conscious inner argument of the form: "Does my commitment to survival make it necessary to go out and jog four miles a day? Does my commitment to social success make it imperative to stay at this boring party?" In these cases a conscious connection is created between an immediate goal and an existing deep commitment; in just this way politicians will make a case for new taxes by referring to existing deep and agreed-upon goals like "national security," "winning the war on poverty," and "bringing back prosperity." By consciously mobilizing the deep Goal Hierarchy one's superficial reluctance may be overcome. These rhetorical connections between local goals and deep goals may be specious, but as long as they allow the conscious goal to be available long enough to be executed they will be effective.

In section 7.8.3 we argue that most normal action is relatively conflict-free; that is, it takes place in the domain of overlap between many deep goals (9.3). But conflict between goals is not unusual. Any new major goal must of course be reconciled with existing priorities.

Thus, much of the time people may carry on an inner argument about their goals. Not all of this inner argument may be fully conscious; some of it may consist of fleeting images that function merely as reminders. Notice an interesting thing about this inner argument: If the ideomotor theory is valid, it is very important to *have the last word* in a train of arguments; the last word, after all, is the one that will be carried out, because it is not followed by competing thoughts. This simple notion has many interesting consequences (e.g., 7.7–7.9).

Inner arguments about goals have many implications. For example, one can define a *belief* as an abstract concept that is not disputed in the stream of thought, although it could be. One can dispute a political or religious belief or a scientific position, but it is quite remarkable how rarely people challenge their own beliefs. Indeed, stable beliefs seem to become contextualized and provide deep goal and conceptual contexts, often lasting for a lifetime. Along these lines, a *belief system* may be defined as a consistent set of such undisputed concepts, one that becomes contextualized and serves to stabilize and direct one's conscious thoughts, feelings, and actions – presumably just by giving the belief system control over the last word in the inner argument, since the last word has the real power by the ideomotor theory; it is the one that controls action without contradiction. Finally, a *closed belief system* may be defined as one that has a ready answer to all apparent counterarguments, so that any possibility of change is minimized (e.g., Rokeach, 1960). Perhaps all ideological, political, philosophical, and even scientific belief systems are closed to some extent. Simple observation should convince us that most people have self-validating closed belief systems about many disputable topics, especially those that are difficult to decide on direct evidence.

7.6.2 Resistance to intended actions, perceived effort, and perceived voluntary control

We have already noted that voluntary control is different from spontaneous problem solving (6.0) in that we usually *know* that our voluntary actions are goal-directed. We have "metacognitive" access to many voluntary goals, and often to mental events that block voluntary goals (e.g., Flavell & Wellman, 1977). Two factors may give us this kind of metacognitive access. The first is obvious: *ex hypothesi*, the ideomotor theory states that voluntary control involves conscious images, which, if they are available long enough, are also available to metacognitive processors. Metacognitive processors are presumably involved in representing, recalling, and describing the fact that we do have a certain conscious goal. Thus readers know that they are reading this book voluntarily, in part because they may be able to recall the conscious goal of doing that.

But there must be many times when we experience an action as voluntary even when we do not remember its controlling goal-image. After all, goal-images are fleeting, their memory may be masked by later events, and so on. By our discussion above, the more automatic the action, the less we can report our intention. Conversely, the more the action encounters resistance, the less automaticity will operate, and the more a decision to act can typically be reported.

This suggests that *resistance* to performing an action, the perception of effort, and perceived voluntary control are all of a piece. Let us examine, for example, the issue of perceived effort, which appears very much as a conflict between expected control and actual control. The author's experience in typing the manuscript of this book may illustrate the point. As a practiced (though errorful) typist, I am normally unconscious of the details of typing. The computer program that displays words on my screen works so quickly that normally I do not notice it at all. But sometimes when I am typing, the computer is simultaneously printing out some other material, and then the screen seems to slow down enormously. The lag time between a finger stroke and a character's appearing on the screen is then very long compared to my expectations, and the relationship between keystrokes and characters on the screen becomes agonizingly conscious. The subjective experience is one of great effort, as if I must forcibly push each character onto the screen. I am acutely aware of the voluntary character of every keystroke.

This example may provide a way to test the hypothesis that perceived voluntary control results from perceived effort. It suggests that a goal context contains information about the length of time an action should take. When this time is delayed, we tend once more to become conscious of both goal-images and feedback, so that many processors can now operate on the conscious components of the action. As the conscious goal-image becomes more available, metacognitive processors can also operate on it to facilitate recall and self-description. In sum, our knowledge that we have a certain goal may depend on violations of "invisible" expectations in attempting to accomplish the goal.

Notice that the increase in conscious access to such a delayed goal gives us four distinct advantages: First, we have more time to edit and change the conscious goal; second, in this process we can improve our voluntary control over the action; third, we can comment on the goal in question metacognitively, which then allows us to recall it, to talk about it, and perhaps to find alternative ways to accomplish the same ultimate end. Finally, as we will see in Chapter 8, access to a conscious goal can also guide *later* conscious contents, as when we make conscious decisions about what to pay attention to next.

7.6.3 Ideomotor control of conceptual thought: A solution to the puzzle of nonqualitative consciousness?

One of our persistent thorny problems has been the relationship between clear, qualitative conscious contents such as percepts, feelings, and images versus nonqualitative conscious events such as concepts, beliefs, expectations, and intentions, which surely can compete for limited capacity, but which are not experienced with qualities like warmth, color, taste, and smell (1.5.4).

We have previously remarked on the fact that human beings have a great tendency to concretize abstract ideas: to think in terms of metaphors that can be visualized, or to reduce an abstract class of events to a concrete prototype. It may be no accident that mathematics and physics really have two separate symbol systems: an algebraic code and a geometric one. The two are mathematically equivalent, but not psychologically, because people can use their visual imagination with geometric figures but not with algebraic formulas.

We do not have to resort to science for examples. All of us clearly represent the meaning of a sentence in an abstract form. To illustrate this, let the reader recall word-for-word the sentence before this one. (No looking!) Most readers will not be able to do this, but they will be able to recall a *paraphrase* of the sentence – that is to say, a semantic equivalent, with different words, different syntax, and even different sensory qualities than the original sentence; but the paraphrase will preserve the abstract meaning of the original. The evidence is very good that educated adults rapidly convert words and sentences into a semantic code that is quite abstract and impossible to experience qualitatively (Bransford & Franks, 1976). The question we must face here is, of course: How do we then manipulate the abstract semantic code through consciousness?

One possibility is that we have ideomotor control over abstractions. Take the complex conceptual structures developed in the course of this book. We have now defined a set of *terms* like "context," and "global workspace," which are perceptual in nature even though they refer to abstract nonqualitative concepts. The more we can manipulate these abstractions accurately, using words we can see and hear, the easier we will find it to understand the theory. Likewise, we have made a great effort in this book to present useful metaphors for our theory, such as the image of a conference of experts, each competing for access to a central blackboard. But every concrete metaphor is really inadequate. For example, the conference image fails to show that expert processors in GW theory are decomposable, while human experts are not (1.4.2). (Human experts have a tendency to stop running when they are decomposed.) This point is quite general: Metaphors are useful but ultimately inadequate representations of a more abstract and complex reality (Lakoff & Johnson, 1980). In science, they must be used with care.

In general, an imageable metaphor seems to serve the function of evoking and recruiting conceptual processes that are more abstract and often more accurate than the image itself. These abstract entities may be impossible to experience qualitatively. Hence the need for visual figures, audible words, and concrete metaphors. These can be made qualitatively conscious when needed, to stand for abstract nonqualitative entities.

All this suggests that we do indeed have ideomotor control over abstract concepts, so that we can always concretize an abstraction, and conversely, we can always abstract from concrete symbols. It is not enough merely to translate the perceptual world into abstractions as we do in comprehending a sentence; in turn, we must be able to retrieve the abstractions in perceptual form, in order to work with them, to resolve conflicts between them, to make predictions from them, and to use them to act on the world. In all these transformations, it is useful to recode the abstractions into some qualitative, imageable form. The ideomotor theory seems to add some real clarity to the puzzling issue of the relationship between qualitative experience and abstract representation.

7.6.4 Fleeting goal-images make accurate source attribution difficult

If it takes time for a goal-image to result in action, then what about goal-images that not only trigger an action, but also require us to talk about them? If we want people to report their own goal-images, they must make the goal-image available long enough not only to trigger the original action, but also to help recruit linguistic systems able to describe the image. This is of course the same problem we encountered before, when we first raised the possibility of fleeting conscious events that pass too fast to describe (1.5.5). The best example, again, is in tip-of-the-tongue states when people experience the missing word fleetingly, and encounter the frustration of trying to hold onto it long enough to say it.

This fundamental problem of metacognitive access may help to explain a number of findings about human self-observation. There is the extensive social–psychological literature showing frequent errors in attribution of personal causation and the common failure of people to know their own reasons for doing things (Nisbett & Wilson, 1977; Weiner, 1986; see 6.0). This common failure may reflect the fact that actions are controlled by fleeting goal-images that last long enough to trigger the actions, but not long enough to permit accurate recall and attribution. Accurate source attribution is very important for metacognitive knowledge and self-control. This is another topic we can not explore in much detail, but we can suggest its relevance to GW theory.

7.6.5 The relationship between a goal-image and the action it evokes may be highly variable

The act of walking to the kitchen may be triggered by many different goal-images. One can imagine a seductive peanut-butter-and-jelly sandwich or leftovers from last night's dinner; one can remember that the stove needs cleaning or imagine the odor of cooking gas. We need not imagine any of these in great detail. A fragment of a related image will do quite nicely to trigger a habitual action. This is very much like the issue of synonymy and paraphrase in language: There are dozens of ways of saying the same thing. In action control, a conscious cue is presumably interpreted by many different context-sensitive lower-level systems. We do not need a detailed conscious plan or command, since the action is carried out by specialists that know more about local conditions than we do consciously. Various unconscious specialists keep continuous track of our posture, balance, and gravity, about salivation and digestive enzymes to prepare for eating, about remembering the route to the kitchen. Greene (1972) has pointed to the simplicity of high-level commands in distributed control systems as a general and very useful property.

This point has important implications for research. We must not fall into the trap of looking for *the* goal-image for walking, or talking, or for any other action that looks the same in different circumstances. This is what misled introspectionists around 1900, who were astonished to find the great range of variation in mental images between different observers (1.5.5). The modern ideomotor theory indicates that many different goal-images can serve to recruit and initiate any given action. Conscious images may seem quite irrelevant and still result in appropriate action. Imagining a sandwich while lost in the desert must not trigger an automatic walk to the kitchen, but it can stimulate new efforts to find food and water. Thus goal-images may vary tremendously between different situations and observers, and yet be quite effective in controlling appropriate, context-sensitive, voluntary action.

7.7 Absorption and hypnosis as ideomotor events

7.7.1 Absorption as a drop in competition for GW access

The ideomotor theory has many interesting implications. For example, it suggests a reasonable account of hypnosis as a state in which ideomotor control operates without effective competition (7.6.7). Before we discuss this, we can define an *absorbed state* – watching a movie, reading a novel, and the like – as a state in which only one coherent stream of events dominates consciousness (viz., Spiegel, 1984; Tellegen & Atkinson, 1974). That is, there is a low level of effective competition between different topics (Dominant Goal Contexts), and there is no voluntary effort to change topics (see Chapter 8).

In principle, it would seem that there are two ways to reach an absorbed state. One is for the number of competing contexts to decrease. This may happen simply when we relax, let go of our current concerns, solve a major preoccupying problem, or enter a state of trust that things will work out without voluntary effort (Klinger, 1971). A second way to enter an absorbed state is to allow one context to become extremely dominant and thereby to exclude alternatives. Shadowing tasks compel one to repeat immediately each word in a coherent stream of words (Broadbent, 1958; Cherry, 1953). This task is so demanding that competing thoughts are simply excluded from conscious experience. Nevertheless, competing thoughts have probably not disappeared (MacKay, 1973; Moray, 1969). Thus we can enter an absorbed state either if consciousness is dominated by a very strong context, or if there is a drop in competition from alternative contexts. In fact, most actual absorbed states have both of these features. In watching a fascinating movie our experience is being structured by the story line, which continually generates new expectations about future events that need to be tested. At the same time we may relax, postpone some pressing concerns, and thus lower the urgency of competing topics.

One implication is that *we are always in an absorbed state relative to our own dominant context*. If we look at the goal hierarchy (4.3.2), we can see that its lower levels can change much more easily than higher goals, which are quite stable over time. Most people do not cease wanting to survive, to be socially accepted and respected, and to pursue other lifelong goals. Adults change their major beliefs and goals quite slowly if at all. Even perceptual and imaginal contexts do not change every instant. This suggests that we are never truly "absent-minded," "mindless," or even "preoccupied" with respect to everything (Reason & Mycielska, 1982). We are always "present-minded" to our *own* dominant preoccupations. Now, if we are driving a car and thinking thoughts of love at the same time, we may run over a pedestrian. *Relative to* the act of driving the car we were preoccupied and absent-minded. But relative to thinking thoughts of love, we were quite present. Taking a bird's eye view of the situation, it would seem impossible to be utterly absent-minded. "Absorption" is only a relative term.

When we are absorbed in one mental topic to the exclusion of others, the other topics must go on automatic. Thus if we were to ask someone to shadow speech while performing a fairly routine task – driving a car along a familiar route – we would see the automatic components of driving emerge with minimal conscious and voluntary overlay. We should then expect to find large numbers of automatic "habit intrusions" into the act of driving (Reason, 1983). Driving a car distractedly may be rather suicidal, but similar experiments can be done under less dangerous circumstances.

7.7.2 Hypnosis as ideomotor control without competition

Absorption has long been thought to be a key element in hypnosis. When we combine the idea of absorption with ideomotor control, we have a possible theory of hypnosis (James, 1890/1983, Chapter 27). The major features of hypnosis seem to flow from the fact that in this state we have only one conscious goal-image at a time, which tends to be carried out because the chances of competition from other elements are reduced. Although we cannot go into hypnosis in great detail, this possibility is worth exploring briefly.

What are the major features of hypnosis? There seems to be good agreement on the following:

1 *Absorption*. Sometimes called "monoideism," or "imaginative involvement" (Ellenberger, 1970; E. Hilgard, 1977; J. Hilgard, 1979; Spiegel & Spiegel, 1978; Tellegen & Atkinson, 1974). Hypnosis seems to create a new, imaginative context that dominates experience for some time to the exclusion of other events (Singer, 1984).

2 *Dissociation*. Good hypnotic subjects show several kinds of spontaneous dissociation. First, there are two kinds of temporal dissociation. A good subject is often spontaneously amnesic for the experience, which is a kind of posthypnotic temporal dissociation. There is also prehypnotic dissociation, since separation from previously dominant trains of thought is common (J. Singer, personal comm.). In addition to temporal dissociation, two kinds of *concurrent* dissociation occur. These may be called "dissociation from effectors" and "dissociation from the normal self." Subjects often report feelings of alienation from their own limbs that are manipulated by suggestion, as if their arms and legs had "a will of their own" (Spiegel & Spiegel, 1978). Further, there is commonly some surprise at *oneself* for allowing the hypnotic actions and experiences to happen, so that there is a kind of dissociation between one's "normal self" and one's "hypnotic self" (viz., 8.5.2). In sum, there is an experienced temporal separation from earlier and later states, and also concurrent separation during hypnosis from one's own normal experience of self and one's own hypnotically controlled actions.

3 *Suggestibility*. This is a defining feature of hypnosis; but can be viewed as a consequence of ideomotor control, plus a kind of dissociation from normal inhibitions. But dissociation from inhibiting thoughts is a property of absorption as a state of low competition for consciousness. If the ideomotor theory is true, and if our normal editing mechanisms are not competing against novel conscious contents, it follows that one will show a great flexibility in obeying the conscious ideas. Thus suggestibility seems to flow from "absorption plus ideomotor control."

4 Strong and stable *individual differences*. Between 10 and 25 percent of the population is highly hypnotizable. These people easily slip into this remarkable state with a very simple, standard induction (E. Hilgard, 1977; Spiegel and Spiegel, 1978).

5 *Hypnotic inductions are arbitrary*. Anything believed by the subject to induce hypnosis will induce hypnosis (James, 1890/1983). However, relaxation and a reasonable feeling of trust for the hypnotist are common features.

These are the positive facts about hypnosis that command a good consensus. At the same time hypnosis has some puzzling "negative" features; properties that we might expect, but that researchers have not found in spite of repeated efforts.

1 No reliable neural correlates of hypnosis have been found so far. Physiologically, hypnosis looks like a normal waking state.
2 There is a puzzling absence of strong and reliable personality correlates, in spite of many attempts to find them (e.g., J. Hilgard, 1979).
3 It is difficult to demonstrate a conclusive difference between hypnosis and pretense (Barber, Spanos, & Chaves, 1974). But this may be in good part because very good "pretenders" are able to experience their pretended states very deeply and realistically – in other words, good pretenders may enter an absorbed state, in which only one train of conscious contents dominates their actions.

There may thus be no real difference between very good play-acting and hypnosis, but this fact may reveal as much about acting as it does about hypnosis. Many professional actors experience deep absorption and identification with the characters they play. The difference between half-hearted acting and Stanislawskian method acting is the difference between being superficially involved and being deeply absorbed in a certain character (Moore, 1960). Stanislawskian method actors may believe for a while that they are the character they are playing. Absorption may be the key both to good hypnosis and to good pretense.

The close connection between absorption, dissociation, and high performance comes out in Spiegel's clinical observation that

> it has been commonly observed that many highly hypnotizable performers, such as actresses and musicians, dissociate their ordinary awareness of themselves when they are performing, and feel strangely disconnected from the results of their performance after it is over. One highly hypnotizable pianist reported that her only memory of her graduation recital was of floating above the piano admiring the grain of the wood. She had to ask a stagehand whether she had in fact completed her program, which she had performed extremely well. (Spiegel, 1984, p. 102)

Hypnosis as absorbed ideomotor control

Several investigators maintain that absorption may be the basic element of hypnosis, the single central fact from which all else flows (e.g., Spiegel & Spiegel, 1978, p. 24). This is a very attractive argument from our point of view. We can simply take James's ideomotor theory – in our modern version – and explain all of the features listed above. That is:

1 *Absorption* or monoideism is simply a low level of competition for access to consciousness between alternative contexts that can sometimes last for hours. Under these conditions of "low editing" the dominant stream of consciousness, which may be quite different from our normal states, should be in control.

2 We can also explain both temporal and concurrent *dissociation*. Spontaneous amnesia after hypnosis is a difficulty in voluntarily reconstructing the hypnotic state in such a way as to easily retrieve information from it. This is not surprising, given the differences in content between the hypnotic, absorbed context and our most usual contexts, those we *call* normal. Thus, spontaneous amnesia would seem to follow quite easily. The same argument applies to the temporal dissociation from the dominant context before hypnosis. We should feel dissociated from it, given the differences in content. If hypnosis is mainly an absorbed state, there should be relatively few shared features between it and our normal state, making recall difficult.

The two kinds of concurrent dissociation also make sense. Dissociation from our own hypnotically controlled limbs may be just the act of noticing the truth of ideomotor control. In our normal waking state we tend to forget that we are *always* unconscious in detail of actions that carry out our conscious goals. That is what the ideomotor theory is all about, after all. Similarly, we are normally unconscious of the controlling contexts of our own actions. In hypnosis we may be surprised to realize that. But in our whole approach in this chapter, the unconsciousness of goal contexts and automatic actions has become a fundamental assumption about normal action. From this point of view, it is not dissociation that is unusual. What is novel in hypnosis is the fact that we *realize* the existence of ideomotor dissociation between conscious events, their consequent actions, and their antecedent goal contexts. Perhaps we recognize this in hypnosis because hypnotically controlled actions are often unexpected; they violate our usual contextual assumptions about ourselves (9.0).

Other features of hypnosis are also consistent with this point of view.

3 *Suggestibility* and flexibility seem to be merely the result of ideomotor control in an absorbed stated, with minimal competition and self-examination.

4 The reasons for the strong and stable *individual differences* in hypnotizability are not clear. Given that the notion of hypnosis as "absorbed ideomotor control" seems to work quite well, the question seems worth exploring from this theoretical perspective.

5 The *arbitrariness* of hypnotic induction techniques is quite understandable, since we know that any conscious experience may trigger a context (4.4.1). Hypnosis involves a context, one of minimal competition for GW access. Relaxation and trust for the hypnotist may be simply different ways of describing this absorbed state.

We can also make sense of some of the negative results, the absence of expected features of hypnosis. Hypnosis appears to be such a spectacularly different state of mind that many researchers expected to find major physiological and personality differences. But if we assume that hypnosis is not an unusual state at all, but is rather a state of low competition for access to consciousness, we should find few if any physiological differences between hypnosis and relaxation. The absence of personality correlates is not surprising either, because we are all absorbed in our own topmost goal context, as suggested in Section 7.7.1. In that sense all personality types involve absorption. Finally, we should find it hard to distinguish between hypnosis and very good pretense, because successful pretense is like excellent performance in any other demanding, complex task. It requires absorption.

In sum, hypnosis may simply be ideomotor control in a state of absorption. But absorbed states are quite normal and, in a general sense, we are all absorbed in our own top-level contexts. The major difference seems to be that highly hypnotizable subjects are quite flexible in the topics of their absorption, while most people are not. Perhaps we should turn the usual question around. Instead of asking what is *different* about hypnosis, we might ask; Why is flexible absorption so difficult for three-quarters of the population? What is it that is added to a "ground state" of absorption, which we all share, that resists flexible ideomotor control? We explore this question in the next few chapters.

7.8   Conflicts between goals

We have already discussed the possibility of competing goals and contexts (4.3.5); here we will explore the implications for conflicting emotions. Goals can encounter conflict, either from other goals or from reality. All emotions involve goals combined with real events: Happiness may result from achieving a wished-for goal, sadness involves loss of a desired object, depression is due to helplessness and hopelessness about significant life goals, anger and frustration occur when obstacles stand in the way of achieving a desired goal, fear is due to the expectation that something will happen that is fervently desired *not* to happen, love involves the goal of being with someone, and so on. All these goals can be represented in GW theory. But all these emotions involve clear, dominant goals that can be consciously achieved, delayed, thwarted, and the like.

The really difficult cases for voluntary control arise when this is not true; when there is competition for access to consciousness between different goals, so that no single goal can dominate. We have already discussed indecision due to conflicts between goals, and the possibility of an "inner argument," in which the final word wins ideomotor control. William James's (1890/1983) discussion of "weakness of the will" and "explosive will" is also relevant here, and can be treated in terms of different patterns of competing goals. Perhaps most intriguing, the discussion so far leads quite naturally to a viewpoint on *unconsciously* conflicting goals, those that may compete with the dominant goal hierarchy by generating a momentary global message that will be carried out by well-prepared systems, but with minimal metacognitive recall. We turn now to such unreportable goal conflicts.

7.8.1 A modern version of psychodynamics: Modeling unconscious goal conflict

Unconscious conflict has been the key assumption in the long tradition of psychodynamic thought, starting with Freud and Janet in the nineteenth century and continuing in an uninterrupted creative stream to the present time (Ellenberger, 1970). While it has been difficult to find solid evidence outside the clinic for many psychodynamic ideas, there is now a growing conviction among many scientific psychologists that these ideas can be tested and modeled in a reasonable cognitive framework (Baars, 1985; Erdelyi, 1985; Luborsky, 1977; Meichenbaum and Bowers, 1984). This discussion is in that spirit.

7.8.2 Disavowed goals can be assessed by contradictions between voluntary (edited) and involuntary (unedited) expressions of the same goal

Suppose one is furious with a friend, but finds it impossible to express this feeling. The goal hierarchy may exclude the goal of expressing anger so completely that the anger – presumably some context competing for access to consciousness – can only create a fleeting global goal image. Thus there will be little if any metacognitive access to the goal image. Suppose the friend asks the angry person whether he would like to meet for lunch next week, and receives the reassuring reply, "I'd like to beat you very madly," instead of "I'd like to meet you very badly." This is one kind of Freudian slip (Freud, 1901/1938), and we have experimental evidence that deep goal conflicts can sometimes produce this kind of meaningful slip (see below). The key notion here is that we can observe an *in*voluntary slip that expresses an emotion, but that subjects will voluntarily disavow the emotion when asked about it. This may be true in general: When there is a deep conflict between goals, and one goal system dominates voluntary action and speech, it may still be possible for the excluded goal to express itself counter-voluntarily when a fleeting global goal triggers a prepared action. Voluntary actions – those that are metacognitively reportable as voluntary – presumably have rather long-lasting goal-images. Since long-lasting goal-images are edited by multiple criteria, a voluntary expression of anger may be vetoed by some part of the goal hierarchy, but a fleeting angry image might gain expression if the appropriate motor systems were ready to express it. It *should* be edited out, but it may not be, due to a lack of editing time. All this suggests that we can use an observed contradiction between voluntary and involuntary expression of the same feeling as a signal that there is a basic goal conflict.

In general, we can suggest that emotional conflict of this kind is marked by a contradiction between voluntary and involuntary expressions of the emotion (Baars, 1985). The person makes an angry slip, but quite honestly disavows any conscious goal of expressing anger because metacognitive access to the momentary angry goal-image is lost. This pattern of self-contradiction between voluntary and involuntary expressions of conflicted emotion has indeed been found with sexual slips made by males who score high on a measure of Sexual Guilt (Motley, Camden & Baars, 1979), and for angry double entendres in subjects who have been given a posthypnotic suggestion of anger (Baars, Cohen, & Bower, 1986). Presumably the same sort of explanation applies to the finding that female High Sex Guilt subjects show more physiological sexual arousal to an erotic tape-recording than do Low Sex Guilt subjects, even though their verbal reports show the opposite tendency (Morokoff, 1987). Further, Weinberger, Schwartz, & Davidson (1979) have identified a group of "repressors" who are marked by high autonomic reactivity to emotional stimuli that they claim have no emotional effect. All these cases are marked by *involuntary expression* of affect along with *voluntary disavowal*.

Presumably conflicted subjects, such as the males who score high on Sexual Guilt, are in conflict between approaching and avoiding sexually desirable people (*A* and ~*A*). This conflict can be modeled as competition for access to a global workspace between goal-images for avoiding and goal-images for approaching sexual goals. Goal-images for avoidance may encounter little competition, so that they are available longer, and are therefore reportable by relatively slow linguistic processors. But goal-images for approach encounter competition from the avoidance goals, and are thus limited to very brief access to the global workspace. Even brief access, however, may be long enough to trigger automatic or prepared responses expressive of the forbidden goal-image. The slip task presumably provides the kind of highly prepared response that allows expression to the fleeting desire to approach the attractive person.

The more these two intentions compete, the more the subject loses control over the unintentional expression of the prohibited goal, because the fleeting goal-image cannot be modified as long as it is available for only a short time (7.6.4). Thus the very effort to avoid thinking of the sexually attractive person may paradoxically trigger the taboo thoughts

(7.5.3). This way of thinking allows us to explain a number of phenomena that have a psychodynamic flavor, in the sense that they involve competition between contrary intentions.

These are not quite the ideas proposed by Freud, because we make no claim that deep underlying conflicts cause these phenomena – rather, they may result from the normal functioning of the system that controls voluntary action by means of conscious goals. However, we cannot exclude the stronger Freudian hypothesis that enduring unresolved goal conflicts may initiate and bias this series of events (Luborsky, 1977). Indeed, the notion of a momentary conscious goal for avoidance resembles Freud's concept of "signal anxiety," a momentary experience of anxiety that signals that there is something to be avoided, but without knowing what and why.

Notice that in this framework the difference between "repression" and "suppression" is only a matter of degree. If the goal-image for inappropriate anger is available long enough, it may be suppressed by competition, but there will be metacognitive access to the taboo thought. But with more automaticity, or greater effort to compete against the taboo goal-image, metacognitive access may be lost and we may disavow the thought quite sincerely because it is no longer accessible. However, it may still influence well-practiced action systems. Thus repression could simply be automatic suppression.

7.8.3 The conflict-free sphere of conscious access and control

If goals can conflict, it makes sense to suppose that our normal, successful actions occur mostly in a domain of minimal competition. Otherwise we would show great hesitation and indecision even with acceptable and highly-practiced actions. There must be thousands of actions that are well within our power that we simply do not carry out because they conflict with other goals. Physically we are quite able to slap a close friend in the face, drop a baby, break a store window, or insult a colleague. We could deliberately break a leg or avoid eating for a month. These possibilities rarely become conscious even fleetingly; they are usually not even considered. Most goals that are consciously considered are not the objects of heavy competition from other goals. Ego psychologists like Hartmann (1958) refer to this domain of minimal competition as the "conflict-free sphere of the ego."

In Chapter 9 we will explore the relations between conflict-free voluntary action and self-attributed action. The conflict-free domain will then appear as one aspect of the notion of self (9.3.1).

7.9   Chapter summary

We began this chapter with a contrastive analysis comparing similar voluntary and involuntary actions. Next, the ideomotor theory of William James was explored and translated into GW theory; this in turn was found to explain the voluntary–involuntary contrasts. Voluntary control is treated as the result of conscious goal-images that are carried out consistent with the dominant goal context; conflicts with the goal context tend to become conscious and are edited by multiple unconscious criteria. Conscious goal-images are impulsive, and tend to be carried out barring competing goal-images or intentions. This perspective on voluntary control has implications for numerous phenomena, including slips, automaticity, psychopathological loss of control, decision making, the question of conscious access to abstract concepts, the issue of fleeting conscious events and source attribution, absorption, hypnosis, and even psychodynamics.

7.9.1 Some testable predictions from Model 5

We have made some strong claims in this chapter, not all of which are supported by direct and persuasive experimental evidence. The ideomotor theory especially needs much more testing.

One approach to testing the ideomotor theory may be to use experimentally elicited slips as actions to be triggered by ideomotor goal-images. A slip such as *darn bore – barn door* may increase in frequency if one shows a rapid picture of a farm immediately before the slip. We know this is true for relatively long exposures of words related to the slip (Motley, Camden, & Baars, 1979), but it may occur even if the exposure is so fast that it cannot be reported accurately, much like the Sperling figure (1.1.2). A further refinement might be to evoke a conscious mental image immediately before the action. In that case, one might be able to study the effects of automatization of the image (1.2.4). Highly automatized actions such as those studied by Shiffrin & Schneider (1977) should execute even with fleeting goal-images. Finally, one might induce a cue-dependent mental image by means of posthypnotic suggestion, with amnesia for the suggestion. Thus a highly hypnotizable subject may be told to feel an itch on his or her forehead when the experimenter clears his throat; one would expect the subject to scratch the hallucinatory itch, even though the subject was not told to scratch, merely to itch. But of course, this should generalize beyond itching and scratching. If the subject is sitting, he or she may be told to imagine on cue how the room looks from the viewpoint of someone who is standing up. If the ideomotor theory is correct, the subject should tend to stand up spontaneously. But since there has been no suggestion to stand up, this tendency cannot be attributed to hypnosis directly. Indeed, the tendency to stand up might be inhibited, so that one could only observe small movements in that direction, perhaps with postural muscle electrodes.

Similarly, one could induce competition against certain goal-images and study the ways in which inhibition of action can be lifted. In social situations, there is a set of prohibitions against inappropriate actions, which may be induced using experimentally evoked slip techniques. If we evoked an aggressive slip directed to the experimenter, such as *yam doo – damn you*, and created a distraction immediately after onset of the slip, would inhibitory restraints be lifted? If subjects were given a posthypnotic suggestion to feel an itch on cue, but to be embarassed to scratch the itch, would the inhibition be lifted by distraction? All these techniques are potentially informative about the ideomotor hypothesis.

7.9.2 Some questions Model 5 does not answer

This chapter has only addressed the issue of voluntary control: We do not yet know how this control is manifested in attention, the control of access to consciousness (Chapter 8). Further, we do not yet have an explicit role for metacognition, which is of course necessary in order to report that some event is voluntary or conscious. And finally, we do not know why voluntary actions are always attributed to the self as agent, and why involuntary actions are not attributed to oneself (Chapter 9). These are important questions for the following chapters.

Part V

Attention, self, and conscious self-monitoring

Common sense makes a useful distinction between conscious *experience* (as a subjectively passive state) and *attention*. The word *attention* implies control of access to consciousness, and we adopt this usage here. This can be readily modeled in the theory, as we see in Chapter 8. Attention in this sense involves access priorities, which must be informed by currently dominant goals. Attention itself can be either voluntary or automatic. This also raises the very central issue of *metacognitive access and control*, as we must often know about our previous conscious decisions to make voluntary choices about future conscious contents.

In Chapter 9, we adapt the method of minimal contrasts from previous chapters to give more clarity and empirical precision to the notion of *self*. A contrastive analysis of spontaneously self-attributed versus self-alien experiences suggests that self can be interpreted as the more enduring, higher levels of the Dominant Context Hierarchy, which create continuity over the changing flow of events. Thus, the self serves to organize and stabilize experiences across many different situations.

Because context is by definition unconscious in GW theory, self in this sense is thought to be inherently unconscious as well. This proposal is consistent with a great deal of objective evidence. However, aspects of self may become known through *conscious self-monitoring*, a process that is useful for self-evaluation and self-control. The results of conscious self-monitoring are combined with self-evaluation criteria, presumably of social origin, to produce a stable *self-concept*, which functions as a supervisory system within the larger self-organization.

299

8   Model 6:
Attention as control of access to consciousness

8.0   Introduction: Attention versus consciousness

Common sense makes a distinction between attention and consciousness. In everyday English we may ask someone to "please pay attention" to something, but not to "please be conscious" of it. Yet we know that when people pay attention to something they do become conscious of it. Likewise, we can "draw," "get," or "call" someone's attention *involuntarily* by shouting, waving, or prodding the person; as soon as we succeed, our subject becomes conscious of us. Nevertheless, we still do not speak of "getting" or "drawing" someone's consciousness.

It seems as if the psychology of common sense conceives of attention as something more active than consciousness, while consciousness itself is thought of as a "state." A similar distinction is implied in pairs of verbs like *looking* versus *seeing*, *listening* versus *hearing*, *touching* versus *feeling*, and so forth. In each case the primary sense of the first verb is more active, purposeful, and attentional, while the second verb refers to the conscious experience itself. Nor is this distinction limited to perception: It also works for memory, as in *recalling* versus *remembering*; even in the case of imagination, the verb *imagining* is more active and purposeful than *daydreaming*.

Of course consciousness is profoundly active, even when it is not experienced as such, and we have previously suggested that superficially purposeless thoughts may in fact serve specific goals (6.0). But the commonsense distinction between attention and consciousness is still important. It embodies the insight that there are attentional control mechanisms for access to consciousness – both voluntary and automatic – that determine what will or will not become conscious. It implies that attention involves metacognitive operations that guide the stream of consciousness.

This belief is backed by good evidence. We can obviously control what we will be conscious of in a number of voluntary ways: We can decide

Table 8.1. *Contrasts between voluntary and automatic control of attention*

Conscious	Unconscious
Voluntary decisions to make things conscious (e.g., being asked to pay attention to something, especially when this is effortful)	Automatic mechanisms for access to consciousness (e.g., one's own name breaking through from an unattended stream of speech)

whether or not to continue reading this book, whether to turn on the television, whether to stop thinking some unpleasant thought, and so on. Prototypically we can treat attention as analogous to the control of eye-movements. We can decide voluntarily to look at an object or to look away from it; in these cases, a conscious, voluntary, reportable decision precedes the act of attending (see Table 8.1). But of course, most eye-movements are not consciously controlled; they are automatically controlled by sophisticated systems that are not normally reportable. Of course the control of eye-movements is only a convenient prototype of attention. There must be analogous access-control systems for all the senses, for memory retrieval, for imagery, knowledge, and indeed for all sources of conscious contents. There is even attentional control in vision without moving the eyes (Posner & Cohen, 1982). Thus attention as access control is not one system but many; nonetheless, we will try to describe common features of all access control systems.

The distinction between voluntary and automatic control is crucial. Without flexible, voluntary access control, humans could not deal with unexpected emergencies or opportunities. We could not resist automatic tendencies when they became outdated, or change attentional habits to focus on new opportunities. Without automatic access control, on the other hand, rapid shifting to known significant events would be impossible. We need both voluntary and automatic attention.

For all these reasons we adopt here the commonsense view of *attention* as *that which controls access to conscious experience*. This chapter aims to enrich GW theory with this capacity.

8.0.1 Attention involves metacognition

The control of access to consciousness is inherently metacognitive. That is, it requires knowledge *about* our own mental functioning, and about the material that is to be selected or rejected. Voluntary attention would seem to require conscious metacognition, or the ability to have conscious access to and control over the different things that can become conscious.

Metacognition is a major topic in its own right, one we can only touch on here. It is widely believed that knowledge of one's own performance is required for successful learning (Flavell & Wellman, 1977). Among students in school, good learners continually monitor their own progress; poor learners seem to avoid doing so, as if fearing that the results might be too awful to contemplate (Bransford, 1979). But by avoiding conscious knowledge of results, they lose the ability to guide their own learning in the most effective way. We have previously maintained that consciousness is especially involved in the learning of new things, those that demand more adaptation (Chapter 5). If that is so, then attention (as metacognitive control of consciousness) seems to be necessary for voluntary, *purposeful* learning.

We have already remarked on the fact that we can only know that someone is conscious of something by a metacognitive act: "I just saw a banana." That is why our operational definition (1.2.1) is unavoidably metacognitive. But this is not the only important link between metacognition and consciousness. Many of the most important uses of consciousness are metacognitive. Normal access to Short Term Memory involves metacognitive control of retrieval, rehearsal, and report (see Figure 8.2). Long Term Memory retrieval is equally metacognitive. One cannot know consciously why or how one did something in the past without metacognitive access. Without metacognition one cannot deliberately repeat an action by evoking its controlling goal, nor can one construct a reasonably accurate and acceptable self-concept (9.0.2) without extensive metacognitive operations. All these functions require sophisticated – and partly conscious – metacognitive access and control, which inevitably becomes a major theme of this book from here on.

One of our main concerns in this chapter is the role of conscious metacognition in voluntary attention. One cannot choose consciously between two alternative conscious topics without anticipating something about the alternatives. That is, one must represent to oneself what is to be gained by watching the football game on television rather than reading an interesting book. Further, one must operate upon one's own system in order to implement that voluntary choice. These are all metacognitive operations. Later in this chapter we propose that human beings have access to something analogous to a computer "directory" or a "menu," which we will call an Options Context. The Options Context makes consciously available whatever immediate choices there are to attend to in sensation, memory, muscular control, imagery, and the like (see Figure 8.2). Voluntary control of attention then comes down to making a conscious decision (7.6.1) about current options. Since Options Contexts are called through the global workspace, control of the global workspace also determines one's ability to control voluntary attention.

8.0.2 *Attention is directed by goals*

We suggest in this chapter that attention is always controlled by goals, whether voluntarily or not. This is obvious in the case of voluntary attention: When we have the conscious, reportable goal of paying attention to the weather rather than to a good novel, we can usually do so. It is not so obvious for automatic attentional mechanisms, but the same case can be made there. If one's own name breaks through to consciousness from an unattended stream of material, while a stranger's name does not, this suggests that significant stimuli can exercise some sort of priority; but significant events are of course those that engage current goals (Moray, 1959). Since there was in this case no conscious decision to pay attention, there must be unconscious mechanisms able to decide what is important enough to become conscious. One's own name must surely be recognizable by the higher levels of the goal hierarchy. Indeed, we have previously touched on the idea that significant input can be defined as information that reduces uncertainty in a goal context; there is thus an inherent relationship between significance and goals (5.2.3). Therefore it seems likely that automatic attention is controlled by the goal hierarchy in such a way that more significant events tend to out-compete less significant ones.

Automatic attentional mechanisms have been widely investigated, in general by training subjects to detect or retrieve some information; but of course training works by teaching subjects that some previously trivial event is now a significant goal in the experiment. That is, in experimental training we always transmute the social and personal goals of the subject into experimental significance. A subject may come into the experiment intending to cooperate, to appear intelligent, to satisfy his or her curiosity, or to earn money; in the course of the experiment, this translates into a good-faith effort to detect tones in auditory noise or to spot faces in a crowd (e.g., Neisser, 1967). Successful performance on this previously irrelevant task is now perceived to be a means to satisfy one's more personal goals. Whatever motivates the subject to participate now becomes the indirect goal of the experimental task as well. In this sense, significance is something we create by the very social conditions of an experiment. Any experiment that trains automatic attention therefore involves a significant object of attention.

Thus attention has to do with the assignment of *access priority* among potentially conscious events. Practicing voluntary attention to the point of automaticity is known to improve the chances of an event becoming conscious (e.g., Neisser, 1967; 8.3.1). But of course in the real world those events that we decide voluntarily to pay attention to most often, and which therefore become highly practiced, are precisely those that are significant. We practice more voluntary attention to the color of a traffic light than to the paint on the pole that holds up the light. In the real world, significance and the amount of attentional practice covary.

8.1 Voluntary and automatic control of access to consciousness

We will maintain in this chapter that voluntary control of attention may be quite flexible, in contrast to automatic attention, which is relatively rigid because unconscious and automatic processes are insensitive to context (2.1). Whereas automatic attentional mechanisms seem to be controlled by the enduring Dominant Goal Hierarchy, there is reason to think that voluntary attention can operate independently of habitual goals to some degree. Even the most compulsive overeater can voluntarily ignore, at least for a while, the presence of delicious, tempting food. But doing this requires voluntary effort – there may be a struggle between the habitual goals of automatic attention and voluntary attention as controlled by recent conscious inner speech and imagery. We now explore these issues in some detail.

8.1.1 Voluntary attention: Conscious control of access to consciousness

According to the last chapter, volition comes down to ideomotor control. That is, it involves a momentary conscious goal-image that serves to recruit unconscious processors needed to carry out the goal. Thus voluntary control requires consciousness, at least briefly. But attention, according to the argument made just above, is the control of *access* to consciousness. It follows that voluntary attention is conscious control of access to consciousness.

This may sound paradoxical, but it is not. We can be conscious of the next thing we want to be conscious of, and display a goal-image to embody that intention. This goal-image in turn can trigger unconscious processes able to fulfill the intention. An obvious everyday example is the intention to watch a news program on television. Once the goal of watching the news becomes conscious, the details of walking to the TV set and turning the channel knob may be mostly automatic. It can be done in a preoccupied state, for example. The conscious attentional goal-image may be broadcast to many processors – for instance, to eye-movement-control nuclei in the brain stem. In the case of the program on television, once the goal of watching television becomes conscious with no competing goal-image or intention, our head and eyes will swivel in the right direction automatically. Thus attentional specialists may simply reside among the other unconscious specialists, and may be triggered into action just like the other action control systems discussed in Chapter 7.

8.1.2 Automatic attention: Unconscious control of access to consciousness

We already have proposed a simple mechanism whereby different unconscious events may access consciousness: namely, competition between input processors (2.2) guided by feedback from receiving processors (5.3). However, this kind of competition is not guided by system goals. Access that is not sensitive to goals may not be harmful when there is no urgency and enough time to allow different elements to come into consciousness to be evaluated for relevance. But random, impulsive access to consciousness becomes maladaptive when quick decisions are needed to survive or to gain some advantage. We would not want a stray thought to enter consciousness just when walking along the very edge of a cliff, or when making split-second decisions to avoid a traffic accident. We need some way in the GW model to connect automatic access control to the goal hierarchy; but we cannot afford to let existing goals control all input automatically, because some information whose significance is not yet known may become very important in the future. As usual, we face a trade-off between rapid, routine access, and flexible but slower access.

The role of significance is not the only thing to be explained; another major factor is practice. There is a sizable research literature on attentional automatization with practice in perceptual search (e.g., LaBerge, 1974; Neisser, 1967; Shiffrin & Schneider, 1977). We know, for example, that scanning a list for a well-practiced word will cause the target to "pop out" of the field. Evidently there are detection systems that present the target word to consciousness quite automatically once they find it. Similarly, items that come to consciousness in automatic memory search have a compelling, unavoidable quality, suggesting that here, too, access control to consciousness has become automatic (Sternberg, 1966; see 1.4.2). The same may be said for the well-known Stroop phenomenon, in which the printed *name* of a color word like "brown" or "red" tends to drive out the act of naming the *color* of the word. In all these cases, access to consciousness has itself become automatic and involuntary, at least in part due to practice. We have previously developed arguments that automaticity can be quite rigid and inflexible (2.1), and this suggests that automatic control of attention, too, can be rigid and dysfunctional in new situations.

The simple word game we have cited before can make the point. We can ask someone to repeat "poke, poke, poke, . . ." ten times, and then ask, "What do you call the white of an egg?" Even those who really know better will answer "the yolk" – presumably the first word that comes to mind. Or we can ask a person to repeat "flop, flop, flop, . . ." and ask, "What do you do at a green traffic light?" Most people tend to answer, "Stop" – which is not correct. Notice that this is a retrieval error, an error in bringing a word from memory to consciousness. Practicing the priming word only five or ten times will set the system to bring rhyming words to consciousness, as if conscious access control is at least momentarily controlled by rigid automatisms (Reason, in Baars, in press, c). Relying on automatic conscious availability is known to lead to errors in reasoning as well (Tversky & Kahneman, 1973).

Outside of the experimental setting, automatic attention must surely work as well. By comparison to the great research literature on voluntary recall there is only a small body of work on spontaneous memories, although in the real world spontaneous thoughts and memories are surely many times more common than deliberate acts of recall. Studies of thought monitoring indicate that the spontaneous flow of thought is highly sensitive to current personal significance, just as we would expect from the evidence discussed above (Horowitz, 1975a, b; Klinger, 1971; Pope & Singer, 1978).

8.2 Modeling voluntary and automatic access control

8.2.1 Model 6A: Automatic attention is guided by goals

Figure 8.1 shows how automatic attention might work in a GW frame-work. Suppose that there are "attentional contexts" – goal contexts whose main purpose is to bring certain material to mind: to move the eyes and head, to search for words in memory and bring them to conscious-ness, and so forth. These are symbolized in the diagram by context frames with the words "get *A*" or "get *B*." We have already discussed how the intention to retrieve a word may operate like this (6.1), so now we are only generalizing this notion. In the figure, two attentional contexts compete to guide mechanisms for bringing different materials to con-sciousness. In the beginning, context *A* dominates the stream of con-sciousness, as it might in listening to a football game on the radio. Stimulus *B* is able to interrupt the flow by virtue of its personal significance: It might be the listener's own name. How can this stimulus interrupt context *A*? The key idea is that the name is detected uncon-sciously (e.g., MacKay, 1973), and that it activates a high level in the Dominant Context Hierarchy in a way that is inconsistent with current

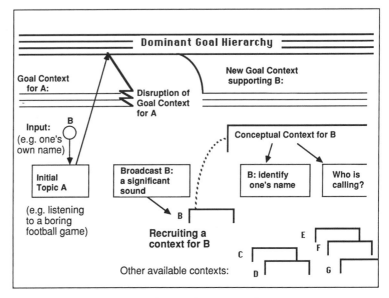

Figure 8.1. Model 6A: Automatic attention is controlled by goals. In automatic attentional control, certain stimuli have high-priority access to consciousness, apparently in line with their personal significance. For example, one's own name will tend to break through to consciousness from an unattended stream of information, even when it is not spoken very loudly. Physically intense or painful stimuli will break through as well. One hypothesis is that the significant stimulus *B* (such as one's name) receives support from high level goals in the Dominant Goal Hierarchy, at the same time disrupting the existing lower-level hierarchy that supported the previous conscious content *A*. This disruption then allows *B* to be broadcast, to recruit a new set of contexts able to interpret and support Topic *B*. This hypothesis allows us to explain how stimuli that are significant but not physically intense can automatically interrupt the dominant flow of conscious contents.

lower levels of the hierarchy. In Figure 8.1, the listener's own name may be recognized as important by high-level goals, which serve to disrupt the Dominant Context Hierarchy that controls the experience of the football game. The hierarchy is then reconstructed so as to take account of the new input *B* in the same way that a goal hierarchy is supposed to reorganize after any surprising event (4.4.1). The change in context may happen quickly enough so that the interrupting name can be identified and become conscious.

The ability to explain interruption by significant stimuli is very important theoretically. In Chapter 1 we noted that the various "filter" models of attention have not successfully explained either the interruption by personal names or the biasing of ambiguous conscious words by unconscious material (1.3.4). These models give rise to a "filter paradox," as follows: Let us suppose, along with conventional models, that attention involves a selective filter that eliminates certain input from consciousness. The filter must process and represent the meaning of an interrupting stimulus in order to keep it from consciousness. But if that is true, then having such a filter would save no perceptual processing capacity, because it takes as much capacity to detect something to eliminate it as it does to detect it in order to make it conscious.[1] But the entire rationale of selective attention by filtering rests on the assumption that it does save processing effort (Broadbent, 1958). Hence the filter paradox.

We have previously suggested that all input, conscious and unconscious, may be processed automatically to identify it; but only conscious material is broadcast systemwide. If that is true, then attention does save processing effort, but not on the input side. If all input, conscious and unconscious, is processed enough to identify it, the savings occur only in the fact that unconscious material is not broadcast systemwide, and therefore does not engage most of one's processing capacity.

We now suggest that unconscious material may either disrupt or shape the conscious stream if the unconscious input is recognized as relevant by the Dominant Context Hierarchy that currently controls the attended stream. *Disruption* of the dominant context can occur if the unconscious input activates higher levels of the goal hierarchy that are incompatible with current lower levels. If we are listening to a boring football game and someone calls our name, that may disrupt the Dominant Context Hierarchy controlling the conscious stream, because our own name is more significant than the boring game. Alternatively, the unconscious input may remain unconscious but help to *shape* the conscious experience (e.g., MacKay, 1973). If the unconscious input is compatible with the Dominant Context Hierarchy, as in the case of disambiguating unconscious words discussed in Section 1.3.4, unconscious input may help to shape the conscious experience. In this way, the unconscious word "river" can bias the conscious interpretation of an ambiguous word like "bank" – even though the unconscious word never becomes conscious. The GW approach therefore suggests a way of resolving the filter paradox for both of these experimentally demonstrated cases.

The main point, again, is that automatic attention is evidently sensitive to the Dominant Context Hierarchy, and particularly to dominant goals. Input that triggers a high-level goal seems to receive higher access priority to consciousness.

---

1   I am grateful to Michael Wapner for clarifying the "filter paradox" for me.

8.2.2 The Options Context for conscious metacognition

Thus far it seems that we can understand automatic attention without adding fundamentally new ideas. Voluntary attention will be somewhat more demanding.

In a computer one can find out the contents of memory by calling up a "directory," a list of files that may be selected. Given the directory, one can choose one or another file of information, and engage in reasoning about the different options: One file may lack the desired information; another may have it in an awkward format; a third may be so long that the information will be hard to find, and so on. Seeing the directory permits one to engage in conscious reasoning about the options. But once a file is selected, its contents will dominate the viewing screen. Exactly the same necessity and solution would seem useful in the nervous system.[2] It would be nice to have rapid conscious access to the alternatives one could pay attention to.

Even a well-known phenomenon such as Short Term Memory (STM) suggests that there is a such "directory" or "menu" of readily available options. We can retrieve information from STM; we can rehearse it, using voluntary inner speech; or we can report its contents. People can do any or all of these separable functions on request. Clearly all of them must be readily available. But how do we represent this fact in GW terms? We could say that certain specialists or contexts are highly active, ready to compete for access to consciousness. However, it seems more convenient to represent the options in a goal context of their own, much like the context of alternatives shown in Model 3 (Figure 5.5). Voluntary control of attention then comes down to ready conscious access to, and the ability to select, the choices defined within such an Options Context. Specialized processors could "vote" for the various options, as shown in Figure 7.3, and the winning option could evoke the appropriate effectors and subgoals by ideomotor control, as in Models 4 and 5 (6.2.1 and 7.3.2). Thus we seem to have all the makings for a mental directory already at hand, as shown in Figure 8.2.

An Options Context shows consciously available options for future conscious contents. It is shown in Figure 8.2 as a rounded frame with the options listed inside. Options Contexts may be evoked from among the receiving processors in the GW system by a conscious event, such as the question, "What should I do next?" Once the Options Context dominates the global workspace it presents a menu or directory of possible con-

---

2 I am grateful to David Spiegel and Jonathan Cohen for suggesting the directory analogy in the context of hypnosis.

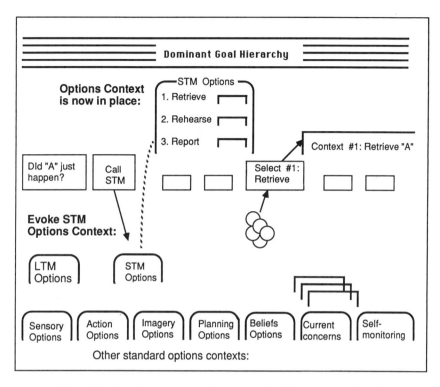

Figure 8.2. Conscious metacognitive access: Recalling an event from Short Term Memory. Voluntary attention requires the ability to access and select among potential alternative streams of consciousness. Thus, in deciding through conscious considerations to read a book rather than watch television, the two alternatives must be made consciously accessible to allow conscious and unconscious support to build up for each one. We propose a new entity, called an Options Context, that makes the alternative topics consciously accessible. It resembles a directory or menu on a computer, showing what can be accessed next. Many routine functions associated with consciousness, such as Short Term Memory (STM), voluntary muscle control, access to the senses, and Long Term Memory (LTM), may involve rapidly available Options Contexts, symbolized by the rounded frames above. Options Contexts seem necessary for conscious metacognition – our ability to access our own processes consciously – which in turn is vitally important for a number of normal mental processes. A critical point is that the Dominant Goal Hierarchy now controls access through the Global Workspace to all Options Contexts, as well as to the specialized processors and potentially dominant contexts.

scious contents; the most relevant one is chosen by a decision process, which may include votes from specialists as well as from the goal hierarchy; and the winning option then evokes a working context by ideomotor control. This may seem complex, but it is difficult to see a simpler way to implement what we know about voluntary attention.

Figure 8.2 shows how an Options Context might work in the case of Short Term Memory. The simplest event that may evoke STM might be a conscious query about some recent event to be recalled – "What just happened?" – but Short Term Memory is obviously used *in the service of* many other functions. For example, if we have a goal of gaining familiarity with a certain psychological theory, STM might be used to connect two recent ideas that were not previously connected. In that case the conscious query that evokes the STM Options Context might be, "How does the idea of 'attention' relate to 'consciousness?' " Options Contexts may be used as subgoals in the service of any dominant goal, including another Options Context. Thus the Self-monitoring Options Context in Figure 8.2 presumably makes routine use of Short Term Memory.

8.2.3 Model 6B: Voluntary attention allows conscious choice

We have previously noted that voluntary attention must be sensitive to the goal hierarchy, but that it cannot be completely controlled by automatic goals. After all, we can consciously work to change our own goals (8.2.4), and even the most habit-driven person can for some time avoid paying attention to habitual conscious contents. This may be quite difficult at times, but if it were impossible, people would lose the ability to change their goals. Flexibility is indeed the only reason to have voluntary attention in the first place, otherwise automatic attentional control would be quite sufficient. Somehow the current model must reflect the evidence that voluntary attention retains some amount of freedom from automatic control by the goal hierarchy.

Inherent in the global workspace, of course, is the notion that multiple sources of information can interact to create new responses to new conditions. Figure 8.2 shows how a coalition of specialized systems can "vote" for one or another option, something that is not possible with automatic attentional contexts as shown in Figure 8.1. Nevertheless, goal contexts can still influence the choice, and indeed, different parts of the goal hierarchy may support different conscious contents. From this point of view, conscious choices may cause the goal hierarchy to decompose; previously cooperating goal contexts may now compete in support of different options. This is indeed the definition of a dilemma – being caught between one deep goal and another. This is of course the stuff of human tragedy, on stage and off.

Conscious inner speech may be very important in maintaining voluntary attentional control when it runs counter to automatic tendencies. We have already cited the evidence from clinical experiments with children

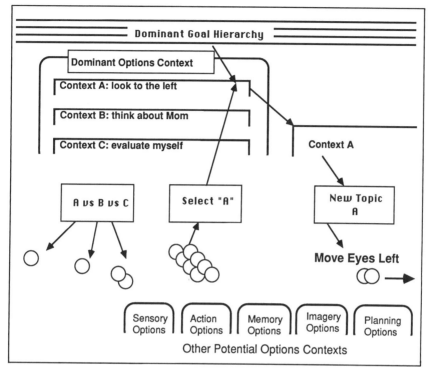

Figure 8.3. Model 6B: Voluntary control of attention: Options Contexts serve as directories of readily available conscious topics. This diagram shows the use of Options Contexts to exercise voluntary control over the selection of conscious contents. The Options Context presents the potential conscious topics; support for one option may come from specialized processors and/or the goal hierarchy. Conceivably, different goals in the Dominant Goal Hierarchy may support different options, leading to goal conflict. Notice that the choices within the Options Context may consist of other Options Contexts. Like ordinary contexts, Options Contexts may be recursive. In the diagram Context *A* wins out, becomes dominant, and then causes Topic *A* to become conscious. This can be compared to Figure 8.1 in which attentional control is automatic, so that no Options Context is necessary.

who have impulse-control problems, showing that teaching them to speak to themselves is helpful in maintaining control (Meichenbaum & Goodman, 1971). On a short-term basis, voluntary inner speech and voluntarily retrieved mental images may also be helpful to fight off automatic attentional tendencies (Figure 8.3). In the model, conscious availability of recent thoughts – for example, "Do your homework, don't think about playing outside!" – may help to control the automatic tendencies, at least for a while. Thus recency may be used to combat automaticity. But a permanent victory for the voluntary control effort presumably requires the creation of a new, coherent context within which the automatic choices are differently defined (4.3.5).

8.2.4 Automatizing voluntary attention

Experimental studies of trained perceptual access may mimic the way in which normal attentional mechanisms become automatic. In a typical experiment, subjects are asked to pay attention voluntarily to something they would normally ignore (e.g., Neisser, 1967). Subjects come into the experiment with their own goals, which range from earning money to impressing the experimenter. In order to achieve these goals, they are asked to do something that was previously quite irrelevant to them. Searching for a conscious stimulus – a famous face in a picture of a crowd, for example – is given very high priority by the experimental instructions. The instructions say, in effect, that in order for the subject to perform satisfactorily, he or she must pay attention to the face in the crowd. The task is repeated over and over again until it becomes automatic – that is, until the alternatives in the voluntary Options Contexts for the task are reduced to one (5.3.1).

If we can generalize from this situation, there are apparently two necessary conditions for creating automatic access to consciousness:

1 A target that has low priority for access is given high priority by a temporary, consciously available goal-image, which may be associated with high levels of the permanent goal hierarchy; for example, social compliance in an experiment.

2 Voluntary attention to the target is practiced until the Options Context has no more degrees of freedom, so that it changes into a single automatic goal context (Figure 8.1).

Presumably one's own name acquires associations early in life with high priority goals, such as one's desire for attention, for protection and care, for food, or for avoiding punishment. And surely paying voluntary attention to one's name occurs many thousands of times. Hence, presumably, the Moray phenomenon of the subject's name breaking through to consciousness by virtue of automatic access control.

We can now consider two important cases of attentional control, directing attention toward something versus directing it away from something. The first is obviously important, and the second raises the classical psychodynamic issues of suppression and repression, which can be easily modeled in GW theory.

8.3 Directing attention *toward* something

Suppose we feel hungry, and have some conscious image of delicious food. Inherently, this image, we have argued, recruits processors able to help achieve the goal, and these must include attentional processors. If we are able to reach for food automatically, little attentional control would seem to be required. But if we must think about how to reach the desired food, to deal with obstacles, or to make choices about equally attractive alternatives, the goal-image should be able to recruit access of these issues to consciousness. Given an interesting conscious goal-image, recruitment of attention should happen automatically along with recruitment of other subgoals. The simplest case of directed attention toward something involves one goal-image that recruits automatic eye-movements, memory search, and so forth, in order to bring up a conscious content.

8.3.1 *Using voluntary attention to create new access priorities*

One way to make an unimportant stimulus important is to associate it explicitly with one's major goals. This is indeed what one does in conditioning. Pavlov's dog was typically deprived of food for a day or so, so that eating became highly significant in the goal hierarchy. Through paired repetition, the famous bell then became a signal for food, so that it functioned as a conscious event that engaged the eating goal. Similarly, in operant conditioning, the act of wiggling one's tail may become a subgoal after which, magically, food appears in the Skinner Box. While one must be cautious in anthropomorphizing animal experience, surely the experience of humans in such a situation is easy to guess. It often involves explicit, conscious association of the conditioned event with a preexisting, significant goal: "Aha! So pushing this button always gives the right answer" (Dawson & Furedy, 1976).

Nor is conscious association of new events with existing high-level goals limited to the laboratory. One extremely common persuasive technique used by all politicians and advertisers is to associate a previously irrelevant event with a major life goal of the audience. Underarm deodorant was not very important before millions of people were consciously reminded that it is a *sine qua non* of social acceptability. For our purpose, this suggests two critical points: one, that the event to be connected to the significant goal must be conscious; and two, that this event can then come to control attentional mechanisms that control access of the previously irrelevant event to consciousness.

8.3.2 *Mental effort due to competition between voluntary and automatic attention*

We have defined "mental effort" as voluntary control against unpredicted resistance (7.6.2). One obvious example involves trying to control one's attention voluntarily against contrary automatic tendencies.

All children know how it feels to have homework when they really want to go outside and play. The process here presumably involves decision making (7.6.1), except that the decision is not in the first instance about *doing* something – it is about *paying attention to* something. That is, it is a struggle whose first outcome is purely mental. The act of paying attention to homework is more novel and effortful and less pleasant, and hence requires more conscious involvement, than the routine and pleasant act of thinking about playing. But once the issue is decided, one may become absorbed in the chosen path, which is itself controlled by unconscious contexts, naturally. Then the experience of struggle and effort may utterly disappear, even for tasks that were initially seen as onerous and boring. Absorption is typically experienced as positive, perhaps because we simply do not monitor our experiences when we are truly absorbed (8.5.1). Or perhaps absorption is inherently pleasant as well (Czikzsentmihalyi & Czikszentmihalyi, 1988).

This kind of mental effort is a struggle between voluntary and automatic attention. Presumably the conscious goal-images of having to do homework serve to recruit additional processors and contexts, which may be able to "outvote" the automatic attentional systems promising fun and adventure by playing outside. This voluntary decision may have to be repeated a number of times at natural choice-points in the task. After taking a break from doing homework, the same struggle may have to be repeated. At each decision point, the intention to think about playing outside will tend to come up automatically, while the intention to continue with homework will have to be raised voluntarily, perhaps with the aid of a powerful motivating goal-image or inner-speech reminder. Each decision point can be viewed as a case of the voting process discussed in section 7.6.1, but one that is *meta*cognitive – that is, it concerns what is to become conscious later.

Obviously some of the recruited voting systems may be more significant than others. If some deep goal context is recruited to support homework – such as the promise of quick approval by a loving parent, or the threat of ridicule by an older sibling – the relevant deeper goal contexts can move the vote in one direction or another (Figure 8.2). During the decision struggle, conscious thoughts related to these deeper goals may aid one or the other side in the process.

We can see this struggle for control especially in vigilance tasks, in which people are asked to monitor a blip on a radar screen, or some other minor perceptual event in an otherwise boring situation. Attentional control drops quite rapidly under these circumstances (Mackworth, 1970), but variation in attentional focus is quite normal even in interesting tasks (Warm, 1984). In all of these cases, one may enter a period of conflict between voluntary tendencies to continue attending with high efficiency and the spontaneous or automatically controlled tendency to attend less well.

8.3.3 The importance of accurate source attribution

For effective metacognitive control, we should be able to refer to previous or future events with accuracy. If we decide to repeat something we just learned, by the arguments in Chapter 7 we should be able to retrieve the relevant goal-image and guiding goal context. Similarly, if we are to answer questions about our own thoughts, we must be able to refer to them. *Accurate source attribution* – knowing why and how we did what we did – seems vital for these tasks. We know, however, that source attribution fails in a number of important cases (Ericsson & Simon, 1984; Langer & Imber, 1979, Nisbett & Wilson, 1977; Weiner, 1986). That is, much of the time we lose track of why and how we did what we did, so that it becomes difficult to report these things accurately.

We have discussed the Langer & Imber (1979) study, in which automaticity in a task undermined the ability of people to report the features of the task and made them more vulnerable to a misleading attribution about their own performance. In terms of the model, we can simply see how with practice, a voluntary Options Context is reduced to a single option (that is, just a single goal context). Further, goal-images should become more fleeting over time if they are predictable. In either case, it should become much more difficult to retrieve the way in which one performed the task.

8.4   Directing attention *away from* something:
Suppression, repression, and emotional conflict

Although there is unresolved controversy in the scientific literature about the existence of repression, there is no real doubt about the existence of some sort of tendentious evasion of conscious contents. Even the most skeptical observers acknowledge that people tend to make self-serving errors and interpretations whenever there is enough ambiguity to permit this. The scientific arguments seem to revolve around the issue of repression, defined as *unconscious* inhibition of troubling conscious contents (e.g., Erdelyi, 1985; Holmes, 1972, 1974). This is of course a terribly contentious issue, because we do not currently have good scientific tools for assessing these zero-point issues (1.1.2). It is very difficult to tell with certainty whether someone really knew, even momentarily, that a thought was sufficiently threatening to avoid. But the fact of avoidance, and even some of the mechanisms of avoidance, are not really in question.

How can we possibly avoid thinking of some topic if the decision to avoid it is itself conscious? Children play a game in which the participants try to avoid thinking about pink elephants, and of course they cannot do so. There is a contradiction between having the guiding goal-image "pink elephants" and trying to avoid it at the same time. Similarly, in clinical hypnosis there is extensive lore suggesting that subjects should not be given negative suggestions. To help someone to stop smoking it is not helpful to say, "You will stop thinking of cigarettes," because the suggestion itself contains the thought of cigarettes. Thus directing attention *away from* something seems to be quite different from directing it *toward* something.

8.4.1 Thought avoidance can occur in many ways

The "pink elephant" game cited above should not be taken to suggest that people simply cannot avoid conscious thoughts in a purposeful way. There is very good evidence for the effectiveness of thought avoidance in experiments with both normal and clinical populations (e.g., Meichenbaum & Bowers, 1984). Several mechanisms may serve to exclude information from consciousness. These range from changes in receptor orientation, as in evasive eye-movements, to deliberate failure to rehearse items in Short Term Memory in order to forget them, or tendentious reinterpretation of experiences and memories (Bjork, 1972; Holmes, 1972; Loftus & Palmer, 1974).

"Directed forgetting" is one example (Bjork, 1972). People in a Short Term Memory experiment are simply told to forget certain items, and they will do so quite well. They probably rehearse only what they need to remember, and the to-be-forgotten items fall by the wayside. That is, one can use the limited capacity of Short Term Memory to load one topic in order to avoid another. This is indeed the principle of distraction: Every human being must engage in some distraction sometimes to avoid pain, boredom, or difficulty. In these cases there is no doubt about the existence of conscious thought avoidance.

In general, we can distinguish between *structural* and *momentary* evasions. A religious belief system may help the believer escape anxiety about death and disease. After all, almost all religions provide reassurance about these things. Once a reassuring belief system is accepted and not challenged it creates a conceptual context for the believers' experience (4.2.2); thus certain anxious thoughts presumably will come to mind much less often. There is a close connection between this common observation and the claim made in Chapter 7 that the ideomotor theory suggests an interpretation of trust and confidence in terms of a low degree of competition between different conscious thoughts (7.7.2). Suppose that thought *A* is anxiety about disease, and not-*A* proclaims that disease is only a trial on the way to heaven; if not-*A*, once thought, is not contradicted, there is a conclusive answer to the source of anxiety. Probably most human beings in the world operate within self-serving belief systems of this kind. Their prevalence suggests that reassuring belief systems are quite effective, often for a period of years.

There are obviously also *momentary* evasions, such as not looking at beggars on the street, avoiding the gaze of dominant or frightening persons, and avoiding recall cues for unwanted memories. In principle any of these mechanisms can come under purposeful control, either voluntary or involuntary.

8.4.2 When we lose voluntary access to avoided thoughts, there is the appearance of repression

In fact, the clinical evidence for repression is just *apparently purposeful but disavowed failure in voluntary access to normally conscious events*. If we fail to recall some painful event that happened just yesterday, even though we remember everything else; or if we cannot remember a thought that challenged a fundamental belief; or if we fail to make an inference that seems obvious but is painful to contemplate; any cases like these are clinically likely to be interpreted as repression. One classical example is the *belle indifférence* of the conversion hysteric, who may be suffering from psychogenic blindness, local anesthesia, or paralysis, but who may deny that this is much of a problem (Spitzer, 1979). Thus the key is failure of voluntary metacognitive access. (*Involuntary* measures of memory may not show any decrement: We know that recognition, skill learning, and savings in recall may survive failures of voluntary recall [Bower, 1986].) But of course we can model such access failure in Model 6 (8.2.3). Figure 8.4 shows how the outward evidence for repression may be modeled in GW theory.

8.4.3 Signal anxiety as ideomotor control of thought avoidance

There is a very interesting connection between these ideas and the psychodynamic notion of anxiety as a signal. GW theory suggests that people may have fleeting quasi-conscious goal-images that may serve to

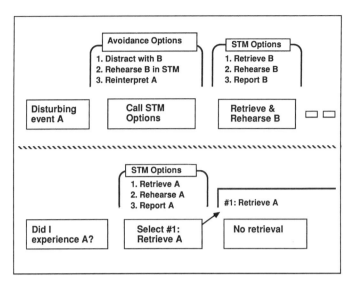

Figure 8.4. Repression as source amnesia for avoided conscious contents. Thought avoidance can happen in many ways: e.g., by distraction from the conscious event *A* that is to be avoided, by failure to rehearse *A*, by reinterpreting it, or by accessing a conceptual context in which *A* does not exist. In this example, topic *A* is avoided simply by retrieving and rehearsing topic *B:* The limited capacity of conscious experience ensures that *A* is not readily available. When memory is queried at a later point, topic *A* cannot be retrieved, perhaps because it was too fleeting, or because in the context of *B* it is very difficult to retrieve voluntarily (e.g., Bower, 1986). Such a sequence of events may suggest purposeful repression to an outside observer, and indeed, it may be under the purposeful control of a goal context. Notice that other, nonvoluntary measures of memory may still reveal the presence of *A*. But accurate voluntary retrieval is necessary for such normal mental functions as spontaneous autobiographical memory; knowing how and why one does something; the ability to repeat an action by retrieving its controlling goal-image; accurate self-attribution of responsibility; maintaining impulse-control; and the construction of an accurate and acceptable self-concept. In sum, successful repression requires no more than a tendentious breakdown in voluntary recall, which can happen in many ways (Erdelyi, 1985).

mobilize attentional mechanisms for avoidance of certain conscious contents. This is precisely the role of signal anxiety. While the notion of signal anxiety may sometimes apply to clearly conscious feelings, some sources suggest that people can have very fleeting images that serve as warnings to avoid certain upsetting thoughts. Thus Freud is quoted as writing that thinking must aim "at restricting the development of affect in thought-activity to the minimum required for acting as a signal" (Freud, 1926/1936, p. 5). In discussing the appearance of "substitutive ideas" in phobia, that is, ideas that may evoke less fear than the original phobic object, Freud writes that "Excitation . . . give[s] rise to a slight development of anxiety; and this is now used as a signal to inhibit . . . the further progress of the development of anxiety." Here is another point of theoretical contact. Note that the same ideas play a role in behavior-modification theory of phobia. For example, one can have a hierarchy of increasingly upsetting mental images about fire. A fire phobic may be able to have the thought of a book of matches with little fear, but the thought of a bonfire may be quite frightening. The image of a matchbook may then act as a safe goal-image, which may trigger avoidance mechanisms that help the person to stay away from the really troubling mental images.

8.5   Further implications

8.5.1 Absorption and suspension of disbelief

Conscious metacognition should of course compete with other limited-capacity events, including the conscious content that is being controlled attentionally. We cannot read this book and at the same time entertain the conscious possibility of doing other things. It follows that absorption in a stream of events, such as a movie or piece of music, should decrease access to metacognitive options. One common observation is that when we become absorbed in a film or novel, we can easily identify with the main characters. In the parlance of the theater, we "suspend disbelief." If disbelief is a conscious disputing of previous conscious contents (7.8.1), this is easy to model in GW theory. We need only suppose that disbelief requires an Options Context of the form, "Is what I just experienced really true or acceptable?" In deeply absorbed states accessing these conscious options may be competed out of consciousness. Suspension of disbelief then presumably liberates our tendencies to identify with attract-ive fictional models, free from inhibition and contradiction. We can allow ourselves for a while to live in wishful fantasy.

8.5.2 Hypnosis may decrease access to Options Contexts

Chapter 7 suggested that hypnosis is reducible to absorbed ideomotor control. If that is true, and if absorption implies a decrease of access to attentional options, then we may be able to explain the extraordinary compliance of hypnotic subjects. We may suggest that self–other differ-entiation often requires a momentary conscious decision: "Did I really want that, or was I persuaded by advertising to want that?" "Did the hypnotist tell me to raise my arm, or did I tell myself to do so?" Compliance in highly hypnotizable subjects may therefore follow from their capacity to be deeply absorbed in the hypnotic situation, to the point where no conscious capacity is available to reflect on the situation from an outside perspective. Previously we were able to account for several other features of hypnosis (7.7.2), but not the remarkable compliance with suggestion, and the lack of resistance of unusual suggestion. We can now fill in this gap.

8.5.3 *The role of attention in motivation and the maintenance of mental stability*

There are thousands of experiments focused on "perceptual defense," the apparent tendency of people to avoid reporting rapidly flashed words that are obscene or conflictful (Erdelyi, 1974). However, these experiments apparently showed two opposite tendencies. People sometimes underreported taboo words ("perceptual defense") and sometimes over-reported them compared to control words ("perceptual sensitization"). This seemed to be a paradox, which led to considerable criticism and disillusionment. However, the coexistence of defense and sensitization may not be just an experimental difficulty, but a fundamental fact about human allocation of attention. After all, we must do two things when presented with something painful, alarming, or ego-threatening: First, we must know that it is there, so that we can cope with it; second, if possible, we try to avoid it. If the event is novel, we presumably need conscious involvement in order to identify it and to learn to avoid it. Thus the existence of both sensitization and avoidance is something one might predict on an a priori basis.

This suggests that attention may have two major functions:

> 1 Allocation of conscious involvement to significant events and problems by making them conscious in proportion to their motivational signifi-cance; this includes painful, alarming, or ego-threatening events. Some examples include the resistance of significant stimuli to habituation; the ability of one's own name to interrupt ongoing streams of conscious events; and our tendency to pay more attention to problems that demand more novel solutions.

This role of attention may be countered by another function, which is,

> 2 Regulating the flow of novel information, so that we do not confront either too much, or the wrong kind of novelty. We can think of this as protecting the Context Hierarchy from too-rapid change. Thoughts that threaten the stability of one's beliefs are avoided by most people.

Notice that in the case of painful sources of information, these two tendencies will run counter to each other: On the one hand, pain or threat is important, and therefore deserves attention; on the other, it may demand such a fundamental change in the Context Hierarchy that it is, rather, avoided.

It is possible that psychodynamic thought-avoidance results from this second role of attention. Excessive novelty, especially emotionally charged novelty, may threaten a fundamental realignment of the Goal Hierarchy. This hierarchy is connected to the notion of self in Chapter 9.

8.5.4 Some further thoughts about the operational definition of conscious experience

Chapter 1 suggested an operational definition for conscious experience, one that we have tried to adhere to quite faithfully. Namely, we were going to consider something a conscious experience if it could be reported accurately, and was claimed by the subject to be conscious. Early in the theoretical development we could not model this phenomenon of accurate retrospective report because it is actually quite complicated. It involves

> consciousness of an event (e.g., 5.3)
> retrospective ability to direct conscious recall voluntarily to the event (e.g., 8.3)
> the ability to recode the event into speech or gestures (e.g., 7.64, 7.65)
> the ability voluntarily to carry out those words or gestures. (e.g., 7.3)

In brief, in order to model the operational definition we first needed a usable conception of consciousness, volition, and attentional access. We had to "bootstrap" upward from the operational definition, until eventually we could hazard a true theoretical account. Ultimately, of course, every theory must explain its own operational definitions. Are we ready to do so now?

Notice that, initially, there is merely a conscious experience of a banana. Numerous systems adapt to this conscious event, including systems able to re-present a later image of the conscious event, voluntarily, on cue, in the context provided by a goal system that is instantiated by the experimental instructions. This goal system, when it is triggered by the question, "What did you just experience?" acts to guide a search for a plausible answer. Miyake & Norman (1978) have pointed out that finding a plausible answer to any question, such as "What was George Washington's telephone number?" requires a complex and sophisticated search, one that we would frame within a goal context. Similarly, a subject who has been instructed to report what he sees while looking at a television screen, and who perceives a banana on the screen, must know that the correct answer is "banana" and not "television screen." So there is a large interpretive component in answering even seemingly obvious questions.

Once it is interpreted properly, it is reasonable to think that one can voluntarily attempt to recall recent events, decide which ones could be meant by the questioner, retrieve it as an image, redisplay it consciously, and allow unconscious verbal systems to search for a lexical match: "a banana." Again, it takes a voluntary act to carry out the verbal report, which involves, by the arguments of Chapter 7, a momentarily conscious goal-image of the distinctive aspects of the action (perhaps the word "banana" in inner speech), the goal-image is rapidly inspected by numerous systems able to check its propriety, and, barring contrary images or intentions, it executes. Complex? Certainly, yes. But probably not too complex in the face of psychological reality.

It is quite satisfying to be able to give a plausible descriptive account of one's operational definition after seven or eight chapters of hard work. It suggests again that we are on the right track.

8.6   Chapter summary

This chapter has explored the topic of attention, defined as access control to consciousness. There is a traditional distinction between voluntary and involuntary attention of which we can make good use. Automatic attention apparently involves unconscious mechanisms for bringing things to consciousness in a way that is controlled by the goal hierarchy, so that significant things have access priority. Voluntary attention requires a new idea: the notion of an Options Context, which presents alternative things one could aim to make conscious next. As before, these comparatively simple ideas have widespread implications for other psychological questions. There is a distinction between calling attention to some topic and steering attention away from some painful or threatening topic. Both kinds of phenomena can be accommodated in the GW framework. Finally, in this chapter we have explored some of the implications for absorption, hypnosis, and the operational definition of conscious experience that was proposed in Chapter 1.

9   Model 7:
Self as the dominant context of experience and action

The total self [is] partly known and partly knower, partly object and partly subject . . . we may call one the *Me* and the other the *I* . . . I shall therefore treat the self as known or the *me*, and . . . the self as knower, or the *I*.

William James, 1892 (p. 189; italics in original)

Unidentified Guest:
There's a loss of personality
Or rather, you lost touch with the person
You thought you were. You no longer feel quite human.
You're suddenly reduced to the status of an object –
A living object, but no longer a person.
It's always happening, because one is an object
As well as a person. But we forget about it
As quickly as we can. When you've dressed for a party
And are going downstairs, with everything about you
Arranged to support you in the role you have chosen,
Then sometimes, when you come to the bottom step
There is one step more than your feet expected
And you come down with a jolt. Just for a moment
You have the experience of being an object
At the mercy of a malevolent staircase.

T. S. Eliot, 1950 (pp. 29–30)

9.0   Introduction

It was not the original intent in this book to deal with "self." However, there are good reasons to think that we cannot discuss consciousness adequately without introducing some reasonable conception of self (e.g., Dennett, 1978; Nagel, 1974; Tulving, 1985). This makes it necessary to explore the question, though "self" really requires a separate book. There is of course a profound literature on the psychology of self and

This chapter has been influenced by ideas proposed by Michael A. Wapner, David Spiegel, Werner Erhard, and David Galin, who are hereby gratefully acknowledged.

other, with major scientific, clinical, and philosophical contributions (e.g., A. Freud, 1938; S. Freud, 1923/1962; Hartmann, 1958; Horowitz & Zilberg, 1983; Kihlstrom & Cantor, 1984; Kohut, 1971; Markus & Sentis, 1982). We cannot deal with this great literature here with any adequacy, but in a tentative way we can outline some ways in which the current theory may make contact with it.

We take the viewpoint here that some notion of "self" in psychological theory is not a luxury, not a metaphysical or artificial issue, but a necessity for any complete psychological framework. In this respect "self" is like consciousness, a core psychological problem that stubbornly survives all attempts to ignore or circumvent it. Self–other differentiation is a central concern in perceptual–motor systems, in mother–child interaction, in the development of autonomy, and even, as recent good evidence indicates, in the workings of the immune system.

Some commentators suggest that consciousness is essentially the domain of access of the self. Thus Dennett writes:

> That of which I am conscious is that to which I have *access*, or (to put the emphasis where it belongs), that to which *I* have access. (Dennett, 1978, p. 149)

This idea has a good deal of intuitive plausibility. It certainly fits our ordinary language: All statements about conscious experience use personal pronouns, as in "I saw a pussycat," "You are only imagining that pain in your tummy," "She smelled a rat," and so forth. Certainly we would be surprised if we were unable to access consciously some vivid recent memory, some sight, smell, or taste in the immediate environment, or some well-known fact about our own lives. The "self" involved in conscious access is sometimes referred to as *the self as observer*. Similarly, all commonsense statements of voluntary control have "self" as the initiator or actor in charge, as in "I told him to go," "He decided to find out more," and "I am responsible for my own actions." Again, we would be surprised and upset if we were unable to move an arm, to stop an intended speech act, or to control a usually controllable conscious desire. The controlling agency for this expected domain of voluntary control is sometimes labeled *the self as agent* (e.g., James, 1890/1983).

A number of behavioral psychologists maintain that the notion of self is a delusion of common sense; perhaps we simply infer a nonexistent agent in charge of our actions and experiences, creating an imaginary entity where there is none. Certainly people sometimes make false inferences. The scientific question is, of course: Is there an underlying reality that can justify the inference? If there is, then "self" is not delusional; it is something we need to understand.

In this chapter we develop the idea that "self" can be operationally defined as *that system whose change or violation is spontaneously interpreted as a loss of the sense of self.* The Jamesian "I," in other words, is only knowable directly by the experiences that take place in moments of challenge and change. This makes sense theoretically because we can interpret self as an enduring Dominant Context, near the topmost levels of the Dominant Context Hierarchy. We have previously cited evidence that contexts can be accessed consciously mainly through mismatch – through change or violation in contextual expectations (4.4.3). In the same way, it may be that self becomes accessible to experience mainly through mismatch.

The idea of "mismatch with self" leads naturally to a contrastive analysis of self versus not-self reports. People report self-alien experiences in many situations that seem superficially just like the normal, self-consistent experiences that most of us have most of the time. Spontaneous self-alien experiences are reported in disorders like depersonalization, psychogenic fugue, and multiple personality (9.1.1). Reliable evidence is available about these conditions, and they are all grist for our mill. We develop a contrastive analysis based on this evidence.

We will conclude that the self can be viewed theoretically as *the enduring higher levels of the Dominant Context Hierarchy, including both conceptual and goal contexts.* Thus the self-system is more than just another knowledge representation – it is knowledge that provides the framework for all conscious experience. Self, in this sense, is a perspective, a point of view, an overarching context for the flow of conscious events. It has perceptual–motor, evaluative, conceptual, motivational, and social aspects. The self-system evidently mediates and creates continuity among more local contexts.

The word "self" will be used as an abbreviation for "self-system," and contrasted to the self-*concept*, which is a set of beliefs *about* oneself. The self-concept corresponds to James's *Me*. Like any context, self has aspects that can be decontextualized and experienced as objects of consciousness (5.3.4). These objectified aspects of self can then be used to construct a model of self; but, contrary to some suggestions, we suggest that this model of ourselves is not the self itself. When T. S. Eliot's Unidentified Guest in the epigraph remarks on the experience of stumbling on the staircase on the way to a party, he is pointing to a moment where an aspect of the self as context comes to be experienced as conscious content or object. Stumbling is a violation of expectations, of course, and suddenly, from being in charge and confident of one's reception at the party, one becomes an object "at the mercy of a malevolent staircase." We humans are often surprised by our own reactions to a new situation, suggesting again that the self (as Dominant

Context) and self-concept (as one's beliefs about oneself) are not the same. However, in the normal course of events we are continually, smoothly switching back and forth between self as context and aspects of self as objects of experience.

Thus our notion of self corresponds to what James called the *I* while the self-concept, insofar as it is consciously accessible, corresponds to James's *Me*. As a set of beliefs about oneself, the self-concept is based on experiences of oneself *as if seen from an outside perspective*. When people are asked about themselves they will express some part of their self-concept, but the self itself is not immediately available to put into words. For this reason it is best to avoid using the beliefs people express about themselves as evidence for the self; it is, of course evidence about their self-concepts.

The self-*concept* may function as a monitoring system within the larger self-system. One's beliefs about oneself, including beliefs about how one *should* be, can serve as a tool to evaluate and control thoughts and actions. In adults, most voluntary activities can be quickly tested against the self-concept. That is, most of the time adults can answer the question, "Is what I am doing right now really what I should be doing?" In the language of psychodynamics, the self-concept includes the ego-ideal (Freud, 1923/1962). Severe violations of the self-concept are experienced as shameful, guilt-provoking, or depressing, as we fall short of our ideal self. Matches with self-concept may be experienced as pride, self-acceptance, and satisfaction.

In sum, in this chapter we explore both a theoretical opportunity and a necessity. The necessity comes from the fact that any discussion of consciousness seems incomplete without appeal to some plausible self-system; the opportunity lies in the fact that we can develop one such concept straightforwardly from what we already know. Indeed, access to a self-system may be a necessary condition for conscious experience. This perspective has implications for motivational conflict, the disruptive nature of emotional upset, impulse control, and attributional ambiguity (Mandler, 1975a; Weiner, 1986; 9.6). We will now develop these ideas in detail.

9.0.1 The self-system is opaque to direct introspection

How could we approach the organization of self? First of all, we can try to pinpoint a set of empirical operations that presumably reflect it. There are a number of reasons to believe that the evidentiary basis of self may be different from the evidence for our readily available *concept* of ourselves. Here are a few reasons for this distinction.

Resistance to self-knowledge

Perhaps the most obvious reason to differentiate between the self-system and self-concept are the psychodynamic barriers to self-knowledge, the extent to which we profit from self-deception (Goleman, 1985; Holmes, 1972, 1974). One does not need to accept all of psychodynamic theory to believe that wishful thinking (and sometimes catastrophic thinking) stands in the way of an accurate self-concept. Indeed, even the scientific skeptics do not question the existence of pervasive self-serving distortions about ourselves (Holmes, 1978). In everyday life we often surprise ourselves with unexpected feelings, actions, and images. If we knew ourselves thoroughly this could not happen. Accurate self-knowledge seems to be culturally and developmentally sophisticated, and rare; it may always be incomplete.

Other sources of incorrect self-knowledge

But we do not have to appeal to wishes and fears, repression, or emotional conflict to note the absence of accuracy in many self-descriptions. A number of social psychological studies show that people often make false claims about themselves when there seems to be little motivational payoff in doing so. These studies emerge from two streams of investigation within social psychology, one focused on errors of attribution, and the second on the induction of cognitive dissonance. In a typical attribution study a subject may be led to believe that the sound of an accelerating heartbeat is the sound of his or her own heart. This false feedback has been shown to affect subjects' perceptions of their own emotional excitement, say, in the context of threatening stimuli (e.g., Valins, 1967; see also Schachter & Singer, 1962). Further, a wide variety of cognitive dissonance studies show that subjects will evaluate an unpleasant event more highly if they are given *in*adequate justification for their involvement in the unpleasant event. Presumably they create a higher evaluation to justify their involvement *post hoc* (Festinger, 1957). In general, these studies show that people are consistently inaccurate in their descriptions of their own motives.

Nisbett & Wilson (1977) claim on the basis of such studies that human beings have no privileged access at all to their own processes. This conclusion has been widely criticized as overstated (e.g., Ericsson & Simon, 1984; White, 1982). The critics have pointed out that there are many persuasive cases of accurate introspection, and that what we really need to know is *under what conditions* we can expect accurate judgments about ourselves. Nevertheless, the evidence remains strong that people cannot tell us about themselves much of the time, even when common sense would expect them to be able to do so. For example, when people choose from a display of identical stockings, they will tend to choose the right-most, or the best-illuminated stockings. Asked to explain their preference, they will generate hypotheses with an air of conviction; but they will not know the reasons for their action. There are numerous examples of this kind, showing that very often people do not know their own motives. The study by Langer & Imber (1979) on misinterpreting one's own automatic performance makes this point very clearly. In general, human beings greatly overestimate the accuracy of their self-knowledge, and seem to freely fabricate answers about their intentions, especially when the information available to make the judgment is inadequate.

Self-concept is typically oversimplified

Another reason for doubting the identity of self-concept and self is the extraordinary oversimplification that seems to characterize our self-concept. The self-concepts seem to be value-laden, reducing the complexities of living to remarkably simple "shoulds" and "wants." These voluntarily accessible beliefs about ourselves often seem to be context-free and absolute. "I'm a likable person. I'm very efficient. I have a lot of friends." In contrast, the organization of the self-system, as we will see below, seems to be highly complex, multilayered, and adaptive. In the overall self-system, the self-concept may play a monitoring or supervisory role (see 9.2.2).

Research on thought monitoring by Singer and his co-workers suggests an explanation for the remarkable oversimplification of the self-concept (e.g., Pope & Singer, 1978). If we were to track every bit of inner speech produced by one person, day after day, we would quickly fill volumes. Even disregarding other conscious events – mental images, evanescent feelings, percepts, and the like – the stream of consciousness is lengthy, constrained by numerous accidental and local factors, often self-contradictory, and complex. When we are asked to characterize ourselves in a phrase or two, we are forced to summarize this rich lode of information. And the fact is that people are often unable to produce accurate summaries for great amounts of diverse information (e.g., Ericsson & Simon, 1980; Newell & Simon, 1972; Tversky & Kahneman, 1973). With the best will in the world, and even absent of all the motivational distortions in self-perception, we simply cannot describe ourselves very well.

This does *not* mean that it is hopeless to ask people about themselves and expect accurate answers. Rather, it is vital to do so under optimal circumstances, and not to expect people to have access to the deeper layers of their own organization. Further, our previous discussions throughout this book suggest that people only learn about contextual representations by failure of those representations; we can check reports of such violations objectively and see whether the results accord with voluntary self-reports. Inferences made about ourselves on the basis of these surprising events may lead to a different understanding of ourselves than our normal self-concept indicates.

9.0.2 Conscious self-monitoring may be guided by the self-concept

In yet different language, we can say that the self-concept as an object of conscious thought and experience may be considered to be *an objectlike analogue of the self-system*. The self-concept represents self as an object of knowledge. But self is not in the first instance an object of knowledge; it is contextual. We can of course monitor many aspects of self at will: our orientation in space, the loudness of our speech, our social acceptance by others. These events are objects of consciousness that are usually compared to some set of criteria: Where are we compared to where we want to go? Should we be speaking louder? Should we curry favor with others? Such criteria are presumably part of one's self-concept. The self-concept is that part that is always looking at ourselves from a real or imagined outside point of view. At the social level, it is as if we are always asking, consciously or automatically, "What will the neighbors say?" If not the neighbors, then parents, peers, siblings, professional colleagues, teachers, or the judgment of history.

Self, on the other hand, may be considered to be the cross-situational context of experience and action. Our consistent expectations about the world are unconscious; the more predictable they are, the less they are likely to become conscious. All of our experience is shaped and defined by these unconscious contextual expectations: perceptual, conceptual, social, communicative, scientific, and so forth (4.2.1). Even our actions are generated and interpreted in a context of goals that are mostly unconscious at the time we perform the actions. One way to think of self is as a contextual organization that seldom encounters contradiction, because it remains largely predictable across the situations we normally encounter. But once the predictable situations of our lives change, aspects of ourselves that previously provided adequate context for our experience are violated and need to be changed; these stable presuppositions may then be perceived as objectlike, even though they were invisible components of self before.

9.1   Contrasting self and not-self experiences

As James points out at the start of this chapter, the "I" is difficult to know directly. Certainly just asking people about it is problematic, because by definition we do not have direct conscious access to it: It is, in Jamesian language, the knower rather than the known. However, we can approach "self as knower" empirically with a contrastive analysis, just as we have with conscious experience and volition (2.0, 7.0). We will find a great range of evidence for self/not-self contrasts in perception and motor control, in social situations, self-evaluative experiences, psychopathology, and the like. The empirical evidence regarding self is actually plentiful and well-studied, once we know where to look.

9.1.1 The wide range of self/not-self contrasts

When the eyeball is gently pressed with a finger, the world seems to jump; but, as Helmholtz noted in the 1860s, this does not seem to happen with normal eye movements (Helmholtz, 1962). Evidently the visual system can distinguish between self-generated and externally induced movements. Somehow self-generated movements are compensated for, so that the experience of the world remains stable in spite of our movement. Self–other differentiation is absolutely necessary not just in the visual system, but in any sensory system, natural or artificial. If a radar dish rotates at a regular rate and detects an apparently moving object, it must differentiate between movements due to its own motion, and those that are due to object itself. Otherwise the moon could be interpreted as a rapidly moving object and a passing flock of birds as a stationary object in space. Thus self–other differentiation is fundamental indeed, even in perceptual–motor systems.

One can easily show the same need for self–other differentiation in the social world, or in the realm of self-evaluation and personality. The point is that we need some conception of self as a multilayered entity with perceptual–motor, social, personality, and other components. We will focus here on the personality realm, contrasting self-attributed and self-alien experiences, but with the clear understanding that the layers of the self-system cannot ultimately be separated. Amputation of a limb will impact perceptual–motor processes most directly, but it may create major changes in personality and the socially defined self as well.

9.1.2 Self-alien experiences as evidence for self as context

Just as we have contrasted comparable conscious and unconscious processes throughout this book, we can also compare cases where "self" is perceived as "not-self," or as "another self." The most radical, well-established cases involve psychogenic fugue, multiple personality, and depersonalization disorder. The standard psychiatric diagnostic manual *DSM-III* is an authoritative source on these conditions (Spitzer, 1979). We will briefly review all three syndromes.

Note that if self can reasonably be viewed as a Dominant Context, we can make some predictions about the effects of violating it. We know well that contexts can be decomposed by events that violate contextual expectations and intentions (4.4.3). These violative events may be either internal or external in origin, but we should certainly expect "shocking" external events, which are easy to observe, to trigger a disruption in the stable Dominant Context. Further, since context helps to shape, control, and evoke conscious experience, some changes in the contents of consciousness may also be expected under these conditions. Fundamental life changes should sometimes evoke surprising alterations in thought, images, inner speech, feelings, and perhaps even perception. Personal values may change, because, after all, values are associated with the Dominant Goal Context – all values posit a claim that one thing is more desirable (hence goal-like) than another. Finally, this point of view predicts that after fundamental life-changing events, people may lose touch with their assumptions about reality as well – these are after all viewed in GW theory as part of the conceptual context. All of these predicted features are found in the following self-alien syndromes.

Depersonalization disorder is described in *DSM-III* as

> an alteration in the perception and experience of the self so that the usual sense of one's own reality is temporarily lost or changed. This is manifested by a sensation of self-estrangement or unreality, which may include the feeling that one's extremities have changed in size, or the experience of seeming to perceive oneself from a distance. . . . The individual may feel "mechanical" or as though in a dream. Various types of sensory anesthesias and a feeling of not being in complete control of one's actions, including speech are often present. All of these feelings are ego-dystonic (self-alien). (Spitzer, 1979, p. 259)

Mild depersonalization is quite common: It is estimated to occur at some time in 30–70 percent of young adults.

Depersonalization has many of the expected features. First, it is often triggered by severe stress – such as military combat or an auto accident – physical pain, anxiety, and depression. A similar syndrome can occur after brainwashing, thought reform, and indoctrination while the captive of terrorists or cultists – all cases in which routine, dominant goals and perspectives are profoundly challenged. These facts are consistent with the notion that disruption of the self involves deep context-violation. Indeed, stress may be defined as a deep violation of expectations and intentions (goal and conceptual contexts) (Horowitz, 1976). *Onset* of depersonalization is therefore likely to be rapid, as is indeed found, while recovery may be slow, because it takes time to reconstruct a disrupted fundamental context. The high incidence of depersonalization in early adulthood is also significant, since people often establish their fundamental goals and expectations during this period of life, while at the same time going through major life changes that may challenge a new, tentative integration.

Second, there are evidently changes in the way victims of depersonalization experience themselves and the world, consistent with the fact that contexts constrain conscious experiences (4.3.2). Along these lines, *DSM-III* states that

> derealization is frequently present. This is manifested in a strange alteration in the perception of one's surroundings so that a sense of the reality of the external world is lost. A perceived change in the size or shape of objects in the external world is common. People may be perceived as dead or mechanical. . . . Other associated features include . . . a disturbance in the subjective sense of time. (p. 259)

Evidently, as the self is challenged, the perceived world may also be estranged.

Psychogenic fugue provides another example of a self-alien syndrome. It involves "sudden, unexpected travel away from home or customary work locale with assumption of a new identity and an inability to recall one's previous identity. Perplexity and disorientation may occur. Following recovery there is no recollection of events that took place during the fugue." This diagnosis is not made if there is evidence for organic disorder.

Again, this disorder can be seen to be a result of deep violations of the normal Dominant Context, followed by an effort to create a new Dominant Context, free from the environment that created insupportable problems for the original identity. Fugue typically "follows severe psychosocial stress, such as marital quarrels, personal rejections, military conflict, or natural disaster (Spitzer, 1979, p. 256)." It seems to be related to *psychogenic amnesia*, in which a loss of memory occurs after severe psychological stress. Amnesia sometimes involves a loss of personal identity, but no purposeful travel and no assumption of a new identity. Note, by the way, that we have encountered spontaneous amnesia before, in our discussion of highly hypnotizable people, who often have spontaneous amnesia for the hypnotic session (7.7.2). This is consistent with the notion that high hypnotizables enter a deep, absorbed state, in which they are guided by a context that differs radically from their posthypnotic context, so that there is relatively little in the way of recall cues available to them afterwards. The issue of spontaneous amnesia and loss of autobiographical memory is indeed a key to the notion of self we are developing here.

The most famous example of self-altering pathology involves *multiple personality* (Hilgard, 1977; James, 1890/1983; Prince, 1908/1957; Spiegel,

1984). Here, too, an eclipsed personality reports a gap afterwards in the flow of experience, just as do victims of amnesia and fugue. "The essential feature," says *DSM-III*,

is the existence within the individual of two or more distinct personalities, each of which is dominant at a particular time. Each personality is a fully integrated and complex unit with unique memories, behavior patterns, and social relationships that determine the nature of the individual's acts when that person is predominant. . . . Studies have demonstrated that different personalities may have different responses to physiological and psychological measurements. One or more subpersonalities may report being of the opposite sex, of a different race or age, or from a different family than the original personality. . . . The original personality and all of the subpersonalities are aware of *lost periods of time*. (Spitzer, 1979, p. 257; italics added)

Subpersonalities may hear each other or speak to each other, but often with a sense that the voice heard is self-alien – outside of the self of the current dominant personality.

Again, we can make an argument for a causal role for some deep challenge to the normal Dominant Context of intentions and expectations. Thus it is said that "transition from one personality to another is *sudden and often associated with psychosocial stress*" (Spitzer, 1979, p. 257, italics added). Spiegel (1984) has made the case that multiple personality syndrome is *invariably* associated with a history of severe traumatic abuse in childhood. He suggests that when abused, children learn to enter a radically dissociated state, which develops over time into a complete, differentiated self. It is easy to interpret these ideas within our current framework.

Recent work with multiple personalities indicates that there is often a "regulator personality," one that keeps track of and mediates between other subpersonalities (D. Spiegel, personal communication, 1986). Spiegel suggests on this basis that the normal self, too, may function as a regulator, integrating experience across different situations (personal communication, 1986). This again is consistent with the notion of the self as a Dominant Context, one that creates continuity across subordinate contexts.

Note the repeated theme of gaps in autobiographical recall in the self-alien syndromes. Autobiographical recall is of course the domain of self-attributed experience, and in a GW framework, if self is identified with deep context, we know that it must shape and select characteristic experiences.

Everyday examples of deeply absorbed states, as in reading a novel or watching a film, reveal the same cluster of phenomena: gaps in autobiographical memory, loss of time, and a changed sense of self. It is often difficult to remember a period of absorption later, and time seems to have gone faster in retrospect, presumably because we can recall fewer details of the absorbed period (Ornstein, 1969). Finally, absorption is strongly associated with identification with fictional characters in movies, plays, and novels – i.e., a change in the sense of self.

Another common theme in the self-alien syndromes is the relationship between a loss of self and losing valued or presupposed conditions of one's life. It seems as if the more we rely upon something in dealing with the world – upon an assumption, a personal capacity, a skill, or a goal – the more its loss will lead to self-alien experiences. This may be particularly true when the lost element is presupposed, so that we no longer even *know that it is there* as an object of experience. If we have assumed all of our lives that we can trust people completely, so that this assumption has simply become part of our dealings with them, a deep violation of trust will have consequences that propagate widely through-out our selves and our experiences. Presumably, if we rely less on this implicit assumption, violations of trust will not be so disruptive.

9.2   Modeling self and self-concept

We will now attempt to model these observations. This will prove surprisingly easy, because we can assimilate all the aforementioned facts to the theory we already have. Figure 9.1 shows how the deep goal contexts and conceptual contexts can be viewed as different aspects of self. This is of course James's self as "I" – as the observer and agent – rather than self as an object of experience. In general, the deeper, more predictable, and more fundamental levels – those that lower levels depend upon – are more self-like, in the sense that their violation will propagate throughout the goal hierarchy and lead to disruptive, surprising, and self-alien experiences and actions.

9.2.1 Self as deep context

Because the context hierarchy can control the Options Contexts dis-cussed in Chapter 8, the self-system has routine access to all sensory modalities – to immediate memory, recent autobiographical memories, routine facts, long-term personal "marker" memories, and future or fantasied images. In addition, we have indirect voluntary access to a host of specialized skills (like English syntax and motor control) which are not conscious in the qualitative sense – we do not experience our syntactic rules directly – but whose unexpected absence would create great conscious surprise. This is of course the point Dennett (1978) remarked upon in the passage quoted at the beginning of this chapter, the notion

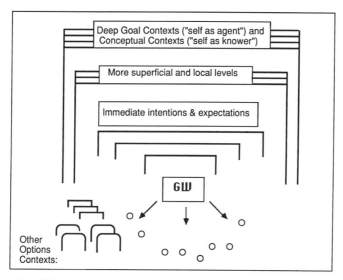

Figure 9.1. Self as the enduring context of experience and action. A study of contrasts between self-attributed and self-alien experiences suggests that "self" can be treated as the deeper levels of the context hierarchy. Self-alien syndromes are typically associated with profoundly violative events and often result in a loss of autobiographical memory. Since voluntary recall is influenced by the Dominant Goal Hierarchy, a fundamental change in the deeper levels of the goal hierarchy may make it difficult to retrieve experiences that were represented within a different organization of self. Experiences that are perceived as self-alien in one deep goal context may be self-attributed in another, as in the case of multiple personality or fugue. Thus, access of a self-system to the global workspace is required for any reportable conscious experience.

that self is that which has access to consciousness. A major, rapid change in the access conditions of any of these domains may be perceived as a self-alien change in one's experience. Thus loss of memory should impact one's sense of self, as should sudden blindness, or even a sudden *increase* in one's ability to imagine things. Any rapid change violates contextual predictability, but changes consistent with one's goals should be relatively more acceptable.

The same may be true on the output side. We expect voluntary control over our skeletal muscles; over many mental functions, like the ability to recall this morning's breakfast or the ability to express our thoughts; over many objects in our environment; over people, to some extent; and, within limits, over some social institutions. We can even control autonomic bodily functions through mental images. A loss in any area of expected control may be perceived as a profound change in self.

These functions are controlled by the goal hierarchy, and are normally self-attributed. Recall that English sentences describing an act of voluntary control always take a personal pronoun as subject (9.0). Hence people should experience a loss of control over one's body, over the social domain, and even over deeply presupposed possessions – such as a car or a house – as a self-alien experience. Notice that such a self-alien experience is not just a sense of loss, sadness, or mourning – these feelings may all be self-attributed. It is rather a sense of things being out of control, of surprising thoughts and feelings and images, that characterize self-alien experiences.

9.2.2 The self-concept system controls conscious self-monitoring

Next, we attempt to model the self-concept. The self-concept presumably emerges from many conscious experiences of self-monitoring, and comparing the results to real or imagined evaluations from other people. It has been said (rather cynically) that conscience is the still small voice reminding us that someone may be looking. It may be the fleeting ideomotor image that says, "What would the neighbors think? . . . What will Daddy say when he comes home? . . . My friends would laugh at me if they saw me now. . . . Any person of the opposite sex simply must admire my looks, strength, wit, and intelligence." Such sentiments are utterly commonplace and must surely have an effect on one's self-concept. Indeed, an effective therapy for depression is based on the assumption that such rapid, nearly automatic thoughts are the key to depressive self-denigration (Beck, 1976; Ellis, 1962).

Figure 9.2 shows a case of such conscious self-monitoring as an Options Context with a variety of subcontexts, including tracking of one's own performance, calling upon the self-concept for comparison, and adjusting the self-concept up or down in value, depending upon the results.

The self-concept system can then be treated as a high-level context, operating within the self-system, and making use of the kind of conscious self-monitoring shown in Figure 9.2 to control and evaluate one's own performance. Over time, conscious self-monitoring experiences, like any other predictable experiences, must become contextualized. Thus self-concept apparently begins to function as a part of the larger self-system. The contextualized aspects of the self-concept are of course less available to voluntary retrieval, just as any other context is hard to recall voluntarily. Further, aspects of oneself that are not acknowledged in the self-concept are notorious for influencing human actions and experiences. The entire psychodynamic tradition of the last hundred years is devoted

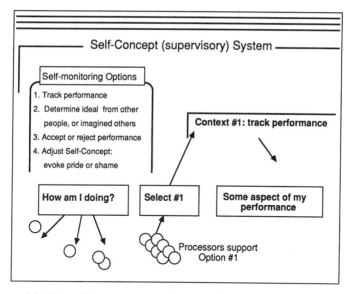

Figure 9.2. The self-concept can evoke conscious self-monitoring. There is extensive evidence that most people continually monitor their own performance against some standard, presumably of social origin. This diagram shows how the self-concept, viewed as a supervisory system, may use conscious self-monitoring to evaluate performance. Since conscious self-monitoring requires control of attention, an Options Context is needed to present the various components of self-monitoring in a "menu" from which one can choose the needed action. In the diagram, "tracking one's own performance" is chosen, evoking systems that present performance information consciously. Results from self-tracking are then compared to some ideal level of performance.

to the study of these phenomena. Perhaps all human beings have potential conflicts between those aspects of the self that match our self-concept, and those that are disavowed. But even parts of oneself that are not disavowed may be difficult to monitor consciously, simply because they have become automatic with practice (Langer & Imber, 1979).

Given reasonable conceptions of self, conscious self-monitoring, and self-concept, we can now show an integration of these ideas in Model 7 (Figure 9.3).

9.2.3 Model 7

As suggested above, the self-concept system can be treated as a goal context that makes use of self-monitoring and evaluation in order to move one's performance closer to the ideal, as shown in Figure 9.3. Notice that this goal encounters competition from other goals; perhaps there is

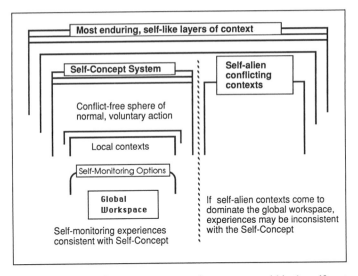

Figure 9.3. Model 7: Self-concept as a supervisory context within the self-system. The self-concept as reflected in the beliefs people express about themselves, may be seen as a goal context within the Context Hierarchy. Ready availability of self-evaluative judgments and standards suggests that the self-concept is much more consciously accessible than the higher-level self-system. The self-concept system presumably makes use of self-monitoring to evaluate and control actions and experiences. But at times, normal self-attributed experiences may be disrupted by experiences controlled by deeper levels of the self-system: for example, in the self-alien images, actions, and feelings of neurotic psychopathology; in multiple personality; in unwanted and self-alien impulses; and so on. These well-established phenomena suggest that the self-concept, as the expressed beliefs about oneself, is governed by a still deeper layer of organization plausibly called the "self-organization" or just "self." The area of overlap between self and self-concept seems to correspond to the "conflict-free sphere of the ego" proposed by Hartmann (1939/1958). Other parts of the system may be much more conflictful; everyone could in principle do things that would violate their self-concept, as symbolized by the conflicting contexts shown above.

resistance to the effort demanded by the self-concept system to reach its goals; perhaps there are goals aiming to obtain more immediate rewards than are allowed by the self-concept; perhaps there are goals expressing impulses that are not consistent with the self-concept. All these goal systems may compete with the self-concept system. The goal hierarchy that is consistent with the self-concept comes very close to the idea of the "conflict-free sphere of the ego" articulated by the ego psychologist Heinz Hartmann (1958). That is, it is a domain in which the system that always tries to control our actions, the self-concept system, coincides in its aims with other major goals. Thus there is no destructive competition between different goal systems. Presumably most of our normal, voluntary actions are guided by this conflict-free sphere of the goal hierarchy.

9.3   Further questions to explore

9.3.1 Normal, voluntary action is largely conflict-free

These considerations create a new perspective on the issues of conscious experience and voluntary control. In particular, the conflict-free sphere provides an executive of sorts that is in control of most voluntary action. That is, there is a set of goals and expectations within the larger self-system that are acceptable to the self-concept, and within this shared domain, actions can be planned and carried out without inner conflict. For example, although we are physically perfectly able to slap our close friends and colleagues in the face, most of us rarely do so. If we were to do so, most likely we would shock not only others but ourselves, and the action would have immediate repercussions for our self-concept. Thus even intense anger is likely to be expressed in a form that is a compromise between fantasy revenge and the self-concept. Voluntary control is profoundly shaped by these considerations. It seems as if we are always attempting to earn our own self-respect first of all.

Now we can reconsider Dennett's remark that consciousness is the domain of access to the self. After all, by means of Options Contexts, the Dominant Context Hierarchy can indeed gain access to all domains of consciousness: to the senses, to immediate memory, to voluntary effectors, to imagination, and the like. The conflict-free sphere as an executive can presumably access any of these domains without internal resistance.

9.3.2 Unresolved goal conflicts may persist outside of the conflict-free sphere

However, outside of the conflict-free domain, competing goal contexts may persist, conceivably for many years. This would allow GW theory to represent typical impulse-control problems, where people may successfully resist the temptation to express anger for a period of years, and then, perhaps when the Dominant Goal Hierarchy becomes less dominant, the suppressed anger may emerge overtly. The research evidence for this type of phenomenon may be controversial, but naturalistic evidence seems persuasive. In any case, the existence of such persistent competition is implied by the fact that goal contexts can compete for access to consciousness. From a theoretical point of view, the possibility of persistent unexpressed goals costs nothing in added theoretical conceptions, and it may allow for future expansion of the theory into an important domain of human motivation.

Multiple personality represents the most spectacular case of such persistent conflict between different selves or, in our earlier terminology, between different context hierarchies. Whenever one goal hierarchy dominates consciousness, it is presumably able to access the senses, immediate memory, voluntary musculature, as well as Options Contexts that allow one to access Short Term Memory, to monitor and evaluate oneself, and so forth. This model also allows us to interpret the evidence cited in Chapter 7 for conflictful states in which people disavow sentiments that they demonstrably hold (7.8.2). Disavowal is a voluntary action based on a lack of voluntary access to the sources of information that still continue to "prime" involuntary phenomena like slips of the tongue or externally attributed projections. If this is a reasonable analysis, then multiple personality syndrome is just a more extreme case of rather normal conflict.

9.3.3 Explaining self-alien intrusions of thoughts and images

Chapter 7 describes the common phenomenon of self-alien, unwanted thoughts and images, as one typical psychopathological event. Multiple personality patients often complain of such self-alien intrusive thoughts coming from a more dominant self. There are nonpathological examples of this as well, as in persistent mental repetition of commercial jingles, which may continue even against our best efforts to stop it. In Model 7 we can explain such self-alien intrusions of internal origin as due to competition between different goal systems, including perhaps the disavowed goals discussed above (9.3.2). Momentarily a competing goal-image may gain access to the global workspace, perhaps especially if the normally dominant hierarchy is preoccupied with other matters.

Since self-alien intrusions are obviously not under voluntary control, they presumably engage the same kinds of automatic attention mechanisms that control any involuntary intrusion. As we noted in 8.2.1, automatic attention can be controlled by the goal hierarchy (a part of the self-system). Thus, the hypotheses about self developed in this chapter seem consistent with the proposals about attention advanced in Chapter 8.

9.3.4 What happens if the highest-level context is disrupted?

Early in this book (4.4.3), we suggested that surprise may disrupt the context hierarchy, and that the disruption will propagate downward to

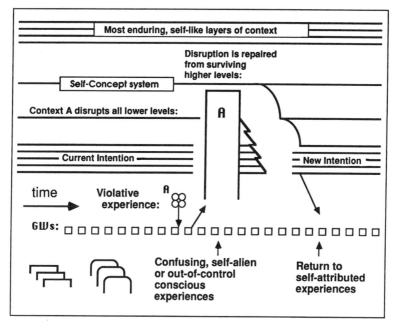

Figure 9.4. Disruption due to competing contexts can propagate downward from the self-system to local intentions. The diagram shows how the system might cope with a fundamental violative experience (e.g., being attacked by a close friend, suffering a stroke that changes perception of reality, losing a valued job or social position, or suffering the death of a close companion). These are classic stressful events, which often lead to temporary self-alien experiences. More extreme cases, such as multiple personality, fugue, and depersonalization can be viewed in much the same way. They too are closely related to major stressful events that violate deep contextual assumptions and goals. For example, there is strong evidence linking multiple personality to a history of consistent childhood abuse. Multiple personality syndrome may involve a deep context like Context A in the diagram, extended over a long time, so that relative to it, the self-alien experiences become self-attributed. Context A may have its own characteristic meta-cognitive access, presumably because the metacognitive Options Contexts must be called through the global workspace. If the GW is dominated by Context A, it can control self-monitoring, voluntary action, voluntary access to the senses, Short Term Memory, etc.

other parts of the hierarchy that depend upon the violated context. Now we can ask another question: If severe surprise can break apart a context, leading to reorganization under a higher-level context, what happens if the *highest*-level context is disrupted? In general, it would seem to be much more difficult to reintegrate the disrupted context hierarchy, because there is no unviolated ''umbrella'' context under which one can reintegrate action and experience (Figure 9.4). If one's car breaks down, one can take the bus. But if one's fundamental assumptions about life break down, all actions, ideas, and experiences that depend upon these assumptions must be reintegrated under a new set of top-level goals. Thus reintegration would take more time, if the violation occurs at a deeper level. This is indeed a model for severe stress and decompensation, for "breakdowns" in the personality.

9.4 Chapter summary

The review of self-alien syndromes lends support to our decision to deal with self at all: It seems clear that alterations in self create changes in conscious experience. That includes the quality of experience but, even more clearly, it is the *continuity* of autobiographical (self-attributed) experience and recall that is affected by the self-system. In multiple personality, fugue, and amnesic loss of identity, there is often a gap in autobiographical memory corresponding to the period in which the recalling self was eclipsed. For this reason we can think of self as a contextual organization that supports voluntary recall (among many other functions). By contrast, the *self-concept*, defined as the beliefs people hold about themselves, seems less fundamental. Many people constantly monitor their actions and experiences by comparison with a set of beliefs and values that show how things should be; this self-concept is evidently a kind of supervisory system operating within the larger self-system. The self-concept seems to guide conscious self-monitoring, which in turn shapes the self-concept. If we feel proud or ashamed of some achievement, the self-concept is adjusted appropriately.

It seems that we can now add another necessary condition for consciousness to the list (see Section 11.3). Consciousness inherently needs to interact with a self-system, at least if its information is to be reportable and usable. This is best expressed in Dennett's dictum, "That of which I am conscious is that to which I have *access*, or (to put the emphasis where it belongs), to which *I* have access" (1978, p. 149; italics in original).

If self is a context, then there is a fundamental difference between self and the objects of consciousness. William James's "me" is the self as viewed from an outside perspective; but the "I" is presumably necessary for the "me" to be experienced at all. Of course, our normal experience moves smoothly from contextualized aspects of self to objectified aspects, just as T. S. Eliot's Unidentified Guest, in this chapter's epigraph, moved smoothly from a contextualized self to a jarring encounter with the bottom of the staircase, which, just for a moment, revealed him to be "an object at the mercy of a malevolent staircase."

Part VI

Consciousness is functional

Contrary to some opinion, we find that conscious experience serves a multitude of vital functions in the nervous system.

10 The functions of consciousness

> The *particulars of the distribution of consciousness*, so far as we know them, *point to its being efficacious* . . . It seems an organ, superadded to other organs which maintain the animal in the struggle for existence; and the presumption of course is that it helps him in some way in the struggle.
>
> *William James*, 1890/1983 (pp. 141–2; italics in original)

> Consciousness would appear to be related to the mechanism of the body . . . simply as a [by-]product of its working, and to be completely without any power of modifying that working, as a steam whistle which accompanies the work of a locomotive . . . is without influence upon its machinery.
>
> *Thomas Henry Huxley*
> (quoted in William James, 1890/1983 (Vol. I, p. 130)

10.0 Introduction

Readers who have come this far may be a bit skeptical about T. H. Huxley's claim that conscious experience has no function whatever in the workings of the nervous system. But the great number of useful roles played by consciousness may still come as a surprise. The eighteen or so functions presented in this chapter provide only one way of grouping and labeling these useful services – some of the labels overlap, and there may be some gaps. But it is doubtful whether any shorter list can do justice to the great and varied uses of conscious experience.

The functions listed in Table 10.1 really belong to the entire GW system, including both conscious and unconscious components. In this architecture, conscious experience represents the jewel in the crown, enabling the whole system to function.

10.0.1 Conscious experience as a biological adaptation

A basic premise of this book is that, like any other biological adaptation, consciousness is *functional*. Many biological mechanisms serve multiple functions: The eyes pick up information in the light, but human eye contact also communicates social messages such as dominance, submission, affection, and plain curiosity. Consciousness, too, has apparently gathered multiple functions in its evolutionary history; we explore some

347

of these functions in this chapter (see also Rozin, 1976; Baars, in press a). But perhaps the most fundamental function is the one we remarked on in Chapter 1: the ability to optimize the trade-off between organization and flexibility. Organized responses are highly efficient in well-known situations, but in the face of novel conditions, flexibility is at a premium. Of course the global workspace architecture is designed to make "canned" solutions available automatically in predictable situations, and to combine many different knowledge sources in unpredictable circumstances.

In another way, consciousness and related mechanisms pose a great challenge to functional explanations because of the paradoxical limits of conscious capacity (1.3.4). Why can't we experience two different "things" at one time? Why is Short Term Memory limited to half a dozen unrelated items? How could such narrow limits be adaptive? Reasoning naively, it would seem wonderful to be able to consciously read one book, write another one, talk to a friend, and appreciate a fine meal, all at the same time. Certainly the nervous system seems big enough to do all these things simultaneously. The usual answers, that the limitations are "physiological" or that we only have two hands and one mouth to work with, are quite unsatisfactory because they simply move the issue one step backwards: Why have organisms blessed with the most formidable brain in the animal kingdom not developed hands and mouths able to handle true parallel processing? And why does our ability to process information in parallel increase with automaticity, and decrease with conscious involvement?

Whenever we encounter a biological phenomenon that seems nonfunctional there are two possible explanations. First, we may be asking the wrong question: Perhaps cultural evolution has simply outpaced biological evolution, and we are now expecting the organism to do things it was not adapted to do. It is a good bet that the human nervous system was not developed for academic study, since universal education is only a few centuries old in almost all cultures. This may be the reason that learning in school seems so hard, while learning to perceive the world, learning to move, or learning one's native tongue seem effortless by comparison. If we then ask why children find it hard to learn arithmetic or spelling, we are asking a culturally biased question, one that may seem natural today, but which is biological nonsense.

A second reason for apparently nonfunctional adaptations may be an invisible "design trade-off" between two different factors (e.g., Gould, 1982). When the mammalian ancestors of the whales returned to the ocean, they must have encountered trade-offs between walking and swimming, and over time lost their legs. This may seem nonfunctional to

Table 10.1. *The major functions of consciousness*

1	*Definition and Context-setting*	By relating global input to its contexts, the system underlying consciousness acts to define the input and remove ambiguities. Conscious global messages can also evoke contexts, which then constrain later conscious experiences.
2	*Adaptation and Learning*	Conscious experience is useful in representing and adapting to novel and significant events.
3	*Editing, Flagging, and Debugging*	Unconscious processors can monitor any conscious content, edit it, and try to change it if it is consciously "flagged" as an error.
4	*Recruiting and Control Function*	Conscious goals can recruit subgoals and motor systems to organize and carry out mental and physical actions.
5	*Prioritizing and Access-control*	Attentional mechanisms exercise conscious and unconscious control over what will become conscious. By relating some particular conscious content to deeper goals, we can raise its access priority, making it conscious more often and increasing the chances of successful adaptation to it.
6	*Decision-making or Executive Function*	When automatic systems cannot routinely resolve some choice-point, making it conscious helps recruit unconscious knowledge sources to make the proper decision. In the case of indecision, we can make a goal conscious to allow widespread recruitment of conscious and unconscious "votes" for or against it.
7	*Analogy-forming Function*	Unconscious systems can search for a *partial* match between their contents and a globally displayed (conscious) message. This is especially important in representing new information when no close models of the input are available.
8	*Metacognitive or Self-monitoring Function*	Through conscious imagery and inner speech we can reflect upon and control our own conscious and unconscious functioning.
9	*Autoprogramming and Self-maintenance Function*	The deeper layers of context can be considered as a "self-system" that works to maintain maximum stability in the face of changing inner and outer conditions. Conscious experience provides information for the self-system to use in its task of maintaining stability. By "replaying" desirable goals, it can recruit processors able to produce solutions and thereby reprogram the system itself.

land animals like ourselves, but the loss was compensated by a great gain in swimming ability. Conscious limited capacity may involve such a trade-off. There may be powerful advantages for a global broadcasting ability that allows access from *any* component of the nervous system to *all other* components. A truly global message, if it is to be available to any part of the nervous system, must come only one at a time, because there is only one "whole system" at any moment to receive the message. Thus vertebrates perhaps evolved a nervous system with two operating modes: a parallel (unconscious) mode and a serial (conscious and limited-capacity) mode. GW theory gives one interpretation of the interaction between these dual operating modes.

Biological adaptations tend to be accretive (Gould, 1982; Rozin, 1976). The speech system, for example, is "overlaid" on a set of organs that in ancestral primates supported breathing, eating, and simple vocalization. Likewise, it may be that the global broadcasting property of the consciousness system is overlaid on an earlier function that is primarily sensory. This may be why human consciousness has such a penchant for sensory, perceptual, and imaginal contents compared to abstract or nonqualitative events (e.g., 2.5.4).

Table 10.1 tells the most plausible story we can posit about the uses of consciousness, based on the foregoing chapters.

10.1   Definitional and Context-setting Function

In looking through a hollow tube at an isolated corner of a room (2.1.1), in listening for the words in a rock song, or in learning to perceive an abstract painting, we engage in conscious observation leading to an experiential transformation. We may experience this transformation directly, simply by attending to the stimulus until it is transformed. But even when we try to understand an easy sentence, rapid transformations are taking place unconsciously: Many different unconscious sources of information combine to build a single interpretation of a focal, rather ambiguous event (2.3.2).

If we were forced to choose one premier function of consciousness, it would be the ability of the consciousness system to combine a variety of knowledge sources in order to *define* a single, coherent experience. Another way to say this is that the system underlying consciousness has the function of relating an event to the three kinds of contexts: to a qualitative context that allows us to experience an event as an object of consciousness, to a conceptual interpretation, and to a goal context that may lead to effective action (Chapters 4, 6, and 7). A word can be experienced as a stimulus without a conceptual context, but such a context is necessary for it to have meaning; and we know that a meaningful word is usually related to some contextual goals, which are not wholly available consciously at the time they guide us. This contextual apparatus is needed to allow even very "simple" things to take place, such as the reader's decision to read the next paragraph. Note that the Definitional Function of consciousness corresponds closely to Mandler's and Marcel's constructivist view of consciousness, emphasizing its capacity to create experiences that go beyond a simple combination of components (Mandler, 1983, 1984; Marcel, 1983a; see 1.3.5, 2.3.2).

A related critical function of consciousness is *context-setting*, the ability to evoke relevant contexts in the first place. This is most obvious in the case of conceptual and goal contexts; for example, in the case of the tip-of-the-tongue (TOT) phenomenon, where the role of a goal context is quite clear (6.1). A TOT state may be evoked by a conscious question or an incomplete conscious sentence (6.0). Given the TOT state, we begin to search (unconsciously) for the correct word; this search process, as well as the goal context for retrieving the word, together will constrain the conscious answers that will come to mind. Context-setting may not be so clear in more complex cases as in meeting a new person, or encountering a new idea, but these conscious experiences do seem to evoke and create new contexts.

10.2 Adaptation and Learning Function

Whether consciousness is *necessary* for learning has led to years of controversy (e.g., Eriksen, 1960; Holender, 1986), but there is little doubt that the more novel the material to be learned, the more time we must typically spend pondering it consciously before learning to cope with it (5.5.3). This is the *learning* function of conscious experience. GW theory suggests that conscious events are broadcast globally to unconscious processors and contexts, which can then *adapt* to this information. If they cannot adapt immediately, they can act to bring the material to mind at some later time, sometimes many times. Several researchers have shown that personally significant information tends to come to mind again and again, until presumably it is absorbed and adapted to (Singer, 1984; Horowitz, 1975a, 1976; Klinger, 1971). Obviously we also adapt to the world by action: We can avoid a threatening predator, approach a new source of food, and explore an unusual situation. Action also requires conscious goal-images, which must, again, be more consciously available the more novel the action is (7.2.2).

10.3 Editing, Flagging, and Debugging Function

Several psychologists have argued that conscious experience plays a role in "*debugging*" faulty processes (e.g., Mandler, 1975a,b). In particular, it seems that conscious events are monitored and edited by numerous unconscious rule-systems that can compete for access to the global workspace if they detect some serious flaw, and that may be able to repair the error cooperatively. Indeed, we have argued in Chapter 7 that voluntary action *is* tacitly edited action (7.3.2). Editing is an automatic consequence of the GW architecture in which many rule systems can simultaneously inspect, interrupt, and help repair a single conscious event. On the other side, conscious experience can also be used to *"flag"* some significant event. The most spectacular example of this is biofeedback training, in which otherwise unconscious events can come under voluntary control simply by having them trigger a conscious feedback signal. In this way we can learn to control apparently any population of neurons, at least temporarily (2.5). Biofeedback training reveals an extraordinary capacity of the nervous system, one that by itself suggests the existence of global broadcasting.

10.4   Recruiting and Control Function

Recruiting has much to do with the Flagging Function – in fact, as soon as we can flag some novel mental event consciously, we may be able to recruit it for voluntary purposes. The ideomotor theory (7.3) suggests that conscious goal-images are necessary to recruit novel subgoals and motor systems that will achieve the goal. But of course conscious goal-images themselves are under the control of unconscious goal contexts, which serve to generate a goal-image in the first place.

The *Control Function* is similar to the notion of recruiting of unconscious systems to help in achieving a goal. But consciousness is useful in setting goals in the first place, and in monitoring action feedback signaling success or failure. To set a goal that is compatible with existing goal contexts, we need to simply become conscious of the goal. Thus: "What is the name of the first president of the United States?" Just being conscious of the question allows the answer to be searched for unconsciously, and candidate answers are returned to consciousness, where they can be checked by multiple unconscious knowledge sources. Feedback checking occurs in essentially all tasks, from striking a tennis ball, to modulating the loudness of one's voice, to word-retrieval, to mental arithmetic. In all these cases it is useful for errors to become conscious in order to recruit unconscious error-detection and correction resources.

10.5   Prioritizing and Access-control Function

Attention involves *access control* to consciousness, and assigning priorities is a core issue in access control. Incomplete conscious thoughts tend to evoke conscious completions. We can apparently use conscious functions to control the likelihood that some piece of information will become conscious more often. Presumably, in the act of voluntarily accessing some information, we also practice the skill of recalling it – that is, of making it conscious again (8.0). In vocabulary development we may want to practice certain words to ensure that they will come to mind readily when needed. Recall, as the skill of bringing material to consciousness, has been studied since Ebbinghaus, but most modern studies ignore the fact that "recall" *means* "bringing memories to consciousness."

We can change the access priority of information in several ways. One is to use associative learning techniques, like paired associate learning. If a neutral conscious event is made to signal a horrifying mental image, the neutral event will take on a higher priority (presumably it has more activation, or it is associated with a higher-level goal context), which will make it more easily available to consciousness.

10.6 Decision-making or Executive Function

While the global broadcasting system is not an executive mechanism, it can be *used by* goal systems in an attempt to control thought and action. Chapters 6–9 are devoted to different aspects of this issue. Consciousness can serve as the domain of competition between different goals, as in indecisiveness and in conscious, deliberate decisions. In a sense, one can broadcast the goal, "Should I . . .?" followed by "Or shouldn't I . . .?" and allow a coalition of systems to build up in support of either alternative, as if they were voting one way or another. The successful coalition presumably supports a goal-image that is broadcast without effective competition, and which therefore gains ideomotor control over the action (7.0). This may be called the *Decision-making* Function of conscious experience.

Goal-images do not have to be recallable as conscious in order to influence action. There is considerable reason to believe that fleeting, hard-to-recall goal-images can trigger off well-prepared automatisms (1.5.5; 7.6.4). These images then act in an *Executive* fashion without allowing conscious decision-making; of course, the executive goal-images are themselves generated by complex unconscious goal structures.

10.7 Analogy-forming Function

Human beings have a great penchant for *analogy* and metaphor, and we use this capacity especially to cope with novel or ill-comprehended situations. Lakoff and Johnson (1980) point out that most everyday idioms involve a metaphorical extension from a well-known concrete situation to one that is abstract or poorly understood. Thus, we find "the mind is a container," "love is a journey," and "consciousness is the publicity organ of the nervous system." Metaphors are both useful and dangerous. In science we use them constantly, and we must be constantly ready to abandon them when they lead us astray. The Rutherford atom of nineteenth-century physics drew an analogy between the planets orbiting the sun and electrons surrounding a heavy nucleus. Here the similarities and differences are obvious in retrospect; but at the time, of course, one did not know how far the metaphor would work, and at which point it would have to be abandoned. But it gave one a place to start. Similarly, whenever we encounter something new, for which our existing knowledge is inadequate, we look for partial matches between the novel case and existing knowledge. Such partial matches invite metaphors. We can best manipulate those metaphors that are familiar and easy to visualize. Thus, we tend to concretize abstract entities and relationships, and thereby transfer our knowledge from one context to another.

The GW system is useful at several points along this path. It helps in detecting partial matches. It allows many systems to attempt to match a global message and to display their partial matches globally. It supports competition between different systems to edit the mental model of the event that is to be understood. And, in its preference for imageable, qualitative experiences, it is probably responsible for the bias for concreteness and imageability that we find in human metaphor.

Indeed even when we have accurate abstract representations of some information, we often still prefer less accurate prototypes and metaphors. We know that the average chair is *not* the prototypical square, brown, wooden, lacquered kitchen chair, yet we continue to use the false prototype, apparently because we have easier conscious access to it than to the more realistic abstraction (Rosch, 1975).

10.8 Metacognitive or Self-monitoring Function

Conscious *metacognition* depends on the capacity of one experience to refer to other experiences. Normally when we speak of consciousness we include the ability to describe and act upon our own conscious contents. Indeed, the operational definition of conscious experience proposed in Chapter 1 is predicated upon this ability (1.2.1). But conscious metacognition *itself* requires the global workspace and consciousness (8.2.3). Another aspect of such a self-referring system is our ability to label our own intentions, expectations, and beliefs, all abstract representations that are not experienced directly the way qualitative percepts or images are.

Nevertheless, people constantly refer to their own intentions as if they were discrete objects in the world.

Conscious *self-monitoring* is perhaps the single most important aspect of metacognition. There is a great deal of evidence for the view that many adults are constantly monitoring their own performance by reference to some set of criteria that can be collectively labeled the "self-concept." We might expect self-monitoring to play a role in the psychology of impulse control – if one has an impulse to do something questionable, and if one can mobilize internal competition against it, to hold the action in abeyance, chances for control are improved. There is direct evidence that impulsive children can be taught to use inner speech in such a self-monitoring fashion, and that this does indeed help to constrain inappropriate actions (Meichenbaum & Goodman, 1971).

10.9 Autoprogramming and Self-maintenance Function

We can ask the reader to pay attention to the period at the end of this sentence. We can ask someone to retrieve a memory, to solve a puzzle, or to wiggle a finger. We can learn new habits. All this implies the ability of the conscious system to engage in self-programming. In *autoprogramming*, goal systems make use of conscious experiences to exercise some control over both conscious and unconscious events. Autoprogramming can encounter obstacles, as in attempts to control smoking, overeating, or other undesired habits, but it is often quite effective. It presumably combines many of the functions discussed before: context-setting, decision making, self-monitoring, and the like.

The smooth functioning of the whole system is dependent upon a stable Dominant Goal Hierarchy, the deeper levels of which apparently correspond to the "self" of commonsense psychology. These deeper levels can be violated by external circumstances, just as any other contextual constraints can be. In addition, there is much clinical experience to suggest that the self can encounter violations of internal origin. *Maintaining the self-system* may be critical for mental and physical survival, and one tool for doing so may be the ability of attentional systems to control access to consciousness. The classical notions of repression would seem to fit in here. The evidence for repression as an unconscious process has been questioned (e.g., Holmes, 1972, 1974), but there is no dispute over the great amount of self-serving ideation and control of access to conscious experience that people engage in. The evidentiary question centers mainly about whether this kind of control is conscious or not. GW theory suggest that this is a secondary issue, since predictable voluntary control tends to become automatic with practice. In any case, self-

maintenance through the control of access of information to consciousness seems to be one central role of the consciousness system.

10.10   Chapter summary

Conscious processes are functional, just as unconscious ones are. Normal
psychology involves a delicate, rapid interplay between conscious and
unconscious events. Our list of eighteen functions does not exhaust the
possibilities: For example, we have not even touched on the uses of sleep
and dreaming. They too must surely have some functional role, probably
even multiple roles, which are likely to be bound up with the systems we
have explored in this book. But this issue must be left for future
exploration, along with so many others.

No doubt there will be some who continue to advocate the curious
doctrine of epiphenomenalism, the idea that conscious experience has no
function whatsoever. All we can do is point to the evidence, and develop
further demonstrations that loss of consciousness – through habituation,
automaticity, distraction, masking, anesthesia, and the like – inhibits or
destroys the functions listed here.

Some epiphenomenalists seem to adopt their position to defend the
special and unique status of conscious experience. They are right.
Consciousness *is* special; but its wonderful qualities are not isolated from
other realities; nor is biological uselessness a special virtue. Consciousness is the vehicle of our individuality, something that makes it of
inestimable significance to each of us. But viewed from the outside, as an
element in a larger system, the marvel of consciousness is one more
wonder in an awesome nervous system, supported by a body that is
scarcely less wonderful, evolved and maintained in a biosphere of endless
complexity and subtlety, in a universe one of whose most miraculous
features, as Einstein has said, is our ability to know it.

Part VII

Conclusion

In the final chapter, we review the flow of arguments in this book and attempt to distill the necessary conditions for conscious experience that have emerged so far. Much remains to be explained. We sketch some ways in which GW theory may be able to accommodate certain unexplained phenomena, and provide some suggestions for future research.

11   A summary and some future directions

11.0 Introduction

We have come to the end of a long journey. For the author, there has been a continual sense of surprise at the fruitfulness of a few fundamental ideas in understanding a topic that has long been thought to be out of bounds for respectable psychologists. Of course, whatever progress we have made is not complete, nor is it conclusive or beyond reasonable dispute. No doubt there are gaps and errors in the story presented here, although there does seem to be a kind of coherence, an underlying simplicity – so many well-established observations fall into place easily, with only a few basic ideas.

A vast amount of experimental and theoretical work is needed to test and clarify the hypotheses developed in this book. That is in the nature of a "framework" theory like this one. It is in many ways an invitation for further work, rather than a monument of indisputable fact.

We cannot claim for the global workspace approach the kind of certainty that one finds in long-established scientific theory. But theory, in the first instance, is not a matter of eternal verities; it is first of all a tool for thinking. A good theory may not be ultimately true. It should, however, aim for the greatest possible empirical adequacy and fruitfulness at this moment, given our limited evidence and imagination. It will be quite satisfactory if the present approach helps to move things in the right direction, as a "scaffolding" for further work, to use Freud's term.

11.1 Overall review

Our theoretical framework has really only a few entities: *specialized unconscious processors*, a *global workspace*, and *contexts*. Indeed, contexts are defined as stable coalitions of specialized processors that have over time gained privileged access to the global workspace (4.3.1). Thus, contexts reduce to sets of specialized processors. Further, there are only a few processing principles: *competition* through the global

359

workspace, which can be viewed as lowering activation levels of global messages, and *cooperation*, which raises those activation levels. "Lowering and raising activation levels" is of course analogous to excitation and inhibition in neurons. There is also local processing within unconscious specialized processors, which does not require the global workspace; but this may also work by means of spreading activation (cooperation) and inhibition (competition) (e.g., Rumelhart, McClelland, & the PDP Group, 1986). In sum, three entities and two processing principles together can explain a vast range of evidence about consciousness, volition, and the organization of self.

11.2   A brief review of the models

Developing a theory is much like tracing a consistent path through a maze of theoretical options. The maze may be quite complex, and certainly the number of *potential* paths is huge, but the most plausible path, given current knowledge, may be relatively short and sweet. We can summarize the basic path we have taken quite simply:

First, we found a way to state empirical constraints that must be met by any adequate theory of consciousness (1.2.2).

Second, this evidence suggested a system architecture in which conscious contents are globally broadcast to a collection of specialized unconscious processors (Chapter 2). This is Model 1.

Third, we explored the neurophysiological evidence and found it broadly consistent with this framework. However, there is evidence not only for global broadcasting, but also for feedback from the recipients of the global messages, and in return to the message source as well.

Fourth, we noticed that some stable coalitions of processors, called contexts, must have privileged access to the global workspace. Like other unconscious specialists, contexts can compete and cooperate with each other to gain global access (Model 2).

At this point the theory suggested that there were two necessary conditions for conscious experience, namely *global broadcasting* and *internal consistency* – the latter because inconsistent global messages inevitably trigger competition that quickly destroys the global message.

Fifth, in order to explain the fundamental general fact that conscious experience fades with practice, we were forced to postulate another major necessary condition for consciousness, namely *informativeness*; this was interpreted in the model as a *choice within a context of alternatives, demanding adaptation by other processors*. This created a functional role for the feedback from the receiving processors to the global workspace, which was already suggested by the neurophysiology (Chapter 3). The whole system now began to behave so as to seek a middle way between novelty and redundancy: too much redundancy, and conscious experience will fade; too much mismatch with established context, and no information can be interpreted (Chapter 5, Model 3).

Sixth, without any further cost in theoretical entities, the framework established so far led naturally to the notion of a goal context or intention, which constrains conscious information processing. This allows an explanation of "incubation" or unconscious problem-solving phenomena, which are extremely common – ranging from word retrieval and the interpretation of ambiguous stimuli to high-level artistic and scientific achievement. The stream of consciousness can indeed be seen as a flow of interacting conscious events and goal contexts (Chapter 6, Model 4).

Seventh, the same ideas led to a modern interpretation of William James's ideomotor theory of voluntary control, suggesting that conscious goal-images can by themselves trigger actions, barring competing goal-images or intentions. This in turn suggested that the conscious component of voluntary action is implicitly edited by multiple unconscious criteria (Chapter 7, Model 5).

We are now able to explain a difficult ongoing puzzle, namely the relationship between concrete qualitative conscious events, such as we find in perception and imagery, and the existence of nonqualitative "conscious" contents such as concepts and immediate intentions to act. We suggested that nonqualitative concepts may be under ideomotor control – that is, that there are in fact fleeting conscious images involved in abstract concepts and intentions, but that the images are difficult to retrieve. They do give rapid access to abstractions that are not qualitative. Thus, ultimately, all conscious events involve qualitative phenomena, even though some may be quite difficult to retrieve. This hypothesis needs further empirical testing, of course.

Eighth, within the GW framework, it made sense to draw a distinction between *conscious experience* as such and *attention* as the control of access to conscious experience. The traditional ideas of voluntary and involuntary attention can then be interpreted as access that is due to previous conscious events versus access that is controlled unconsciously (Chapter 8, Model 6).

Ninth, along the way, and much to the author's surprise, it also became natural to interpret notions of "self" and "self-concept" as the deeper parts of the Context Hierarchy (Chapter 9, Model 7). A set of empirical constraints contrasting self-attributed versus self-alien phenomena seemed consistent with this approach.

Tenth, given the development so far, we were able to suggest eighteen

basic adaptive functions of consciousness (Chapter 10). The most fundamental one is the ability to support cooperative interaction between
multiple knowledge sources, so as to cope with novelty.

A number of empirical predictions were made along the way. Explanations emerged quite naturally for unexpected topics like mental absorption, absent-mindedness, hypnosis, the existence of self-alien symptoms
in the clinic, involuntary slips, mental effort, decision making and
indecisiveness, emotional upset as a deep disruption of context, and
surprise as a momentary "erasure" of the global workspace. There was a
continual sense of surprise that new domains of evidence appear to flow
quite spontaneously from the developing theory in the most natural way.
This repeated esthetic experience – of surprising simplicity underlying the
apparent complexity – remains for the author the single best argument for
the current approach.

11.3   What are the necessary conditions for conscious experience?

We can now summarize five necessary conditions without which conscious experience of an event is lost. They are as follows:

1   Conscious events involve globally broadcast information
This is quite a strong claim to make, but there is considerable evidence in
its favor (2.5). Further, a number of the theoretical claims made throughout this book are based on it. For example, the ideomotor control of
action would not work unless conscious messages were made available to
potentially all effectors and action schemata (Chapter 7). The notion of
universal editing of conscious goal-images (7.3.2) would not work unless
any editing criterion could compete against a globally broadcast goal-
image; and so on.

2   Conscious events are internally consistent
Again, the evidence for this idea from both perception and cognition is
quite good (2.1). Chapter 2 presented the argument that other features,
like limited capacity and seriality, follow from the internal consistency
constraint.

*3   Conscious events are informative – that is, they place a
demand for adaptation on other parts of the system*
Chapter 5 was devoted to pursuing this claim, and the complementary
hypothesis that conscious events that become predictable fade from
consciousness, though they do not disappear – in fact, faded conscious

events may create the context for later conscious events. These facts imply that consciousness requires a global message to be available long enough for many local processors to adapt to it, to reduce their uncertainty relative to the conscious message. That is to say, this condition may imply that conscious events must have some *minimal duration*, as suggested in section 2.4.2.

4   Conscious events require access by a self-system

The deeper layers of context may be "self-like" (Chapter 9), in that strong violations of these deeper layers are experienced as self-alien. These deeper layers may respond adaptively to conscious events, either by generating a voluntary response to do something about the event, or simply by recording that it has happened, much like conventional Long Term Memory. Thus, access to GW contents by a self-system seems to be required for reportable conscious experiences.

5   Conscious experience may require perceptual or imaginal events lasting for some minimum duration

Perception, imagery, bodily feelings, and inner speech seem to be involved in the conscious components of thought and action, not merely in input processes (1.2.5). Even abstract conscious concepts may involve rapid quasi-perceptual events. This suggests that perception may be closer to the mind's *lingua franca* than other codes. The evidence is good that images become automatic with practice, and thus fade from consciousness, though they continue to serve as a processing code (1.2.4). Further, many sources of evidence suggest that the perceptual code must be broadcast for at least 50–250 msec (Blumenthal, 1977;2.4.2).

What is unconscious?

If these are *necessary* conditions for conscious experience, it follows that anything that violates just one necessary condition is unconscious. That is, events that are globally broadcast but internally inconsistent are presumably not conscious; perhaps they last for so short a time before their competing parts destroy the global message that they fail to trigger an informative demand for adaptation. Similarly, it is conceivable that contextual information could be globally broadcast without being informative because the system at large has *already* adapted to contextual constraints. There are thus many ways in which information may be unconscious: habituation and automaticity, distraction by high-priority contextually incompatible events, the absence of a context needed to interpret some event, inconsistent events, and so on. It is possible that motivational mechanisms may employ such ways of making things unconscious in order to avoid conscious thoughts that might evoke intense shame, fear, or guilt (8.4).

In sum, we find again that surprising simplicity emerges from the apparent complexity. The evidence discussed throughout this book seems to converge on only five necessary conditions for conscious events: global broadcasting, internal consistency, informativeness, access by a self-system, and perceptual or quasi-perceptual coding.

11.4   Some practical implications of GW theory

Nothing, it is said, is as practical as a good theory. If that is true, and if the present theory is reasonably good, it should have some practical uses. Consider the issue of self-control for example. Self-control is vital in psychopathology, but also in children's learning to control socially undesirable impulses or in the desire of adults to control unwanted habits. The ideomotor theory suggests that *if* one can be exclusively conscious of a desired action without effective competition for a long enough time (probably on the order of seconds) – that the desired behavior will take place, and undesirable behavior will be avoided. The tricky question is, of course, how to avoid competing goal-images – the images of eating compulsively, of smoking, of expressing inappropriate hostility, and so on – without becoming caught in an active struggle for access to consciousness. GW theory suggests that one way may be to use a strong context: something that already structures a flow of conscious contents in an effortless way. For instance, mnemonic techniques or stories might be used to structure a flow of constructive conscious images, lasting long enough to eliminate an undesirable conscious goal. Or a dominant belief system may create the proper context for action. Whatever the method, this temporary control of consciousness, long enough to exclude the unwanted goal-image, becomes the key to constructive change.

These suggestions are merely illustrative, of course. We cannot explore them here in detail. No doubt such difficult practical problems will not be instantly solved within the theory developed so far; but it may be able to provide a useful framework for addressing them.

11.5   Topics not covered in this volume

This book has slighted certain topics that may yet be addressed from the GW perspective. It is worth remembering what we have not tried to explain. For instance, we have said little about time perception, even though it is clearly related to the flow of conscious thought (Blumenthal, 1977; Fraisse, 1963; Ornstein, 1969). We do not at this point have a satisfactory explanation of the "seven plus or minus two" size limit on

Short Term Memory. We have scarcely begun to address the question of reflective thought, a major concern in much psychological research (e.g., Newell & Simon, 1972). Except for our discussion of hypnosis and absorbed states (7.7, 8.5), we have not dealt at all with altered states of consciousness. All over the world there seem to be universal similarities in mystical experiences, spanning the length of recorded history (Huxley, 1970; Naranjo & Ornstein, 1971). In principle, we should be able to say something useful about this topic too. Finally, we have not really addressed the important issues surrounding sleep and dreaming. If the present framework proves viable, it will be worthwhile to explore the implications of GW theory for such significant questions.

11.6   Philosophical implications: The mind–body problem revisited

Some philosophical questions may be so basic that they are never wholly settled. Several scientists have argued that the mind–body problem may be one of these, and that in fact "mind" has emerged in modern science in the guise of "information," which plays a central role in physics, biology, and the information sciences (e.g., Baars, 1986a; Bakan, 1980; Shannon & Weaver, 1949; Szilard, 1929/1964; Wiener, 1961). Information is said to be irreducible to physical quantities. As Norbert Wiener has written, "Information is information; it is neither matter nor energy" (1961 p. 8). If the claim that consciousness must be informative can be developed (5.3), we might add psychology to the list of sciences for which the concept of information is central. Further, information and control are two sides of the same mathematical coin (Wiener, 1961), just as consciousness and volition are two sides of the same psychological coin (7.0). We can only mention these intriguing hints in passing, but they may be well worth following up.

11.7   Future directions for research and theory

There is a great need to model the ideas developed in this book more explicitly. This is not very difficult; in fact, there have been simulations of "blackboard systems" since the 1970s (see Chapter 2). We have begun to explore a simple simulation intended to capture some central features of GW theory, using the techniques of "connectionist" models (Cohen, Galin, & Baars, 1986); but much more needs to be done.

Further, we need more critical experiments. One basic prediction from GW theory was apparently confirmed even before this book went to press (Greenwald & Liu, 1985, 5.6). But a framework theory like this one clearly requires more than a single critical experiment. We could easily imagine a comprehensive research program to rigorously test the empirical predictions presented in this book and to improve the precision and consistency of the theoretical claims.

The work is never done, of course. Nevertheless, in glancing back to the beginning of this book we can take some satisfaction in the thought that many difficult and confusing issues now seem clearer, and that a great number of facts seem to fit this simple framework surprisingly well. Whether this sense of clarity and integration will endure or whether it is destined to fade in the face of new evidence and theory, only time will tell.

Glossary and guide to theoretical claims

All entries and cross-entries are *in italics*. Relevant sections are cited in parentheses.

absent-mindedness. See *absorbed state*.

absorbed state (7.7). Empirically, a state like fantasy, selective attention, absent-minded day-dreaming and probably hypnosis, in which conscious experience is unusually resistant to distraction. Theoretically, a case in which access to the *global workspace (GW)* is controlled by a coherent *Context Hierarchy*, giving little opportunity for outside information to compete for conscious access (4.3.2). See also *ideomotor theory, access, and Options Context*.

access, attentional control of access to consciousness. Following commonsense usage, a distinction is made between *consciousness* and *attention*, where attention is treated as the set of mechanisms that control access to consciousness (8.0). See also *voluntary attention, automatic attention*.

Access-control Function of the GW system. Repeated conscious access to an event can increase the likelihood of accessing the event in the future (8.0). One of the 18 or so distinguishable functions of the cognitive architecture developed here. See also *Prioritizing Function (10.5)*.

accommodation. In Piagetian theory, a process of adaptation that requires new mental structures. In the present perspective, the pole of the adaptation dimension in which new *contexts* are needed to deal with input (5.1). See also *assimilation–accommodation dimension*.

acontextual (4.1.2). A coined term, along the lines of Markus and Sentis's (1982) "aschematic," to mean the absence of the appropriate *Dominant Context* needed to interpret some potentially conscious input. *Selective attention* may operate by making nonattended information acontextual, *fixedness* in perception and cognition may have this effect, and perceptual learning may be viewed as the acquisition of a context for interpreting the perceptual input, thus going from an acontextual to a contextual state.

action fiat. In William James's *ideomotor theory*, the momentary conscious decision to carry out a previously prepared action, a notion that can easily be interpreted in *GW theory* (7.1, 7.3).

367

action schema. One of the structural components of action, as shown, for example, by action errors, which often cause actions to decompose along structural lines (1.4.4). See also *goal context*.

activation. A widely used theoretical mechanism in which numbers are assigned to nodes in a semantic network. Each node typically stands for an element of knowledge, such as a phoneme, a letter feature, or a concept. Activation numbers associated with each node are typically allowed to spread to neighboring nodes, a process that can model priming phenomena and associative learning. In *GW theory*, activation numbers can be used to represent the likelihood that some event will become conscious. However, activation cannot be the only necessary condition for consciousness because of the *Redundancy Effects*, which show that repeated conscious contents fade rapidly from consciousness even though they clearly continue to be highly active by other criteria (1.3.1, 2.3.3).

activation, spreading (2.3.3). See *activation*.

Activation Hypotheses. A set of proposals about conscious experience going back to F. Herbart in the early nineteenth century, suggesting that ideas become conscious when they cross some threshold of activation (1.3.1).

adaptation. In the narrow sense used in Chapter 5, the ability to match and predict input. In a broader sense, adaptation also includes the ability to solve problems (6.0) and to act upon input (7.0). In the first sense it is treated as a gain in *information*, that is, a reduction of uncertainty about the input within a stable context. Apparently, all neural structures adapt selectively to stimulation. This may be called local adaptation. The fact that repeated predictable conscious events fade from consciousness suggests a kind of global adaptation as well (5.0). See also *Redundancy Effects*.

adaptive system. Any system that works to match informative input. Information processing can be viewed in terms of *representations* and their transformations, or alternatively in terms of adaptive systems. As theoretical primitives, "representation" and "adaptation" are quite similar.

Adaptation Function of consciousness. It is argued that the premier function of consciousness is to facilitate adaptation to novel and informative input (10.2).

Adaptation Level Theory. A theory developed by Helson and others, still the major effort to date to deal with the way experience is shaped by previous experiences along the same dimension. In *GW theory* this is thought to work by means of conscious experiences that modify related *contexts* (4.0, 5.0).

ambiguity. The existence of at least two different interpretations of the same event. Local ambiguity is one of the basic environmental conditions the nervous system must cope with. It is rife in language, vision, conceptual thinking, the social world, the interpretation of bodily feelings, and in understanding any novel event. The prevalence of ambiguity necessitates a neural mechanism that can combine many knowledge sources to arrive at a single interpretation of the input. *Global Workspace theory* describes such a mechanism (2.3, 4.1.3).

Analogy-forming Function of consciousness. Human beings have a powerful capacity for creating analogies and metaphors, focusing on similarities between otherwise different experiences or concepts. This requires mental representations of these different events to interact. The *global workspace* may provide the mechanism for this interaction. Certainly novel analogies and metaphors seem to require consciousness to be understood (10.0).

"any" arguments (2.5). A set of arguments for the existence of a truly *global* workspace, based on phenomena in which "any" event of one kind can be demonstrated to interact with "any" event of another kind. These phenomena include cross-modality matching, *biofeedback training*, conditioning (within biological limits), the *context-sensitivity* of conscious experiences, etc.

assimilation–accommodation dimension of adaptation (5.1). As Piaget points out, adaptive processes may or may not be structurally prepared for some event. If they are highly prepared, they require little adaptation to detect or learn the event, the case of assimilation. If they are unprepared for the input, deep accommodative changes (see *accommodation*) may be demanded in existing structures. *GW theory* suggests that accommodative changes require a change in the relatively stable *contexts* of conscious experience.

attention. In *GW theory*, the control of *access* to consciousness by reference to long-term or recent goals (8.0). Attention may be *voluntary* or *automatic*. See also *Prioritizing Function*.

attentional access to information-processing resources. Some psychologists have suggested that the role of attention is to control access to knowledge and skills (e.g., Navon & Gopher, 1979). This is one motivation for the theory developed in this book (1.3.2).

attentional context (8.2.1). A *goal context* designed to bring material to consciousness, for example by recruiting receptor orientation (e.g., eye movements). See also *context*, *Options Context*, *automatic control of attention*, *voluntary attention*.

attributional ambiguity. Given the fact that the thoughts, emotions, and intentions of other people are invisible, and that we sometimes do not know our own intentions either, there is much room for attributional error and variability. A particularly interesting case is the issue of self–other ambiguity, in which the identical event may be self-attributed or other-attributed under different circumstances (9.0).

automatic attention. Automatic mechanisms can control access to consciousness (8.1). With practice, voluntary attentional strategies tend to become automatic and involuntary. See also *attention*, *voluntary attention*, and *Prioritizing Function*.

automaticity, automatization. The tendency of practiced, predictable skills, concepts, mental images, and perceptual stimuli to fade from consciousness. Automatic processes tend to be dissociated from each other (see *dissociation*), they take up little *central limited capacity*, and resist voluntary control (1.4.4, 2.1, 5.1.3, 5.3). See also *deautomatization*, *habituation*, *Redundancy Effects*.

Autoprogramming Function of consciousness. *GW theory* suggests that consciousness is needed to develop new operating capacities in the nervous system (10.9). See also *Self-maintenance Function*.

bandwidth question. (2.7.3.) For the sake of simplicity we assume that in any single 100-msec integration period of the global workspace only one internally consistent message can gain access. However, the evidence on this point may be arguable, so that we mark this as a *theoretical choice-point*. See *minimum integration time*.

behaviorism. Influential physicalistic philosophy of psychology, some forms of which commonly deny the existence or functionality of consciousness.

belief. 7.6.1. An abstract concept that is not disputed in the stream of thought, though plausibly it could be. A belief *system* may be defined as a consistent set of such undisputed thoughts, which may serve as a *Dominant Context* for many conscious thoughts, feelings and actions. A *closed belief system* is one that has a ready answer to all apparent counter-arguments, so that any possibility of change is minimized (Rokeach, 1960). See also *Decision-making Function*, *ideomotor theory*.

biofeedback training. There is evidence that any neural system can come under voluntary control, at least temporarily, by arranging for a conscious feedback signal whenever the target system is active. This remarkable capacity provides one argument for truly global broadcasting of conscious information (2.5). See *"any" arguments*.

bi-stable perceptual events. Many stimuli can be interpreted in more than one way. Some involve reversible bi-stable stimuli, like the Necker Cube or figure-ground illusions. Much more common are nonreversible cases. Perceptual learning typically shows non-reversible bi-stability. The "Dalmatian" demonstration in 5.1.1 provides one example. See also *ambiguity*.

"blind sight." Damage to the primary visual cortex sometimes leads to a condition in which the victim can recognize visual objects without a sense of their being conscious. This is an interesting and important phenomenon, but we argue that such difficult cases are not to be used for constructing an adequate theory in the first instance (1.1.2). They are, however, a challenge for a theory built upon more common phenomena.

brain duality. The two cerebral hemispheres are well known to have a major division down the midline, connected only by the corpus callosum. In fact, there are midline divisions even in the midbrain and possibly the brain stem. This is a puzzling feature from the viewpoint of *GW theory*, which emphasizes unity rather than duality. One possibility is that brain duality has a primarily developmental role (3.3).

broadcasting. See *global distribution*.

central limited capacity. Consciousness is associated with a central "bottleneck" in information processing, as shown by *selective attention*, *dual-task measures*, and the limitations of immediate memory. (1.3.4). By contrast, unconscious specialized processors, taken together, have much greater processing capacity. See also *automaticity*.

Chevreul pendulum. A classic demonstration of ideomotor control (7.4.1).

coalition formation. See *cooperative processing*.

cognitive architectures. Cognitive theories that focus on the entire human information-processing system, rather than on particular subsystems such as *Short Term Memory*, language, or vision (1.3.6).

coma. Damage to parts of the brain delimited by the *Extended Reticular-Thalamic Activating System* (ERTAS) seems to lead to coma. This can be interpreted as damage to the neural equivalent of a *global workspace* system (3.1.2).

common sense (1.3.1). Originally, the general sense modality that is presumed to provide common ground between the special senses like vision and hearing. This traditional idea has much in common with a *global workspace*. The common sense explained the interaction between the special senses and their ability to share certain features like location, causality, and time of a single event. Aristotle proposed a set of modern-sounding cognitive arguments for the common sense, but this concept is also known in Eastern philosophy.

competition for access to consciousness. There are two kinds of competition, either between potentially conscious stimuli (e.g., in a *dual-task* paradigm), or between different controlling *contexts* when the input is the same (e.g., switching between two interpretations of a stimulus in binocular rivalry or in linguistic ambiguity). Most cases of competition seem to involve both (2.3, 4.3.5, 6.5.1, 7.8).

computational inefficiency of conscious processes (2.1.1). Conscious processes are generally much less efficient than comparable unconscious ones. Consciously controlled skills are slower, involve more mutual interference, and are more prone to error than the same skills after *automatization* (see also *automaticity*).

conceptual context. Unconscious constraints on conscious *access* to abstract concepts. Specifically, the conceptual *presupposed knowledge* needed to use conscious concepts, but which is itself difficult to access.

conceptual Redundancy Effects. Repetitive concepts become more difficult to access consciously. See also *semantic satiation, Redundancy Effects*.

conceptual versus perceptual conscious contents. See *qualitative conscious experiences, nonqualitative conscious events*.

conflict-free sphere of conscious access and control (7.8.3.). A term borrowed from ego psychology to denote the domain in which deep *goal contexts* are not in conflict, so that a variety of conscious contents can be accessed with minimal *mental effort*.

conscious access versus conscious experience. We speak of *qualitative conscious experiences*, as in perception, mental imagery, inner speech, or feelings. All these events have experienced dimensions: color, taste, texture, discrete boundaries in space and time, etc. We speak of conscious *access* in cases such as accurately reported, currently "conscious" concepts, beliefs, and intentions where there are generally no reported conscious qualities (1.5.4, 4.0.0, 6.5.2, 7.6.3). See also *perceptual bias* of conscious experience.

conscious contents. Either qualitative *conscious experiences* or readily accessible *nonqualitative conscious events* that are reported as being conscious.

conscious experience. See *qualitative conscious experiences, conscious access.*

conscious moment (2.4.2). See *minimum integration time.*

consciousness. Operationally defined as the set of events that can be reported with verifiable accuracy and are claimed to be conscious under optimal reporting conditions (1.2.1). It includes qualitative contents (see *qualitative conscious experiences*), such as percepts, mental images, inner speech, and feelings of pleasure, pain, and affect; as well as nonqualitative contents (see *nonqualitative conscious events*), such as currently accessible concepts, beliefs, intentions, and expectations (1.2.5). The operational definition provides a workable starting point about which other properties can accrue, such as the fact that conscious contents load *central limited capacity.* Theoretically, a conscious event is defined in *GW theory* as a mental representation that is broadcast globally (see *global distribution*), that is *internally consistent, informative*, and tends to be expressed in perceptual code (see *perceptual bias*) (11.4). See *necessary conditions* for conscious experience and access, *conscious access versus conscious experience.*

consistency. See *necessary conditions for consciousness.*

content. See *conscious content.*

context. One of the three main constructs of GW theory, operationally defined as a system (or set of systems) that constrains conscious contents without itself being conscious (1.5.3, 4.2). Context effects are well known in virtually all psychological domains, including perception, imagery, action control, learning, and conceptual knowledge. Theoretically, contexts are groups of *specialized processors*, some quite long-lasting, that serve to evoke and shape global messages without themselves broadcasting any message (4.3.2, 5.1.1). Contexts can *compete* or *cooperate* to jointly constrain conscious contents. See also *Context Hierarchy, attentional context, Options Context.*

Context Hierarchy (4.3.2). A nested set of contexts that cooperatively constrain conscious contents. Conscious events are always constrained by the multiple layers of a Context Hierarchy. Because contexts can be thought of as recursively defined entities (see *recursive organization*), a set of contexts is also a context (4.3). See also *Dominant Context Hierarchy.*

context of communication. For communication to work, the speaker and listener must share a great amount of knowledge that is not conscious at the moment of communication (4.2.4).

context-sensitivity (2.1). A major property of conscious experience, which is always shaped and evoked by systems that are not conscious. See also *context.*

constructivism (1.3.5, 2.3.2, 10.1). The view that conscious experience involves a constructed reality that goes beyond its component inputs (Mandler, 1983, 1984; Marcel, 1983a).

Context-setting Function of consciousness. One major role of conscious experience is to create or evoke the context needed to interpret later experiences (10.1).

contextualization (5.34). The process by which a conscious content becomes unconscious (due to practice and adaptation), and thereby becomes part of a new context – it serves to constrain future conscious contents. See also *context*, *objectification*, *decontextualization*.

contrastive analysis. The empirical evidence for GW theory is summarized in several sets of paired contrasts between similar conscious and unconscious events (see Index of Tables and Figures). For example, novel tasks tend to be much more conscious in the beginning than they are after practice, even though their physical and psychological role may be quite similar. These contrasts are analogous to experiments in which consciousness is the independent variable (1.2.2–1.2.4, 2.1).

Control Function of consciousness. In *GW theory*, conscious *goal-images* serve to control action (10.4). See also *ideomotor theory*.

cooperation (cooperative processing, coalition formation). Specialized processors can work together in pursuit of some consciously broadcast goal. Cooperating systems can, over time, come to constitute new specialized processors (2.3.2.). When contextual systems cooperate in this fashion they can be represented as a *Context Hierarchy* (4.3.2).

cortical arousal. Electrical activity in the cerebral cortex that is typically fast, low-amplitude, and desynchronized. It is associated with waking consciousness and mental activity. Stimulation of the *Extended Reticular-Thalamic Activating System* (ERTAS) leads to widespread cortical activation (3.1).

countervoluntary actions. See *involuntary actions*.

deautomatization. The tendency of automatic skills after disruption to break apart into more consciously accessible components, as in attempting to read material that is printed upside-down (1.4.4).

Debugging Function of consciousness. People tend to become conscious of violated expectations. Conscious error detection may be necessary for such errors to be mended ("debugged"), though the details of repair are of course unconscious (10.3).

Decision-making Function of consciousness. GW theory suggests that voluntary decisions may involve a "voting procedure" in which competing sets of specialized processors add *activation* to alternative global messages. Those receiving the most votes tend to remain conscious longest and thus have the "last word." The *ideomotor theory* suggests that the last in a series of conscious experiences will tend to recruit effective action, so that having the last word in the mental dialogue is extremely important (7.6.1, 10.6).

decontextualization (4.1.4). See *objectification*.

default execution of goal-images. The *ideomotor theory* states that conscious goal-images tend to be executed "impulsively" or by default, unless competing *goal-images* or *intentions* prevent execution (7.3).

Definitional Function of consciousness. In GW theory, conscious contents are shaped and evoked by unconscious *contexts*, interacting through the *global workspace*. Thus multiple knowledge sources interact to define the conscious contents, by bringing the proper context to bear, and by resolving ambiguities of interpretation (2.3.2; 4.2; 10.1). See also *Context-setting Function*.

depersonalization. A type of *self-alien experience* in which the victim feels estranged from him- or herself. This condition is apparently very common in late adolescence and early adulthood, and places constraints on the notion of *self* (9.1).

derealization. A condition in which the world is perceived accurately, but is felt to be unreal (9.1). See also *depersonalization*.

Diffuse Thalamic Projection System (3.12). See *Extended Reticular-Thalamic Activating System*.

disambiguation (2.3.2, 4.1.3). In the GW framework, a major function of consciousness is to allow multiple knowledge sources to interact in order to remove ambiguity in focal contents. See also *Definitional Function* of consciousness.

disavowed goals or emotions (7.82). In many cases people can be shown to disavow goals or emotions which, by other empirical criteria, they clearly have. This suggests a conflict between voluntary and involuntary expression of goals and a breakdown of *metacognitive access*. The *ideomotor theory* suggests one account of these conflict phenomena (7.8).

dissociation. Normally unitary functions are sometimes decomposed; conscious access to these functions may be lost, at least for some time. Decomposability is one source of evidence for *specialized processors*. Dissociation is observable in memory access, knowledge representation, motor control, perception, and self-states (1.4, 9.1).

distributed system. A decentralized information-processing system, in which many *specialized processors* work *cooperatively* to solve shared problems. GW theory describes one such system. (1.3.6, 2.2).

Dominant Context. See *Dominant Context Hierarchy*.

Dominant Context Hierarchy. A coherent set of *contexts* that controls current access to the *global workspace*. Both *conceptual* and *goal contexts* seem to be hierarchically organized, although competing contexts can disrupt any given level of the Dominant Context Hierarchy (4.3.2, 6.4.2).

Dominant Goal Context. A goal context that dominates the global workspace, thereby controlling access to the *limited-capacity system*. A nested set of Dominant Goal Contexts make up a *Dominant Goal Hierarchy*.

Dominant Goal Hierarchy. One kind of *Dominant Context Hierarchy*, consisting of nested *goal contexts* that together constrain access to the *global workspace*. It is particularly important in *problem solving, voluntary control,* and the *self-system* (4.32, 6.42, 9.22).

dual-task measures of central limited capacity. Two simultaneous tasks will interfere with each other if they involve consciousness or *mental effort,* even though they may be very different from each other. This is one source of evidence for *central limited capacity* (1.3.4).

editing. The *Dominant Goal Hierarchy* shapes normal, *voluntary action* (7.0). Conscious components of the goal structure are broadcast globally, so that unconscious specialized processors can compete against (edit) those goal-images they find flawed. Since the most *informative* components typically become conscious (i.e., those that are novel, significant, or conflictful), it follows that these components of voluntary action must have been tacitly edited prior to execution if there was enough time to do so (7.3.2).

Editing Function of consciousness (10.3). Conscious events are broadcast to multiple unconscious systems, which can compete against it if it violates their criteria. See also *Flagging Function, Debugging Function.*

editing time (7.5.1). In the GW version of the *ideomotor theory* of voluntary control, the time between the onset of a *goal-image* and its interruption by unconscious *receiving processors* able to spot errors. See also *horse-race model, execution time.*

effort, mental. See *mental effort.*

ego-dystonic. See *self-alien experiences.*

ego-syntonic. See *self-attributed experiences.*

emotional conflict. See *goal conflict.*

empirical constraints on any theory of conscious experience. See *contrastive analysis.*

Enduring Dispositions. A term used by Kahneman (1973), corresponding to long-term *contexts* in GW theory (e.g., 9.2).

episodic memory. The repository of conscious, autobiographical experiences, which, judged by sensitive memory measures such as recognition tasks, appears to be extremely large (Tulving, 1972, 1985; Bransford, 1979). See also *semantic memory.*

event identity after learning, the problem of. If conscious events create new *contexts,* and contexts shape later conscious experiences of the same event, it follows that the event should be experienced differently at a later time. Thus the experienced identity of the event changes with learning. This seems paradoxical, but it may be a characteristic feature of the growth of knowledge, as Kuhn notes in the case of science (5.7).

execution time (7.5.1). The time from the onset of a *goal-image* to the execution of an action recruited by the image. If execution time is shorter than *editing time,* a slip of speech or action is likely to occur (7.3.2, 7.5). See also *horse-race model, ideomotor theory.*

Executive Function of consciousness. In GW theory, consciousness is associated with a *global workspace* in a *distributed system* consisting of many *specialized processors*. This architecture does not involve executive systems in the first instance, just as a television broadcasting station does not necessarily involve a government. However, the global workspace may be utilized by executive *goal contexts* to control a great variety of activities in the nervous system. See *biofeedback training, voluntary control* (2.7.2, Chapters 6–10).

executive ignorance in voluntary control. In the *ideomotor theory*, the claim that executive systems do not track the details of effector control. (All normal people can wriggle their fingers, but very few know that the muscles needed to do this are not located in the hand, but in the forearm.) (7.3).

expectation. A nonqualitative, future-directed mental representation regarding external events that can dominate *central limited capacity.* See also *conceptual context.*

Extended Reticular-Thalamic Activating System (ERTAS). A convenient label for the set of nuclei and pathways extending from the brain stem *Reticular Formation* to the outer layer of the *thalamus* and the *Diffuse Thalamic Projection System* leading to the cortex. ERTAS is closely associated with sleep, waking, coma, and *cortical arousal* – all aspects of conscious processes. This system has many of the features of a *global workspace* (3.1.2).

fading of conscious experience with redundancy. See *Redundancy Effects.*

failure-driven retrieval of contextual knowledge. Presupposed knowledge that rarely becomes conscious can become conceptually available when it runs into a severe contradiction (4.1.4). See also *deautomatization, decontextualization.*

feature-integration view of attention. A recent theory suggesting that consciousness can act as a "glue" to integrate separable features in perception. (1.3.2).

feedback. Two kinds of feedback may exist in a *global workspace* system. First, a global message may be fed back directly to its input processors. Second, *receiving processors* may feed back their interest in some global message, in order to support continued broadcasting of the message. Probably both kinds of feedback exist (3.2).

filter theory of attention. The hypothesis, associated in modern psychology with Broadbent (1958), that the role of attention is to select some aspects of the stimulus world for processing and to exclude others. The role of attention is therefore to conserve processing capacity for the most important things.

Filter Paradox. There is good evidence from *selective attention* experiments that unattended (unconscious) stimuli are analyzed under some conditions to quite a high level. This suggests that unattended input involves as much input processing as attended input, and thus vitiates the claim that attention saves processing capacity. *GW theory* resolves the problem by suggesting that all input is highly analyzed, but only conscious input is widely distributed to a multitude of specialized unconscious *processors* (2.2, 1.4).

fixedness. In perception, problem solving, and action, being blind to what is obvious to an outsider. Explained in *GW theory* as an effect of the *Dominant Goal Context* (4.1).

Flagging Function of consciousness. Conscious (global) display of information can mobilize many specialized processors to work on a common topic. This may happen in *biofeedback training*, for example (10.3). See also *Editing Function, Debugging Function.*

fleeting conscious events. Rapid, potentially conscious, limited-capacity-loading events, which may be quite important in controlling voluntary action, among other things but which may be difficult to report under ordinary circumstances. However, they are often reported in *tip-of-the-tongue* states (1.5.5). While such fleeting events pose evidentiary difficulties, their presence is strongly suggested by *GW theory* (1.5.5, 6.5.2, 7.6.4).

focal consciousness. Usually contrasted with *peripheral consciousness* the part of conscious experience that allows for the clearest discrimination.

fugue, psychogenic. Literally, a "flight" from reality in which the victim travels away from home, adopts a new identity, and may suddenly rediscover his or her old identity. A syndrome relevant to the issue of self (*self-system*) in relation to conscious experience (9.1). See also *depersonalization, self-alien experiences.*

functions of conscious experience. Like other major biological phenomena, consciousness plays more than one significant adaptive role. Some 18 separable functions can be specified (10.0).

functional equivalents of a global workspace system (2.6.1). *Global Workspace theory* claims that consciousness is associated with something like a *global workspace*, but that many system architectures can behave in a functionally equivalent way. One can think of the system as a "searchlight" rather than a "blackboard," for example, or even as a series of mental senses, only one of which can operate at a time. All these systems seem to operate in much the same way.

functional unity of specialized processors. In the act of riding a bicycle, steering, peddling, balance, and visual perception are closely coordinated in a single processing coalition. This coalition may be decomposed and reorganized when one steps off the bicycle and begins to walk. In the same sense, perhaps any *specialized processor* can be functionally unitary in a given task, but may be decomposed and reorganized for some other task. (1.4.5). See also *dissociation, cooperative processing.*

global access. The ability of many *specialized processors* to place or support messages on the *global workspace*. The input side of *global distribution*.

global broadcasting. See also *global distribution*.

global distribution of conscious information (*global broadcasting*). The ability of conscious signals to be made available very widely to numerous *specialized processors*. The output side of *global access*. (2.5)

Global Input Processors. (2.6.4) It may be that only some processors can provide input to the *global workspace,* and that others merely act as *Global Receiving Processors*. The evidence for the *perceptual bias* of conscious contents suggests that perceptual and imaginal system may indeed be special and that global input might be limited to perceptual or quasiperceptual events. Effector control systems, for example, may only be able to receive global information, but not to access the *global workspace* directly. On this question our current evidence is not decisive, so that we merely define a *theoretical choice-point* to define the alternatives, leaving the answer open for the time being.

Global Receiving Processors. (2.6.4) See *Global Input Processors.*

global variable. In computer science, a variable that is defined for more than one subsystem of a larger system.

global workspace. A memory that can be accessed by numerous *specialized processors*, whose contents are widely *broadcast* or distributed, in principle to all specialists in the nervous system. One of the three major constructs of *GW theory* (2.2).

Global Workspace System (2.3). The entire set of theoretical entities postulated in *GW theory*, including specialized processors, the *global workspace*, and contextual systems.

Global Workspace (GW) theory. The theory developed in this book, which associates conscious experience with a rather simple architecture of the psychological system. GW theory has three basic constructs: a *global workspace*, a set of *specialized unconscious processors*, and a set of unconscious *contexts* that serve to shape, evoke, and define conscious contents (2.2).

globally informative (5.3.1). See *informativeness.*

goal. A representation of a future state that serves to recruit and guide subgoals and motor systems needed to reach that state. Classically, behavioral persistence in working towards an end-state in the face of obstacles, has been taken as operational evidence for the existence of a goal.

goal addressability. Some *specialized processors* seem to be responsive to goals, especially conscious goals (1.4.5, 7.2, 7.3). See *biofeedback training, ideomotor theory.*

goal conflict. A state in which two or more goal contexts compete for the ability to dominate the *global workspace.* See also *Dominant Context Hierarchy, Dominant Goal Hierarchy.*

goal context. A future-directed, nonqualitative mental representation about one's own actions that can dominate *central limited capacity.* A *context* that constrains conscious *goal-images* without itself being conscious. Also called an intention (4.2.3, 6.4, 7.3). See also *Dominant Goal Hierarchy, expectation.*

goal-image. In the GW version of James's *ideomotor theory*, a mental image of a future state which serves to recruit processors and *subgoals* that work to achieve the future state. *Goal-images*, if they are conscious long enough to recruit an action, are generally consistent with the *Dominant Goal Hierarchy.* The ideomotor theory suggests that conscious goal-images are inherently impulsive; i.e., they tend to result in action unless they are rapidly contradicted by another conscious event, or by a *goal context* (see *default execution*). It is conceivable however that very fleeting goal-images may trigger *involuntary* actions by well-prepared systems before they have been *edited* or controlled by the *Dominant Goal Hierarchy* (7.3). This loss of control may explain slips of speech and action, and even psychopathological symptoms.

goal structure. See *Goal Hierarchy*.

Goal Hierarchy. A multileveled goal structure consisting of goals and subgoals. Each level may be considered a *goal context*. It seems likely that people become conscious of underdetermined choice-points in any *Dominant Goal Hierarchy* (6.1.3, 7.3, 9.2).

habituation. Most generally, decrease of information-processing activity upon repetition of input (1.2.4, 5.1.3). All neural structures habituate *selectively* to repetitive stimulation. That is, they will decrease their activity to the repeated input, but not to novel input. Sokolov (1963) has argued that habituation of the *Orienting Response* (closely associated with conscious surprise) cannot be a fatigue effect, since fatigue would not operate selectively. Instead, he suggests that habituation reflects a learning process in which the nervous system maintains a model of the stimulus even when it has become habituated (and hence is unconscious). *Global Workspace theory* considers habituation as a *Redundancy Effect*.

habituation of awareness is one kind of selective decrease in responsiveness, in which functions associated with consciousness habituate, including the *Orienting Response*, perceptual awareness, etc. (1.2.4, 5.1.3). See also *Redundancy Effects*.

higher-level contexts. The higher levels of a *Context Hierarchy*, which are more stable and are presupposed by lower levels (4.3.2). Thus higher-level changes in a Context Hierarchy propagate more widely to all lower levels than do low-level changes (4.4.3, 9.4.4).

horse-race, countervoluntary errors, as a losing (7.3.2). Unwanted errors occur in the case of slips of speech and action, *psychopathology*, and voluntarily resisted automaticity (7.5). It is attractive to suppose in these cases that a *goal-image* tends to be executed by *default* unless it is interrupted by other *editing* systems. If editing takes too long, the erroneous goal will be executed. Thus one can imagine a horse-race between *editing time* and *execution time*.

hypnosis. True hypnosis, of the kind found in the highly hypnotizable fraction of the population, is interpreted in *Global Workspace theory* as an *absorbed state*, in which the *Dominant Context Hierarchy* allows very little outside competition for access to consciousness. As a result, conscious *goal-images* can exercise great ideomotor control over thought and action (7.7).

ideomotor theory. In William James and others, the notion that conscious goals are inherently impulsive, and tend to be carried out by *default* unless they are inhibited by other conscious thoughts or intentions. This theory can be straightforwardly incorporated into *Global Workspace theory*, and helps to explain aspects of *voluntary action*, the problem of *nonqualitative conscious events*, and a number of other puzzles (7.3).

imaginal experience (1.2). A conscious, internally generated, quasi-perceptual representation, including visual and auditory images, and perhaps somatically experienced emotions (Mandler, 1975a).

imageless-thought controversy. About the beginning of the twentieth century, an intense controversy about the status of quasi-conscious events that seem to accompany the "set" of solving a problem, and abstract thoughts in general. This controversy was thought by many behaviorists to discredit the entire psychology of the nineteenth century; in fact, it was quite substantive, and raised central issues about the role of consciousness (1.2.5, 7.6.4).

implicit comparison (5.3.4). All conscious events are said in GW theory to be *informative*, implying that they reduce uncertainty in an implicit set of alternatives to the conscious event.

informativeness. In *Global Workspace theory*, one of the necessary conditions for a conscious event (5.0, 5.4, 11.4). Conscious input is always interpreted in an implicit context of alternatives, and results in a reduction of uncertainty among these alternatives. If a stimulus is redundant, consciousness of the input is lost because its information content is now zero (see *Redundancy Effects*). Even the *significance* of a conscious event, which clearly affects the chances of its remaining conscious, can be interpreted as *information* provided by the event within a *Dominant Goal Context*.

information. Formally, the case of a sender, a receiver, and message channel, in which a signal sent to the receiver serves to reduce uncertainty among the receiver's preexisting alternatives (Shannon & Weaver, 1949). The mathematical measure of information based on this definition has been extraordinarily influential in computer science, communication engineering, and even theoretical physics and biology. In psychology there has been debate about its usefulness, though it has been successfully applied in a number of cases. We claim that a somewhat broader conception of information is central to the understanding of consciousness (5.0). See also *informativeness, Redundancy Effects*.

inhibition. See *activation*.

inner dialogue. See *inner speech*.

inner speech (inner dialogue) (1.1.2, 1.3.4, 1.5.4, 8.1.6). Clearly one of the most important modalities of conscious experience. It has been widely proposed that inner speech is often abbreviated, and we suggest that, insofar as individuals share a great deal of the *context of communication* with themselves, only those elements that distinguish between alternatives in this context need to become conscious in inner speech (4.2.4).

input (into the *global workspace*). Input into the *global workspace* allows *global access* by many different cooperating and competing processors (2.4, 1.4). There is considerable evidence for a *minimum integration time* of about 100 milliseconds between separate inputs. The output of the *global workspace* is *globally distributed* (2.5).

intention. See *goal context*.

internal consistency. See *necessary conditions for consciousness.*

involuntary actions. Voluntary actions are mainly automatic (see *automaticity*) in their details, except for certain novel and informative aspects (7.2). Yet even the automatic components of normal action are perceived as voluntary if they are consistent with the *Dominant Goal Hierarchy.* Other automatic actions are unwanted, or *countervoluntary*, such as slips of the tongue, voluntarily resisted automatisms, and psychopathological symptoms (7.1, 7.5). It is important therefore to use the term "involuntary" with care, since it can mean either "automatic and wanted" or "unwanted" (countervoluntary). See also *self-attributed experiences* and *self-alien experiences.*

learning. *Global Workspace theory* claims that consciousness inherently involves adaptation and learning. While it is difficult to demonstrate that consciousness is a necessary condition for learning, the theory suggests that there is an upward monotonic function between the amount of *information* to be learned and the duration of conscious involvement necessary to learn it. See also *informativeness*, *zero-point problem.*

learning without awareness. See *zero-point problem.*

Learning Function of consciousness. See *learning* (10.2).

limited adaptability of *specialized processors.* By virtue of the fact that they are specialized, each of these systems can only deal with a limited range of input (1.4.5, 2.1).

limited capacity. See *central limited capacity.*

lingua franca. A trade language, such as Swahili or English in many parts of the world. By extension, a common language for different neural structures that may do their preferred processing in separate codes (1.5.4). Given the perceptual bias of conscious contents, one likely possibility is a spatio-temporal code (3.2). Many neural structures are indeed sensitive to spatio-temporal information.

linguistic hierarchy. The standard view that language is represented structurally in a series of levels, going from acoustic analysis or motor control to more abstract levels such as phonemics, morphemics, words, syntax, semantics, and pragmatics (2.3.2). Each of these levels can be treated as a *specialized processor*, or a collection of them.

logical positivism. Probably the most influential philosophy of science in the first half of the twentieth century; it discouraged free theoretical construct formation in psychology, and the study of consciousness in particular (1.1.1). See also *behaviorism.*

Long Term Memory (LTM). The store of permanent memory, generally said to include episodic memory, an autobiographical record of conscious experience, and semantic memory, a store of abstract rules and knowledge (Tulving 1972, 1985). LTM could also plausibly include permanent skills, the lexicon, and even long-lasting attitudes and personality features. See also *Short Term Memory.*

meditation. Meditative practices seem almost universally to involve repetition of short words, phrases, or visual input over a long period of time. They therefore seem to evoke *Redundancy Effects*, which are known to directly influence conscious experience (5.7.2).

mental effort (7.6.2, 8.15, 9.2.2). The subjective experience of resistance to current goals. Mental effort takes up central limited capacity, suggesting that it involves the *global workspace*. Effortful action may involve an implicit comparison between the predicted and actual time to the goal (see also *execution time*). The perception of effort may be a key to the experience of voluntary control (7.6.2).

mental workload. *Dual-task measures* can be used to assess the degree to which a task takes up *central limited capacity*. To the extent that doing one task degrades another, this loss of efficiency may be used to measure the workload imposed by the first task (1.3.4).

metacognition. Knowing one's own mental processes. One kind of metacognition involves *self-monitoring*, the conscious comparison of one's performance with some set of criteria (9.3; see *self-concept*). Metacognitive self-monitoring may be degraded in *absorbed states* like *hypnosis*, which may dominate central limited capacity to the exclusion of the conscious components of self-monitoring (7.7). The operational definition of *consciousness* is unavoidably metacognitive at the present time (1.2).

metacognitive access. The ability to retrieve one's own conscious contents. There are clear cases of conscious experiences that are difficult to retrieve, such as the Sperling phenomenon (1.1.2). But metacognitive access is indispensable to the commonly used operational definition of consciousness. See also *metacognition*, *source attribution*, *source amnesia*.

minimal contrasts, method of. See *contrastive analysis*.

minimum integration time of conscious experience. The time during which different inputs are integrated into a single conscious experience (2.4). Blumenthal (1977) provides numerous sources of evidence suggesting a minimum integration time of 50–250 milliseconds, centering at about 100 milliseconds.

Mind's Eye. The domain of visual imagery, which has many resemblances to visual perception. (2.6.2)

Momentary Access Hypothesis (2.4.3, 5.3.2). The notion that processors competing for access to the global workspace may be able to gain momentary, nonconscious access to send brief global messages in order to recruit more supportive systems. See also *Threshold Paradox*, *Waiting Room Hypothesis*.

Momentary Intentions. Kahneman's (1973) term, equivalent to short-term *goal contexts* in *Global Workspace theory*.

necessary conditions for conscious contents. *Global Workspace theory* suggests that consciousness involves mental *representations* that are *globally distributed*, *internally consistent*, and *informative*. In addition, consciousness may require interaction with a self-system, and has a *perceptual bias* (11.4).

nonqualitative conscious events (1.2.5, 6.5.2, 7.6.3, 7.6.4). Immediately accessible concepts, beliefs, intentions, and expectations that are reported as conscious but that do not have clear perceptual qualities like color, taste, texture, and clear figure–ground boundaries in space and time. (See also *qualitative conscious experiences*).

nonspecific interference. Simultaneous events tend to interfere with each other if they are conscious and voluntary, even if they involve apparently quite different systems: Visual imagery will interfere with action control, mental arithmetic with tactile reaction time. Nonspecific interference declines when the competing tasks become automatic with practice (1.3.4).

objectification. Conscious contents tend to be objectlike; even abstract consciously accessible concepts tend to be reified and treated as objects (1.5.3, 4.1.4, 5.3.4). But the same events after *habituation* are not objectlike, and can be said to have become *contextualized*. When contextual representations are disrupted, and become objectlike again, one can speak of decontextualization.

objectlike nature of conscious contents. See *objectification*.

operational definition of consciousness. See *consciousness*.

Options Context. A particular kind of *goal context* that allows two or more potential conscious contents to be compared, so that one can be selected voluntarily (8.2). An Options Context is comparable to a menu or directory on a computer. See *voluntary attention*, *Decision-making Function*.

organization versus flexibility. The nervous system encounters a trade-off between responding in an organized way to predictable input (which is fast and efficient), and dealing with novel situations in a flexible way (which is slow and adaptive). The *global workspace* architecture works to optimize this trade-off (2.7.2, 10.01).

Orienting Response (OR). The bodily reaction to novel stimuli, first detailed by Pavlov. The OR includes orienting of receptors, desynchronization in the EEG, pupillary dilation, autonomic changes in heart rate, skin conductivity, and dilation or constriction of blood vessels. Recently the P300 component of the evoked cortical potential has been added to this list.

parallel processing (1.4.4, 2.1). In principle, different specialized processors can act simultaneously with respect to each other (in parallel), except insofar as they must use the limited-capacity *global workspace*. See also *seriality*.

perceptual bias of conscious experience (2.4.1). The fact that qualitative experiences in perception, imagery, bodily feeling, etc., are perceptual or quasi-perceptual in nature. Even conscious experiences associated with abstract thought, such as prototypes and metaphors, tend to be quasi-perceptual (7.2.2). It is possible that abstract conceptual events and voluntary controls, which we speak of in terms of *conscious access* rather than *conscious experience*, may operate through momentary, quasi-perceptual images (7.6.3). See also *necessary conditions for consciousness*, *qualitative*, *nonqualitative*, and *ideomotor theory*.

perceptual context. Unconscious systems that shape conscious perceptual experiences, e.g., the vestibular system. See *context*.

peripheral consciousness. The quasi-conscious "fringe" of conscious experience associated with the periphery of the visual field and other sensory domains, and with the temporal horizon of focal experiences that are just about to fade; more generally, any borderline conscious experience. Peripheral consciousness is usually contrasted with *focal consciousness* (1.1.2).

potential contexts (4.3.5). *Contexts* that may be available among the *specialized processors*, and that may be evoked in a variety of tasks. For example, since all actions require detailed temporal control, different actions may use a common preexisting context for this purpose. This is not just a specialized processor, since potential contexts, when they are evoked and begin to dominate the *global workspace*, can act to influence conscious contents without themselves being conscious. See also *context* (4.3.1, 6.4, 7.3.2), *Options Context*.

preattentive processing. A term used by Neisser (1967) and others to describe rapid hypothesis-testing of perceptual input before it becomes conscious (1.24, 2.3.2).

presupposed knowledge. The context that shapes conceptual thought, but is not readily consciously accessible when it does so (4.2.2).

priming (4.1). Conscious events increase the chances of related events becoming conscious; they decrease reaction time to related material, and can sway the interpretation of related ambiguous or noisy stimuli. See also *Context-setting Function* of consciousness.

Prioritizing Function of consciousness. *Attentional* systems, which control access to consciousness, are very sensitive to *significance*. A stimulus such as one's own name is apparently made significant by conscious association with high-level goals. Voluntary attentional control can be used to rehearse this association until it becomes routine and automatic, thus guaranteeing automatic access priority to the stimulus (8.0.2, 8.2, 10.5).

problem solving, spontaneous. Incomplete or unresolved conscious events tend to trigger unconscious problem solving, even if these events are not reported to involve deliberate attempts to solve the problem (6.2).

process. A set of transformations of a *representation* (1.4).

processor. A relatively unitary, organized collection of *processes* that work together in the service of a particular function (1.4).

psychopathology. A state of mind characterized by severe and disabling loss of *voluntary* control over mental images, inner speech, actions, emotions, or percepts. *Global Workspace theory* suggests an approach to this loss of control through the *ideomotor theory*. See also *involuntary*.

psychodynamics. In the general sense used here, the study of goal conflicts, especially when one of the goals is not consciously or *metacognitively* accessible (7.8.1, 9.4). A complete psychodynamics presupposes an adequate theory of volition and metacognition. See also *ideomotor theory*.

publicity metaphor. The main metaphor of *Global Workspace theory*, motivated by the need of specialized processors to communicate globally with others to solve novel problems cooperatively (2.2, 2.5).

qualitative conscious experiences. Experiences like mental imagery, perception, and emotional feelings, which have perceptual qualities like color, texture, and taste. Contrasted with nonqualitative concepts, beliefs, etc. that are often described as conscious. See also *perceptual bias* of conscious events and *conscious access versus conscious experience* (1.5.4, 2.4.1, 7.6.3).

qualitative context. The unconscious shaping *context* of *qualitative conscious experiences.* An example in visual perception is the automatic assumption that light comes from above, a contextual expectation that shapes the experience of visual depth without being conscious (4.1).

range of conscious contents (2.1.2). The enormous range of possible conscious contents contrasts sharply with the apparently limited range of any single *specialized unconscious processor.* Presumably a syntax processor cannot handle motor control or visual input, but consciousness is at times involved in all of these functions.

receiving systems. Specialized processors that receive a certain global message. Chapter 5 develops the argument that receiving systems must feed back their interest in the global message, thus joining the coalition of systems supporting global access for the message (5.3).

recursive organization of processors and contexts. Specialized processors may be made up of other processors, and can join a coalition of others (see *cooperative processing*) to create a superordinate processor, depending upon the current function that needs to be served. Thus a tightly organized set of processors is also a processor (1.4.5). Similarly, a consistent set of contexts constitute a context (4.3.1). The properties of recursively defined entities have been worked out in recent mathematics and computer science. (4.3.1).

Recruiting Function of consciousness. The ability of global messages to gain the cooperation of many receiving systems in pursuing their ends (7.3, 10.4).

Redundancy Effects. After an event has been learned, repetition causes it to fade from consciousness (1.2.3). This phenomenon is found at all levels of conscious involvement: in all sensory systems, in motor control, and in conceptual representation as well (5.1.3). Redundancy Effects provide the strongest argument for the notion that *informativeness* is a *necessary condition for conscious contents.* Apparent exceptions can be handled in the same framework (5.4). See also *habituation of awareness.*

relational capacity of consciousness. The nervous system's impressive ability to relate two conscious events to each other in a novel way (2.1, 5.1.1, 6.2). See also *context-sensitivity.*

reminders. In order to maintain the unconscious *contexts* that constrain conscious experience, we may need conscious reminders. This is especially true for contexts that encounter competition, that are effortful to maintain, or that involve choice-points with some degree of uncertainty (4.4.2). The need for reminders may explain the role of social symbols like membership tokens, rituals, periodic festivals, and rites of passage, some of which seem clearly designed to create an intense conscious experience to strengthen largely unconscious contexts.

representation. A theoretical object that bears an abstract resemblance (isomorphism) to something outside of itself, and which is primarily shaped by this resemblance (1.4.1). Operationally, a representation is often inferred if an organism can accurately identify matches and mismatches between current and past experience. Representation is currently an axiomatic notion in cognitive science; it shares many features with the idea of an *adaptive system.*

repression. Motivated exclusion from consciousness, especially when the process of exclusion is itself unconscious. Some patterns emerging from *Global Workspace theory* resemble Freudian "repression proper," sometimes called after-expulsion. This is the case when fleeting conscious *goal-images* trigger actions before they can be properly *edited* by processors that would normally compete against them. *Metacognitive access* to these events may be minimal, since the goal-images are fleeting. They may nevertheless trigger *involuntary* actions such as slips (7.5.1, 7.8, 8.5). See also *psychodynamics.*

residual subjectivity. The argument made by some (e.g., Natsoulas, 1978b) that we can never fully explain the subjective component of conscious experience (1.2.7).

Reticular Formation (RF). A densely interconnected core of the brain stem that extends to part of the thalamus. Ablation of the Reticular Formation generally leads to coma, and stimulation leads to waking and improved perceptual discrimination. Parts of the RF are described here as belonging to the *Extended Reticular-Thalamic Activating System (ERTAS),* a convenient label for the set of neural structures involved in waking consciousness, sleep, and coma (3.1).

selective attention. A situation in which two or more separate, densely coherent streams of input exist. In this case the subject can only be conscious of one stream at a time. *GW theory* treats selective attention as a contextual *fixedness* effect (4.1.2). See also *filter theory, Filter Paradox, acontextual.*

self. See *self-system.*

self-alien experiences (also called ego-dystonic). A large set of normal and pathological experiences in which people report some form of loss of self (9.1). These may vary from severe depersonalization, to making a disavowed statement or an involuntary slip of the tongue. Self-alien experiences can be contrasted to closely comparable *self-attributed* experiences, leading to a contrastive analysis that places empirical constraints on the notion of self (see *self-system*).

self-attributed experiences (also called ego-syntonic). Most experiences are attributed to a "self" as observer, and control of voluntary action is attributed to a "self" as agent (9.1). However, there are important cases where experience and control is perceived to be *self-alien.* A *contrastive analysis* comparing similar self-alien and self-attributed experiences strongly suggests that the concept of self (see *self-system*) is scientifically necessary, and provides empirical constraints on this notion.

self-concept. An abstract representation of oneself, presumably accumulated over many experiences of *self-monitoring*. The self-concept may involve *objectification* or an external perspective on oneself, and is presumably used primarily to control and evaluate performance (9.3). Compared to the great complexity and subtlety of the *self-system*, the self-concept as it is most often expressed by people seems simplistic and tendentious.

self-consciousness. See *Self-monitoring Function*.

Self-maintenance Function of consciousness. (9.4.4, 10.9). Conscious experiences serve to update the *self-system*, and at times may severely violate its deeper contextual levels. Attentional control (see *attention*) of consciousness then becomes a major tool for maintaining stability of the self-system.

Self-monitoring Function of consciousness. (10.8) One major role of consciousness is to track aspects of one's own performance, to see if they match one's *self-concept*.

self-monitoring, conscious. tracking one's own performance by comparison to some set of criteria (8.01, 9.02, 9.31). See also *self-concept, self-system, objectification*.

self-system (self). A *contrastive analysis* between self-attributed and self-alien experiences suggests that the self can be treated as the overarching *context* of experience (9.2). In Jamesian terms, this involves the "self as I," rather than the "self as me" – the latter involves a conception of self as an object of experience. See also *self-concept, necessary conditions for conscious contents*.

semantic memory. Memory for abstract, nonqualitative, and probably unconscious rules and facts. See also *episodic memory*.

semantic satiation (5.1.3). The apparent loss of meaning when a word or phrase is repeated perhaps a dozen times. See also *Redundancy Effects, Verbal Transformation Effect*.

seriality. Events that are conscious or under voluntary control are constrained to occur one after the other, in the limited-capacity bottle-neck of the nervous system. (2.1.5). The same events after *habituation* or *automaticity* may occur in parallel.

Short Term Memory (STM). Immediate, rehearsable memory, which seems limited in size to 7 plus or minus 2 separate elements, if rehearsal is permitted (1.3.4). The elements or "chunks" of STM are typically letters, numbers, words, or judgment categories, which are themselves quite complex. This suggests that the chunks of STM involve knowledge from *Long Term Memory* (LTM), so that STM and LTM cannot really be segregated.

significance. Not all stimuli are equal: Some are far more important than others, biologically, socially, or personally. *Global Workspace theory* treats significant stimuli as information that serves to reduce uncertainty in a *Goal Context* (5.2.3, 9.2.2).

snowballing access to consciousness (3.21). There are both empirical and theoretical reasons to think that *access* of some input to consciousness is not immediate, but may involve a circular flow of feedback between potential conscious contents and numerous *receiving processors*, which are needed to support *global access* for the potential content (5.3).

source amnesia. In *metacognition*, the failure to attribute conscious experiences to the correct event in the past. Posthypnotic amnesia for a hypnotic suggestion is a good example. Source amnesia occurs in normal states of mind when people forget their reasons for having made even a major decision, in part because decisions often change the context of experience, so that the predecision context is lost. This makes recall difficult. Source amnesia is indeed the norm, not the exception, in human development, and is a major source of error in *self-monitoring*. See also *source attribution* (7.6.4, 8.5.2, 9.5.2).

source attribution. In *metacognition*, the problem of assigning events to their proper sources (7.6.4, 8.5.2), especially in attributing the sources of one's own actions to previous conscious goals or conditions. One's own goals may be difficult to make conscious; if the *goal-images* that control novel aspects of one's actions are quite *fleeting*, they may be difficult to retrieve, leading to systematic misinterpretation of one's own goals and motives. There is much evidence for such failures of source attribution, even when the lost information is not particularly painful or embarassing. See also *source amnesia, Self-monitoring Function.*

specialists. See *specialized processors.*

specialized processors (specialist) (1.4.5). One of the three main constructs of *Global Workspace theory.* Specialized processors can be viewed as relatively autonomous, unconscious systems that are limited to one particular function such as vertical line detection in the visual system, noun phrase identification in syntax, or motor control of some particular muscle group. Specialists are said to be *recursively organized,* so that they consist of other specialists and can make up even larger specialized processors. That implies that they can be decomposed and reorganized into another specialist if some other function becomes dominant (1.4.5, 4.4.3, 9.4.4). When a set of specialists provides routine control of GW contents without becoming conscious, it begins to act as a *context* (4.3.1).

specialized unconscious processors. See *specialized processors.*

stimulation versus information (5.1, 5.2). There is much evidence that the nervous system is not sensitive to physical stimulation as such, but is instead highly sensitive to *information.* For example, the absence of an expected stimulus can be highly informative. See also *Redundancy Effects.*

stopped retinal images (5.1.3). The eye is usually protected from excessively repetitive input by eye movements, especially the rapid automatic tremor called physiological nystagmus. Nystagmus can be defeated by moving a visual stimulus in synchrony with the eye; under these circumstances, visual input fades quickly and tends to be transformed. See also *Redundancy Effects*.

stream of consciousness. The apparently unsystematic "flights" and "perches" of conscious ideation, in the words of William James. Explained in *Global Workspace theory* as an ongoing interplay between *conscious contents* and unconscious contextual systems, especially *goal contexts* in the process of solving spontaneously posed problems. See also *problem solving* (6.4).

subgoals. To solve a problem or execute an action, conscious goal images can recruit specialized processors such as muscular effectors. However, in most cases the goal cannot be achieved directly and subgoals must be recruited. These can be viewed as *goal contexts* that can become part of the *Dominant Goal Hierarchy* (6.4, 7.2.2). Novel components of these subgoal contexts may be broadcast to recruit new resources to work toward achieving the subgoal (7.2.2).

subliminal perception. See *zero-point problem*.

suggestibility (7.7.2, 8.2.4, 9.3.1). Highly hypnotizable subjects apparently treat the hypnotist's suggestions the way others treat their own *inner speech*, with a great deal of trust and credibility. The *ideomotor theory* suggests that hypnosis is an *absorbed state* in which there is minimal competition against *goal-images*. In addition, *metacognitive* self-monitoring seems to be limited, perhaps because it requires *central limited capacity* that is not available during absorption. Under these circumstances, unusual conscious contents are presumably not *edited*. Credulity and trust may simply result from an absence of this *Editing Function*.

surprise. The fact that surprise seems to erase *conscious contents* has been pointed out by several writers. In *Global Workspace theory*, surprise can be treated as a momentary erasure of the global workspace by competing contents and contexts. The *Dominant Context Hierarchy* is disrupted as a result, and works to limit damage to its lowest levels (4.4.3). Surprising disruption of high-level Goal Contexts can be stressful and lead to pathology (9.4.4).

thalamus (3.1.2). Traditionally viewed as a "way station" to the cortex, parts of the thalamus resemble a *global workspace* with mutually competitive input from a great number of sources and widely broadcast output through the *Diffuse Thalamic Projection System*. The outer shell of the thalamus (the nucleus reticularis thalami) seems especially well-suited to this task. See also *Extended Reticular-Thalamic Activating System*.

Theater Hypothesis of conscious experience. The view, found in both modern and traditional thought, that conscious experience is much like the stage of a theater in which the audience cannot see the management of the actors on stage. A modern equivalent is the "searchlight" metaphor; an ancient version is the *common sense* of Aristotle and Eastern thought (1.3.1).

theoretical choice-points (e.g., Preface, 1.5.4, 1.5.5, 2.6.1, 2.6.3, 2.6.4, 6.5.2, 7.6.4). *Global Workspace theory* generates a number of strong hypotheses, which are stated as clearly as possible to make them empirically testable. Where we cannot support plausible hypotheses we at least state the alternatives as clearly as possible, without giving even a tentative answer.

Threshold Paradox. When does something become conscious? If any global message is conscious, then global broadcasting cannot be used to recruit the coalition of processors that is needed to gain global access for it in the first place. But if a global message is not necessarily conscious, what then are the necessary conditions for consciousness? There are two theoretical alternatives, labeled the *Waiting Room Hypothesis* and the *Momentary Access Hypothesis* (2.4.3). The former suggests a hierarchy of increasingly global workspaces, which a potentially conscious content must follow to become truly global and conscious, accumulating supporting coalitions along the way. The latter suggests that all systems may have brief global access in order to recruit supportive coalitions, but that such brief global messages are not experienced or recalled as conscious. See also *fleeting conscious events, snowballing access.*

Tip-of-the-Iceberg Hypothesis of conscious experience. The view that consciousness is only the visible tip of a very large and invisible iceberg of unconscious processes (1.3.1).

tip-of-the-tongue (TOT) phenomenon. The process of searching for a known but elusive word, which clearly involves a set of criteria for the missing word, though these criteria are not *qualitatively* conscious. The criteria are said to constitute an *intention* or *goal context*. Further, people often report a fleeting but unretrievable mental image of the missing word, indicating that there may indeed be *fleeting conscious events* (6.1, 7.6.4, 8.5.2).

top-down contextual influences (4.1). The conscious experience of sensory input is always shaped by unconscious contexts.

triadic pattern. Many types of spontaneous *problem solving* show a conscious stage of problem assignment, followed by unconscious incubation of routine problem components, and culminating in conscious display of the solution (6.2, 6.4).

unconscious, operational and theoretical definitions of. When people are asked under optimal conditions to retrieve some information that is clearly represented in the nervous system, and they cannot do so, we are willing to infer the existence of unconscious events (1.2.1, 1.4.1). Examples are the regularities of syntax and the properties of highly automatic tasks. *Global Workspace theory* suggests that we are unconscious of anything that does not meet all the *necessary conditions* for conscious experience. This implies that there are several ways for something to be unconscious (11.4).

unconscious choice-points in the flow of processing. Complex processes involve many choice-points between alternative representations. For example, in speech perception the linguistic system must often choose between two alternative meanings of a word. Which choice is made can often be influenced by previous conscious experiences (4.1.3, 7.7.2). See also *priming.*

underdetermined choice-points in the control of action (7.7.2). Choice-points in the control of action may be quite uncertain; consciousness may be necessary to help resolve the uncertainty. Underdetermined choice-points are likely to become conscious because they involve points of high uncertainty. See also *ambiguity*.

universal editing (7.3.2). A conscious goal-image is thought to be broadcast globally to all specialized processors in the system. This suggests that perhaps all processors can also compete against conscious goal-images and thus interrupt execution of a planned action. See also *editing*.

updating. Many unconscious *specialized processors* may simultaneously track conscious experiences in order to update each of their special domains in the light of current circumstances (5.1.4).

variable composition of specialized processors. See *recursive organization*.

Verbal Transformation Effect. The perceived phonetic shift in words that are presented to a passive listener over and over again for an approximate duration of 30–60 seconds. Treated here as a shift in *perceptual context* (5.4.1).

vigilance. The task of monitoring conscious signals, often quite repetitive ones. A difficult task that declines in accuracy in a matter of minutes. See also *Redundancy Effects*.

violations of context. *Context* can be treated as a set of expectations about conscious experiences, and of course expectations can be violated. Often violation of contextual expectations causes them to become consciously accessible (4.1.4). In the *Context Hierarchy*, deeper violations propagate more widely and demand more extensive *adaptation* to rebuild a functioning Context Hierarchy (4.4.3, 9.4.4). See also *surprise, failure-driven retrieval of contextual knowledge*.

voluntary action (7.00). Action that is consistent with one's *Dominant Goal Hierarchy*, and hence is generally *self-attributed*. Because the conscious components of the *Goal Hierarchy* are globally broadcast, so that many systems have access to them; hence these conscious components are tacitly *edited* by multiple criteria. Developmentally one can argue that at some point in one's history, all informative and significant components of a voluntary action must have been edited. See also *ideomotor theory*.

voluntary attention. *Attention* is defined here as the control of access to consciousness. Since *Global Workspace theory* claims that voluntary control involves conscious (though often fleeting) *goal-images*, it follows that voluntary attention is conscious control of access to consciousness (8.1.2). This can be accomplished through the use of an *Options Context*, comparable to a menu or directory on a computer, which allows different conscious options to become readily available, so that one can choose voluntarily between them.

voluntary control. See *voluntary action*.

Waiting Room Hypothesis (2.4.3, 5.3.2). The notion that a hierarchy of workspaces with increasingly widespread broadcasting ability may be required to allow processors attempting to gain GW access to compete before becoming conscious. See also *Threshold Paradox, Momentary Access Hypothesis*.

wakefulness. In *Global Workspace theory*, a state in which the global workspace is operating. Parts of the *ERTAS* system are known to be involved in the maintenance of wakefulness and sleep (3.1). See also *cortical arousal.*

working memory. See *Short-Term Memory.*

zero-point problem. It is remarkably difficult to find indisputable evidence about events near the threshold of conscious experience, such as subliminal perception, learning without awareness, and the problem of "blind sight." Because zero-point evidence is so controversial, the present approach is based initially on *contrastive analysis* of clear cases that are not disputed. Much can be accomplished in this way. Only after establishing a reasonable framework based on agreed-upon evidence do we suggest hypotheses about the zero point (Preface, 1.1.2, 7.6.4). See also *fleeting conscious events.*

References

Abelson, R. P., Aronson, E., McGuire, W. J., Newcomb, T. M., Rosenberg, M. J., & Tannenbaum, P. H., (1968). *Theories of cognitive consistency: A sourcebook*. Chicago: Rand McNally.

Abrams, K., & Bever, T. G. (1969). Syntactic structure modifies attention during speech perception. *Quarterly Journal of Experimental Psychology, 21*, 280–90.

Ach, N. (1905/1951). Determining tendencies: Awareness. Eng. trans. in David Rapaport (Ed. and Trans.), *Organization and pathology of thought* (pp. 15–38). New York: Columbia University Press.

Allport, F. H. (1954). *Theories of perception and the concept of structure*. New York: Wiley.

Ames, A., Jr. (1953). *Reconsideration of the origin and nature of perception*. New Brunswick, NJ: Rutgers University Press.

Amster, H. (1964). Semantic satiation and generation: learning? adaptation? *Psychological Bulletin 62*, 273–86.

Anderson, J. R. (1983). *The architecture of cognition*. Cambridge, MA: Harvard University Press.

Arbib, M. A. (1980). Perceptual structures and distributed motor control. In V. B. Brooks (Ed.), *Handbook of physiology* (Vol. III). Bethesda, MD: American Physiological Association.

Atkinson, R. C., & Juola, J. F. (1974). Search and decision processes in recognition memory. In R. C. Atkinson, D. H. Krantz, & P. Suppes (Eds.), *Contemporary developments in mathematical psychology*. San Francisco: Freeman.

Atkinson, R. C., & Shiffrin, R. M. (1968). Human memory: A proposed system and its control processes. In K. W. Spence & J. T. Spence (Eds.), *Advances in the psychology of learning and motivation: Research and theory* (Vol. 2). New York: Academic Press.

Azrin, N. H., Nunn, R. G., & Frantz, S. E. (1980). Habit reversal vs. negative practice treatment of nervous tics. *Behavior Therapy, 11*, 169–78.

Baars, B. J. (1980). The competing plans hypothesis: An heuristic viewpoint on the causes of errors in speech. In H. W. Dechert & M. Raupach (Eds.), *Temporal variables in speech. Studies in honour of Frieda Goldman-Eisler* (pp. 39–50). The Hague: Mouton.

   (1983). Conscious contents provide the nervous system with coherent, global information. In R. Davidson, G. Schwartz, & D. Shapiro (Eds.), *Consciousness and self-regulation* (Vol. III, pp. 45–76). New York: Plenum.

393

(1985). Can involuntary slips reveal a state of mind? With an addendum on the conscious control of speech. In M. Toglia & T. M. Shlechter (Eds.), *New directions in cognitive science* (pp. 242–61). Norwood, NJ: Ablex.

(1986a). *The cognitive revolution in psychology.* New York: Guilford Press.

(1986b). What is a theory of consciousness a theory of? The search for criterial constraints on theory. *Imagination, Cognition, and Personality, 1,* 3–24.

(1987). Biological implications of a Global Workspace theory of consciousness: Evidence, theory, and some phylogenetic speculations. In G. Greenberg & E. Tobach (Eds.), *Cognition, language, and consciousness: Integrative levels* (pp. 209–36). Hillsdale, NJ: Erlbaum.

(in press a). What is conscious in the control of action? A modern ideomotor theory of voluntary control. In D. Gorfein & R. R. Hoffman (Eds.)., *Learning and memory: The Ebbinghaus Centennial Symposium,* Hillsdale, NJ: Erlbaum.

(in press b). Momentary forgetting as an erasure of a conscious global workspace due to competition between incompatible contexts. In M. J. Horowitz (Ed.), *Psychodynamics and cognition* (pp. 263–87). Chicago: University of Chicago Press.

(in press c). *The experimental psychology of error: A window on the mind.* New York: Plenum, Cognition and Language Series.

Baars, B. J., Motley, M. T., & MacKay, D. G. (1975). Output editing for lexical status in artificially elicited slips of the tongue. *Journal of Verbal Learning and Verbal Behavior, 14,* 382–91.

Baars, B. J., & Mattson, M. E. (1981). Consciousness and intention: A framework and some evidence. *Cognition and Brain Theory, 4*(3), 247–63.

Baars, B. J., Cohen, J., & Bower, G. H. (1986). Non-accessed emotional meanings of ambiguous phrases are chosen more often by subjects hypnotically induced to experience matching emotions. Unpublished paper, Stanford University.

Baddeley, A. D. (1976). *The psychology of memory.* New York: Basic Books.

Bakan, D. (1980). On the effect of mind on matter. In R. W. Rieber (Ed.), *Body and mind: Past, present, and future* (pp. 117–29). New York: Academic Press.

Banks, W. P., & White, H. (1982). Single ordering as a processing limitation. *Journal of Verbal Learning and Verbal Behavior, 21,* 39–54.

Barber, T. X., Spanos, N. P., & Chaves, J. F. (1974). *Hypnosis, imagination, and human potentialities.* New York: Pergamon.

Barsalou, L. W. (1983). Ad hoc categories. *Memory and Cognition, 11,* 211–27.

Basmajian, J. V. (1979). *Biofeedback: Principles and practice for the clinician.* Baltimore, MD: Williams & Williams.

Beck, A. T. (1976). *Cognitive therapy and the emotional disorders.* New York: New American Library.

Berlyne, D. (1960). *Conflict, arousal, and curiosity.* New York, McGraw-Hill.

Bernstein, L. (1976). *The unanswered question: Six talks at Harvard.* Cambridge, MA: Harvard University Press.

Bjork, R. (1972). Theoretical implications of directed forgetting. In A. W. Melton & E. Martin (Eds.), *Coding processes in human memory.* Washington, DC: Winston.

Blumenthal, A. L. (1977). *The process of cognition.* Englewood Cliffs, NJ: Prentice-Hall.

(1979). Wilhelm Wundt, the founding father we never knew. *Contemporary Psychology, 24*(7), 547–50.

Boring, E. G. (1953). A history of introspectionism. *Psychological Bulletin, 50,* 169–89.

Bower, G. H. (1986). Temporary emotional states act like multiple personalities. Paper delivered at the Conference on Multiple Personality and Dissociative Disorders, Chicago, Sept.

Bower, G. H., & Cohen, P. R. (1982). Emotional influences in memory and thinking: Data and theory. In M. S. Clark & S. T. Fiske (Eds.), *Affect and cognition* (pp. 291–331). Hillsdale, NJ: Erlbaum.

Bransford, J. D. (1979). *Human cognition.* Belmont, CA: Wadsworth.

Bransford, J. D., & Franks, J. J. (1976). Toward a framework for understanding learning. In G. H. Bower (Ed.), *The psychology of learning and motivation: Advances in research and theory* (Vol. 10). New York: Academic Press.

Broadbent, D. E. (1958). *Perception and communication.* New York: Pergamon Press.

Brodal, A. (1956). *The reticular formation of the brain stem: Anatomical aspects and functional correlates.* Springfield, IL: Thomas.

Brown, R., & MacNeill, D. (1966). The "tip of the tongue" phenomenon. *Journal of Verbal Learning and Verbal Behavior, 5,* 325–37.

Bruner, J. S. (1957). On perceptual readiness. *Psychological Review, 64,* 123–52.

Bruner, J. S., & Potter, M. (1964). Interference in visual recognition. *Science, 144,* 424–25.

Buchwald, J. S. (1974). Operant conditioning of brain activity – an overview. In M. M. Chase (Ed.), *Operant conditioning of brain activity.* Los Angeles: University of California Press.

Carterette, E. C., & Friedman, M. (1973–78). *Handbook of perception* (Vols. 1–20). New York: Academic Press.

Case, R. (1985). *Intellectual development: Birth to adulthood.* New York: Academic Press.

Chafe, W. L. (1970). New and old information. In W. L. Chafe, *Meaning and the structure of language* pp. 210–33. Chicago: University of Chicago Press.

(1980) The development of consciousness in the production of narrative. In W. L. Chafe (Ed.), *The pear stories: cognitive, cultural, and linguistic aspects of narrative production* (pp. 9–50). New York: Ablex.

Chase, M. H. (Ed.). (1974). *Operant control of brain activity.* Los Angeles: University of California Press.

Cheesman, J., & Merikle, P. M. (1984). Priming with and without awareness. *Perception and Psychophysics, 36*(4), 387–95.

Chen, J.-Y., & Baars, B. J. (in press). General and specific factors in "Transformational Errors." An experimental study. In B. J. Baars (Ed.), *The psychology of human error: A window on the mind.* New York: Plenum.

Cherry, E. C. (1953). Some experiments on the recognition of speech, with one and with two ears. *Journal of the Acoustical Society of America, 25,* 975–9.

Chomsky, N. (1957). *Syntactic structures.* The Hague: Mouton.

(1965). *Aspects of the theory of syntax.* Cambridge, MA: MIT Press.

Clark, H. H., & Carlson, T. B. (1981). Context for comprehension. In J. Long &

A. Baddeley (Eds.), *Attention and performance IX* (pp. 313–30). Hillsdale, NJ: Erlbaum.

Clark, H. H., & Clark, E. V. (1977). *Psychology of language: An introduction to psycholinguistics*. New York: Harcourt, Brace, Jovanovich.

Clark, H. H., & Haviland, S. E. (1977). Comprehension and the given–new contract. In R. O. Freedle (Ed.), *Discourse production and comprehension*. Norwood, NJ: Ablex.

Cohen, J., Galin, D., & Baars, B. J. (1986). A connectionist blackboard model. Unpublished paper, Langley Porter Psychiatric Institute, UCSF.

Cooper, L. A., & Shepard, R. N. (1973). Chronometric studies of the rotation of mental images. In W. G. Chase (Ed.), *Visual information processing*. New York: Academic Press.

Crick, F. (1984). Function of the Thalamic Reticular Complex: The searchlight hypothesis. *Proceedings of the National Academy of Sciences USA, 81*, 4586–93, July.

Czikzsentmihalyi, M., & Czikzsentmihalyi, I. S. (1988). *Optimal experience: Psychological studies of flow in consciousness*. New York: Cambridge University Press.

Danziger, K. (1979). The positivist repudiation of Wundt. *Journal of the History of the Behavioral Sciences, 15*, 205–26.

Dawson, M. E., and Furedy, J. J. (1976). The role of awareness in human differential autonomic classical conditioning: The necessary-gate hypothesis. *Psychophysiology, 13*(1), 50–3.

Dell, G. S. (1986). A spreading-activation theory of retrieval in sentence production. *Psychological Review, 93*, 283–91.

Dennett, D. C. (1978). Toward a cognitive theory of consciousness. In D. C. Dennett (Ed.), *Brainstorms* (pp. 149–73). New York: Bradford Books.

Dixon, N. F. (1971). *Subliminal perception: The nature of a controversy*. London: McGraw-Hill.

(1981). *Preconscious processes*. New York: Wiley.

Donchin, E., McCarthy, G., Kutas, M., & Ritter, W. (1978). Event-related potentials in the study of consciousness. In R. Davidson, G. Schwartz, & D. Shapiro (Eds.), *Consciousness and self-regulation* (Vol. III, pp. 81–121). New York: Plenum.

Drowatsky, J. N. (1975). *Motor learning: Principles and practice*. Minneapolis, MN: Burgess.

Duncker, K. (1945). On problem solving. *Psychological Monographs*, No. 270.

Dunlap, K. (1942). The technique of negative practice. *American Journal of Psychology, 55*(2), 270–3.

Edelman, G. M., & Mountcastle, V. B. (1978). *The mindful brain: Cortical organization and the group-selective theory of higher brain function*. Cambridge, MA: MIT Press.

Eimas, P. D., & Corbitt, J. (1973). Selective adaptation of speech feature detectors. *Cognitive Psychology, 171*, 303–6.

Einstein, A. (1949). "Autobiographical Notes." In P. A. Schilpp (Ed.), *Albert Einstein – Philosopher–Scientist* (Vol. I). New York: Harper & Row.

Ekman, P. (1984). Expression and the nature of emotion. In K. R. Scherer & P. Ekman (Eds.), *Approaches to emotion*. Hillsdale, NJ: Erlbaum.

Eliot, T. S. (1950). *The cocktail party*. New York: Harcourt, Brace.

Ellenberger, H. F. (1970). *The discovery of the unconscious: The history and evolution of dynamic psychiatry.* New York: Basic Books.

Ellis, A. (1962). *Reason and emotion in psychotherapy.* New York: Lyle Stuart.

Encyclopedia Britannica. (1957). "Common sense," London: Encyclopedia Britannica.

Erdelyi, M. H. (1974). A new look at the New Look: Perceptual defense and vigilance. *Psychological Review, 81,* 1–25.

——— (1985). *Psychoanalysis: Freud's cognitive psychology.* San Francisco: Freeman.

Ericsson, K. A., & Simon, H. A. (1980). Verbal reports as data. *Psychological Review, 87,* 215–51.

——— (1984). *Protocol analysis: Verbal reports as data.* Cambridge, MA: MIT Press.

Eriksen, C. W. (1960). Discrimination and learning without awareness: A methodological survey and evaluation. *Psychological Review, 67,* 279–300.

Eriksen, T. D., & Mattson, M. E. (1981). From words to meaning: A semantic illusion. *Journal of Verbal Learning and Verbal Behavior, 20,* 540–51.

Erman, L. D., & Lesser, V. R. (1975). A multi-level organization for problem solving using many, diverse, cooperating sources of knowledge. *Proceedings of the 4th Annual Joint Computer Conference* (pp. 483–90). Georgia, USSR.

Esposito, N. J., & Pelton, L. H. (1971). Review of the measurement of semantic satiation. *Psychological Review, 75*(5):330–46.

Festinger, L. (1957). *A theory of cognitive dissonance.* Evanston, IL: Row, Peterson.

Finke, R. (1980). Levels of equivalence in imagery and perception. *Psychological Review, 87*(2), 113–32.

Flavel, J. H., & Wellman, H. M. (1977). Metamemory. In R. V. Kail, Jr., and J. W. Hagen (Eds.), *Perspectives on the development of memory and cognition.* Hillsdale, NJ: Erlbaum.

Fodor, J. A. (1979). *The language of thought.* Cambridge, MA: Harvard University Press.

——— (1983). *The modularity of mind: An essay on faculty psychology.* Cambridge, MA: MIT Press.

Foss, D. J. (1982). A discourse on semantic priming. *Cognitive Psychology, 14:* 590–607.

Fraisse, P. (1963). *The psychology of time.* New York: Harper & Row.

Franks, J. J., & Bransford, J. D. (1971). Abstraction of visual images. *Journal of Experimental Psychology, 90*(1), 65–74.

Freud, Anna. (1938). *The ego and the mechanisms of defense.* English Translation, New York: International Universities Press, 1946.

Freud, S. (1895/1966). Project for a scientific psychology. In J. Strachey (Ed.), *The standard edition of the complete psychological works of Sigmund Freud* (Vol. 1, pp. 45–61). London: Hogarth Press.

——— (1901/1938). *The psychopathology of everyday life.* In A. A. Brill (Ed.), *The basic writings of Sigmund Freud* (pp. 35–178). New York: Modern Library.

——— (1923/1962). The ego and the id. In J. Strachey (Ed.), *The standard edition of the complete psychological works of Sigmund Freud* (A. Strachey, Trans.). London: Hogarth Press.

——— (1926/1936). *Inhibition, symptoms and anxiety.* In J. Strachey (Ed.), *The standard edition of the complete psychological works of Sigmund Freud* (A. Strachey, Trans.). Hogarth Press.

Fromkin, V. A. (Ed.). (1973). *Speech errors as linguistic evidence*. The Hague: Mouton.

——— (1980). *Errors in linguistic performance: Slips of the tongue, ear, pen, and hand*. New York: Academic Press.

Galin, D. (1977). Lateral Specialization and Psychiatric Issues: Speculations on Development and the Evolution of Consciousness. *Annals of the New York Academy of Sciences, 299*, 397–411.

Garcia, J., and Koelling, R. A. (1966). Relation of cue to consequence in avoidance learning. *Psychonomic Science, 4*, 123–4.

Garner, W. R. (1974). *The processing of information and structure*. Potomac, MD: Erlbaum.

Gastaut, H. (1958). The role of the reticular system in establishing conditioned reactions. In H. M. Jasper, L. D. Proctor, R. S. Knighton, W. C. Noshay, & R. T. Costello (Eds.), *The reticular formation of the brain*. Boston: Little, Brown.

Gazzaniga, M. (1985). *The social brain: Discovering the networks of the mind*. New York: Basic.

Gelb, A. (1932). Die Erscheinungen des simultanen Kontrastes und der Eindrück der Feldbeleuchtung. *Zeitschrift für Psychologie, 127*, 42–59.

Gelfand, I. M., Gurfinkel, V. S., Fomin, S. V., & Tsetlin, M. L. (1971). *Models of the structural–functional organization of certain biological systems*, trans. C. R. Beard. Cambridge, MA: MIT Press.

Geschwind, N. (1979). Specializations of the human brain. *Scientific American, 241*(3), 180–201.

Ghiselin, B. (1952). *The creative process*. New York: Mentor.

Gilchrist, A. (1977). Perceived lightness depends upon perceived spatial arrangement. *Science, 195*, 185–7.

Gluck, M. A., & Bower, G. H. (1986). From conditioning to category learning: An adaptive network model. *Proceedings of the 8th Cognitive Science Conference*.

Gluck, M. A., & Corter, J. E. (1985). Information and category utility. In *Proceedings of the 7th Cognitive Science Conference* (pp. 283–7).

Goffman, E. (1974). *Frame analysis: An essay on the organization of experience*. New York: Harper & Row.

Goldman-Eisler, F. (1972). Pauses, Clauses, and Sentences. *Language and Speech, 15*, 103–13.

Goldstein, L. M., & Lackner, J. R. (1975). Alterations of the phonetic coding of speech sounds during repetition. *Cognition, 2*, 279–97.

Goleman, D. (1985). *Vital lies, simple truths: The psychology of self-deception*. New York: Simon & Schuster.

Gould, S. J. (1982). *The Panda's thumb: More reflections on natural history*. New York: Norton.

Greene, P. H. (1972). Problems of organization of motor systems, *Journal of Theoretical Biology*, 303–38.

Greenwald, A. G., & Liu, T. J. (1985). Limited unconscious processing of meaning. Twenty-seventh annual meeting of the Psychonomics Society, Boston, MA.

Gregory, R. L. (1966). *Eye and brain: The psychology of seeing*. New York: McGraw-Hill.

Grossberg, S. (1982). *Studies of mind and brain*. Boston: Reidel.

Hadamard, J. (1945). *The psychology of invention in the mathematical field.* Princeton, NJ: Princeton University Press.

Harlow, H. F. (1953). Motivation as a factor in the acquisition of new responses. In *Current theory and research in motivation: A symposium.* Lincoln: University of Nebraska Press.

Hartmann, H. (1958). *Ego psychology and the problem of adaptation.* New York: International Universities Press.

Hasher, L., & Zacks, R. T. (1979). Automatic and effortful processes in memory. *Journal of Experimental Psychology: General, 108*(3), 356–88.

Haviland, S. E., & Clark, H. H. (1974). What's new? Acquiring new information as a process in comprehension. *Journal of Verbal Learning and Verbal Behavior, 13*, 512–21.

Hayes-Roth, B. (1985). A blackboard model of control. *Artificial Intelligence, 16*, 1–84.

Helmholtz, H. von (1962). *Treatise on physiological optics* (3 vols.). J. P. C. Southall, trans. New York: Dover.

Helson, H. (1947). Adaptation-level as a frame of reference for prediction of psychophysical data. *American Journal of Psychology, 60*, 1–29.

(1964). *Adaptation-level theory: An experimental and systematic approach to behavior.* New York: Harper.

Herbart, J. F., (1824/1961). Psychology as a science, newly founded upon experience, metaphysics and mathematics. Reprinted in T. Shipley (Ed.), *Classics in psychology* (pp. 22–50). New York: Philosophical Library.

Hick, W. E. (1952). On the rate of gain of information. *Quarterly Journal of Experimental Psychology, 4*, 11–26.

Hilgard, E. R. (1977). *Divided consciousness: Multiple controls in human thought and action.* New York: Wiley.

Hilgard, J. R. (1979). *Personality and hypnosis: A study of imaginative involvement.* Chicago: University of Chicago Press.

Hinton, G. E., & Anderson, J. A. (1981). *Parallel models of associative memory.* Hillsdale, N.J.: Erlbaum.

Hobson, J. B., & Brazier, M. A. (Eds.) (1982). *The reticular formation revisited.* New York: Raven.

Hochberg, J. (1964). *Perception.* Englewood Cliffs, NJ: Prentice-Hall.

Holender, D. (1986). Semantic activation without conscious identification in dichotic listening, parafoveal vision, and visual masking: A survey and appraisal. *Behavioral and Brain Sciences, 9*, 1–66.

Holmes, D., (1967) Closure in a gapped circle figure. *American Journal of Psychology, 80*, 614–18.

(1968). The search for closure in a visually perceived pattern. *Psychological Bulletin, 70*, 296–312.

(1972). Repression and interference: A further investigation. *Journal of Personality and Social Psychology, 22*, 163–70.

(1974). Investigations of repression: Differential recall of material experimentally or naturally associated with ego threat. *Psychological Bulletin, 81*(10), 632–53.

(1978). Projection as a defense mechanism. *Psychological Bulletin, 85*, 677–88.

Horowitz, M. (1975a). Intrusive and repetitive thoughts after experimental stress. *Archives of General Psychiatry, 32*, 1457–63.

(1975b). Disasters and psychological responses to stress. *Psychiatric Annals, 15*(3), 161–7.

(1976). *Stress response syndromes*. New York: Aronson.

Horowitz, M. J., & Zilberg, N. (1983). Regressive alterations of the self-concept. *American Journal of Psychiatry*, *140*, 284–9.

Hubel, D. H., & Wiesel, T. N. (1959). Receptive fields of single neurons in the cat's striate cortex. *Journal of Physiology*, *148*, 574–91.

Hull, C. L. (1937). Mind, mechanism, and adaptive behavior. *Psychological Review*, *44*, 1–32.

Hutchins, E. (1980). *Culture and inference: A Trobriand case study*. Cambridge, MA: Harvard University Press.

Huxley, A. (1970). *The perennial philosophy*. New York: Harper & Row.

Hyman, R. (1953). Stimulus information as a determinant of reaction time. *Journal of Experimental Psychology*, *45*, 188–96.

Izard, C. E. (1980). The emergence of emotions and the development of consciousness in infancy. In J. M. Davidson & R. J. Davidson (Eds.), *The psychobiology of consciousness* (pp. 192–216). New York: Plenum.

Jackendoff, R. (1987). *Consciousness and the computational mind*. Cambridge, MA: MIT Press / A Bradford Book.

Jacoby, L. L., and Witherspoon, D. (1982). Remembering without awareness. *Canadian Journal of Psychology*, *36*(2), 300–24.

James, W. (1890/1983). *The principles of psychology* (New York: Holt, 1890). Reprint, Cambridge, MA: Harvard University Press.

(1904/1977). Does "Consciousness" exist? in J. J. McDermott (Ed.), *The writings of William James*. (pp. 169–83) Chicago: University of Chicago Press.

John, E. R. (1976). A model of consciousness. In G. Schwartz & D. Shapiro (Eds.), *Consciousness and self-regulation* (pp. 6–50). New York: Plenum.

John-Steiner, V. (1985). *Notebooks of the mind*. Albuquerque: University of New Mexico Press.

Kahneman, D. (1973). *Attention and effort*. Englewood Cliffs, NJ: Prentice-Hall.

Kaidel, W. D., Kaidel, U. D., & Weigand, N. E. (1960). In W. A. Rosenblith (Ed.), *Sensory Communication* (pp. 319–38). Cambridge, MA: MIT Press.

Keele, S. W. (1973). *Attention and human performance*. Pacific Palisades, CA: Goodyear.

Kihlstrom, J. F., & Cantor, N. (1984). Mental representations of the self. In L. Berkowitz (Ed.), *Advances in experimental social psychology* (Vol. 17). New York: Academic Press.

Kimble, G. A. & Perlmuter, D. (1970). The problem of volition. *Psychological Review*, *77*(5), 361–84.

Kinsbourne, M., & Hicks, R. E. (1978). Mapping cerebral functional space: Competition and collaboration in human performance. In M. Kinsbourne (Ed.), *Asymmetrical function of the brain* (pp. 267–73). London: Cambridge University Press.

Klapp, S. T., Greim, D. M., & Marshburn, E. A. (1981). Buffer storage of programmed articulation and articulatory loop: Two names for the same mechanism or two distinct components of short-term memory? In J. Long & A. Baddeley (Eds.), *Attention and Performance IX*, (pp. 459–72). Hillsdale, NJ: Erlbaum.

Klinger, E. (1971). *The structure and function of fantasy*. New York: Wiley.

Klos, D. S., & Singer, J. L (1981). Determinants of the adolescent's ongoing thought following simulated parental confrontation. *Journal of Personality and Social Psychology*, *41*, 168–77.

Köhler, W. (1929). *Gestalt psychology*. New York: Liveright.

Kohut, H. (1971). *The analysis of the self*. New York: International Universities Press.

Kosslyn, S. M. (1980). *Image and mind*. Cambridge, MA: Harvard University Press.

Kosslyn, S. M., & Schwartz, S. P. (1981). Empirical constraints on theories of visual mental imagery. In J. Long & A. D. Baddeley (Eds.), *Attention and performance* (Vol. IX, pp. 241–260). Hillsdale, NJ: Erlbaum.

Kuhn, T. S. (1962/1970). *The structure of scientific revolutions*. Chicago: University of Chicago Press.

LaBerge, D. (1974). Acquisition of automatic processing in perceptual and associative learning. In P. M. A. Rabbitt & S. Dornic (Eds.), *Attention and Performance V*. London: Academic Press.

  (1980). Unitization and automaticity in perception. In J. H. Flowers (Ed.), *1980 Nebraska Symposium on Motivation* (pp. 53–71). Lincoln: University of Nebraska Press.

Lackner, J. R., & Goldstein, L. M. (1975). The psychological representation of speech sounds. *Quarterly Journal of Experimental Psychology, 27,* 173–85.

Lakoff, G., & Johnson, M. (1980). *Metaphors we live by*. Chicago: University of Chicago Press.

Langer, E. J., & Imber, L. G. (1979). When practice makes imperfect: Debilitating effects of overlearning. *Journal of Personality and Social Psychology, 37*(11), 2014–24.

Levicki, P. (1986). *Nonconscious social information processing*. New York: Academic Press.

Levine, F. M., Ramirez, R. R., & Sandeen-Lee, E. E. (1982). Contingent negative practice as a treatment of stuttering. Unpublished manuscript, Department of Psychology, State University of New York, Stony Brook.

Levine, M. (1971). Hypothesis theory and nonlearning despite ideal S–R-reinforcement contingencies. *Psychological Review, 78*(2), 130–40.

Levine, M., & Fingerman, P. (1974). Non-Learning: The completeness of the blindness. *Journal of Experimental Psychology, 102*(4), 720–1.

Liberman, A. M., Cooper, F., Shankweiler, D., & Studdert-Kennedy, M. (1967). Perception of the speech code. *Psychological Review, 74,* 431–59.

Libet, B. (1978). Neuronal vs. subjective timing for a conscious sensory experience. In P. A. Buser & A. Rougeul-Buser (Eds.), *Cerebral correlates of conscious experience* (pp. 69–82). INSERM Symposium No. 6. Amsterdam: North Holland/Elsevier.

  (1981). Timing of cerebral processes relative to concomitant conscious experiences in man. In G. Adam, I. Meszaros, & E. I. Banyai (Eds.), *Advances in Physiological Science* (Vol. 17, pp. 313–17). Elmsford, NY: Pergamon.

  (1985). Unconscious cerebral initiative and the role of conscious will in voluntary action. *Behavioral and Brain Sciences, 8,* 529–66.

Lindsay, P. H., & Norman, D. A. (1977). *Human information processing: An introduction to psychology* (2nd edition). New York: Academic Press.

Lindsley, D. B. (1958). The reticular system and perceptual discrimination. In H. H. Jasper, L. D. Proctor, R. S. Knighton, W. C. Noshay, & R. T. Costello (Eds.), *The reticular formation of the brain* (pp. 513–34). Boston: Little, Brown.

Livingston, R. B. (1958). Central control of afferent activity. In H. H. Jasper,

L. D. Proctor, R. S. Knighton, W. C. Noshay, & R. T. Costello (Eds.), *The reticular formation of the brain* (pp. 177–86). Boston: Little, Brown.

Loftus, E. F., & Palmer, J. C. (1974). Reconstruction of automobile destruction: An example of the interaction between language and memory. *Journal of Verbal Learning and Verbal Behavior, 13*, 585–89.

Luborsky, L. (1977). Measuring a pervasive psychic structure in psychotherapy: The core conflictual relationship theme. In N. Freedman & S. Grand (Eds.), *Communicative structures and psychic structures* (pp. 367–95). New York: Plenum.

(in press). Recurrent momentary forgetting: Its core content and symptom-context, 1–39. In M. Horowitz (Ed.), *Psychodynamics and cognition.* Chicago: University of Chicago Press.

Luborsky, L., & Mintz, J. (1974). What sets off momentary forgetting during a psychoanalysis? Investigations of symptom-onset conditions. *Psychoanalysis and Contemporary Science, 3*, 233–68.

Luchins, A. S. (1942). Mechanization in problem-solving. The effect of *Einstellung. Psychological Monographs, 54*(6), No. 248.

Luria, A. R. (1980). *Higher cortical functions in man* (2nd. edition). New York: Basic. (Russian language edition, 1969)

McClelland, J. L., & Rumelhart, D. E. (1981). An interactive activation model of context effects in letter perception: Part 1. An account of basic findings. *Psychological Review, 88*, 375–407.

McClelland, J. L., Rumelhart, D. E., & the PDP Research Group, (1986). *Parallel distributed processing. Vol. 2: Psychological and biological models.* Cambridge, MA: Bradford Books/MIT Press.

MacKay, D. G. (1973). Aspects of a theory of comprehension, memory and attention. *Quarterly Journal of Experimental Psychology, 25*, 22–40.

(1981a). Speech errors: Retrospect and prospect. In V. A. Fromkin (Ed.), *Errors in linguistic performance* (pp. 319–32). New York: Academic Press.

(1981b). The problem of rehearsal or mental practice. *Journal of Motor Behavior, 13*, 274–85.

Mackworth, J. F. (1970). *Vigilance and attention: A signal detection approach.* Harmondsworth, UK: Penguin Books.

McNeill, D. (1966). Developmental psycholinguistics. In F. Smith and G. A. Miller (Eds.), *The genesis of language: A psycholinguistic approach.* Cambridge, MA: MIT Press.

Magoun, H. W. (1962). *The waking brain* (2nd edition). Springfiled, IL: Thomas.

Malcolm, N. (1967). Wittgenstein. In P. Edwards (Ed.), *The Encyclopedia of Philosophy* (Vol. 8). New York: Macmillan/Free Press.

Mandler, G. (1967). Organization in memory. In K. W. Spence & J. T. Spence (Eds.), *The psychology of learning and motivation: Advances in research and theory.* New York: Academic Press.

(1983). Consciousness: Its function and construction. Presidential address to the General Psychology Division of the American Psychological Association.

Mandler, G., & Shebo, B. J. (1982). Subitizing: an analysis of its component processes. *Journal of Experimental Psychology: General, 111*, 11–22.

Mandler, G. A. (1975a). *Mind and emotion.* New York: Wiley.

(1975b). Consciousness: Respectable, useful, and *probably* necessary. In R.

Solso (Ed.), *Information processing and cognition: The Loyola Symposium.* Hillsdale, NJ: Erlbaum.

(1984). *Mind and body: Psychology of emotion and stress.* New York: Norton.

Marcel, J. (1983a). Conscious and unconscious perceptions: An approach to the relations between phenomenal experience and perceptual processes. *Cognitive Psychology, 15,* 238–300.

Marcel, A. J. (1983b). Conscious and unconscious perception: Experiments on visual masking and word recognition. *Cognitive Psychology, 15,* 197–237.

Marks, L. E. (1978). *The unity of the senses: Interrelations among the modalities.* New York: Academic Press.

Markus, H., & Sentis, K. (1982). The self in social information processing. In J. Suls (Ed.), *Psychological perspectives on the self* (Vol. I, pp. 41–70). Hillsdale, NJ: Erlbaum.

Marr, D. (1982). *Vision.* San Francisco: Freeman.

Marslen-Wilson, W. D., & Welsh, A. (1978). Processing interactions and lexical access during word recognition in continuous speech. *Cognitive Psychology, 10,* 29–63.

Maslow, A. (1970). *Motivation and personality* (2nd. ed.). New York: Harper & Row.

Mednick, S. A. (1962). The associative basis of the creative process. *Psychological Review, 69,* 220–32.

Meichenbaum, D. H., & Bowers, K. S. (1984). *The unconscious reconsidered.* New York: Wiley.

Meichenbaum, D. H., & Goodman, J. (1971). Training impulsive children to talk to themselves: A means of developing self-control. *Journal of Abnormal Psychology, 77*(2), 115–26.

Merleau-Ponty, M. (1964). *The primacy of perception* (J. M. Edie, Ed. and Trans.). Evanston: University of Illinois Press.

Miller, G. A. (1953). What is information measurement? *American Psychologist, 8,* 3–11.

(1955). The perception of short bursts of noise. *Journal of the Acoustical Society of America, 20,* 164–70.

(1956). The magical number seven, plus or minus two: Some limits on our capacity for processing information. *Psychological Review, 63,* 81–97.

(1986). Interview with George A. Miller. In B. J. Baars (Ed.), *The cognitive revolution in psychology.* New York: Guilford Press.

Miller, G. A., Galanter, E. H., & Pribram, K. (1960). *Plans and the structure of behavior.* New York: Holt.

Miller, G. A., & Johnson-Laird, P. N. (1976). *Language and perception.* Cambridge, MA: Harvard University Press.

Milne, R. W. (1982). Predicting garden-path sentences. *Cognitive Science, 6,* 349–74.

Milner, B. (1959). The memory defect in bilateral hippocampal lesions. *Psychiatric Res. Reports, 11,* 43–52.

Minsky, M. A. (1975). A framework for representing knowledge. In M. Winston (Ed.), *The psychology of computer vision* (pp. 211–277). Boston: MIT Press.

(1986). *A society model of the mind.* New York: Simon & Schuster.

Miyake, N., & Norman, D. A. (1978). To ask a question, one must know enough to know what is not known. Center for Human Information Processing, UCSD.

Moore, S. (1960). *The Stanislawsky Method: The professional training of actors.* New York: Viking.

Moray, N. (1959). Attention in dichotic listening: Affective cues and the influence of instructions. *Quarterly Journal of Experimental Psychology, 11,* 56–60.

—— (1969). *Attention: Selective processes in vision and hearing.* London: Hutchinson.

Morokoff, P. (1981). *Female sexual arousal as a function of individual differences and exposure to erotic stimuli.* Unpublished doctoral dissertation, Dept. of Psychology, State University of New York, Stony Brook.

Moruzzi, G., & Magoun, H. W. (1949). Brain stem reticular formation and activation of the EEG. *EEG and Clinical Neurophysiology, 1,* 455–73.

Motley, M. T., Baars, B. J., & Camden, C. T. (1983). Syntactic criteria in pre-articulatory editing: Evidence from laboratory-induced slips of the tongue. *Journal of Psycholinguistic Research, 10*(5), 503–22.

Motley, M. T., Camden, C. T., and Baars, B. J. (1979). Personality and situational influences upon verbal slips. *Human Communication Research, 5*(3), 195–202.

—— (1983a). Polysemantic lexical access: Evidence from laboratory-induced double-entendres. *Communication Monographs, 50,* 193–205.

—— (1983b). Experimental verbal studies: A review and an editing model of language encoding. *Communication Monographs, 50,* 79–101.

Mountcastle, V. B. (1978). An organizing principle for cerebral function: The unit module and the distributed system. In G. M. Edelman & V. B. Mountcastle (Eds.), *The mindful brain.* Cambridge, MA: MIT Press.

Murphy, G. L., & Medin, D. L. (1985). The role of theories in conceptual coherence. *Psychological Review, 92,* 289–316.

Murray, D. J. (1983). *A history of Western psychology.* Englewood Cliffs, NJ: Prentice-Hall.

Nagel, T. (1974). What is it like to be a bat? In N. Block (Ed.), *Readings in philosophy of science* (pp. 159–70). Cambridge, MA: Harvard University Press.

Naranjo, C., & Ornstein, R. E. (1971). *On the psychology of meditation.* New York: Viking.

Natsoulas, T. (1978a). Consciousness. *American Psychologist, 33,* 906–14.

—— (1978b). Residual subjectivity. *American Psychologist, 33,* 269–83.

—— (1982a). Conscious perception and the paradox of "blind-sight." In G. Underwood (Ed.), *Aspects of consciousness* (pp. 79–110). London: Academic Press.

—— (1982b). Dimensions of perceptual awareness. *Behaviorism, 10*(1), 85–112.

Navon, D., & Gopher, D. (1979). On the economy of the human-processing system. *Psychological Review, 86*(3), 214–55.

Neisser, U. (1967). *Cognitive psychology.* New York: Appleton-Century-Crofts.

Newell, A., & Simon, H. A. (1972). *Human problem solving.* Englewood Cliffs, NJ: Prentice-Hall.

Nisbett, R. E., & Wilson, T. D. (1977). Telling more than we can know: Verbal reports on mental processes. *Psychological Review, 84,* 231–59.

Norman, D. A. (1968). Toward a theory of memory and attention. *Psychological Review, 75,* 522–36.

—— (1976). *Memory and attention.* New York: Wiley.

Norman, D. A., & Shallice, T. (1980). Attention and action: Willed and automatic control of behavior. Unpublished paper, Center for Human Information Processing, UCSD, La Jolla, CA.

Olds, J., & Hirano, T. (1969). Conditioned responses of hippocampal and other neurons. *EEG and Clinical Neurophysiology*, *26*, 159–66.

Olson, D. R. (1970). Language and thought: Aspects of a cognitive theory of semantics. *Psychological Review*, *77*, 257–73.

Ornstein, R. E. (1969). *On the experience of time*. London: Penguin.

Oswald, I. (1960). Falling asleep open-eyed during intense rhythmic stimulation. *British Medical Journal*, *112*, 1450–55.

Paivio, A. (1971). *Imagery and verbal processes*. New York: Holt, Rinehart & Winston.

Pani, J. R. (1982). A functionalist approach to mental imagery. Paper presented at the twenty-third annual meeting of the Psychonomic Society, Baltimore, MD.

Penfield, W., & Roberts, L. (1959). *Speech and brain mechanisms*. Princeton, NJ: Princeton University Press.

Peterson, L. R., & Peterson, M. J. (1959). Short-term retention of individual verbal items. *Journal of Experimental Psychology*, *58*, 193–98.

Piaget, J. (1952). *The origins of intelligence in children*. (M. Cook, Trans.). New York: International Universities Press.

(1973). The cognitive unconscious and the dynamic unconscious. *Journal of the American Psychoanalytical Association*, *21*(2), 249–61.

Pichert, J. W., & Anderson, R. C. (1977). Taking different perspectives on a story. *Journal of Educational Psychology*, *69*, 309–15.

Pope, K. S., & Singer, J. L. (1978). *The stream of consciousness: Scientific investigations into the flow of human experience*. New York: Plenum.

Posner, M. I. (1978). *Chronometric explorations of mind: The third Paul M. Fitts lectures*. Hillsdale, NJ: Erlbaum.

(1982). Cumulative development of attentional theory. *American Psychologist*, *37*(2), 168–79.

Posner, M. I., & Cohen, Y. (1982). Components of visual orienting. In K. Bouma & D. Bouwhuis (Eds.), *Attention & performance* (Vol. X). Hillsdale, NJ: Erlbaum.

Prince, M. (1957). *The dissociation of personality: A biographical study in abnormal psychology*. New York: Meridian.

Pritchard, R. M., Heron, W., & Hebb, D. O. (1960). Visual perception approached by the method of stabilized images. *Canadian Journal of Psychology*, *14*, 67–77.

Rapaport, D. (Ed.). (1951). *Organization and pathology of thought*. New York: Columbia University Press.

Razran, G. (1961). The observable unconscious and inferrable conscious in current Soviet psychophysiology: Interoceptive conditioning, semantic conditioning, and the orienting reflex. *Psychological Review*, *68*, 81–147.

Reason, J. (1983). Absent-mindedness and cognitive control. In J. Harris & P. Morris (Eds.), *Everyday memory, actions and absentmindedness* (pp. 113–32). New York: Academic Press.

(1984). Lapses of attention in everyday life. In R. Parasuraman & D. R. Davies (Eds.), *Varieties of attention* (pp. 515–49). New York: Academic Press.

Reason, J., & Mycielska, K. (1982). The Freudian slip revisited. In J. Reason & K. Mycielska (Eds.), *Absent-minded? The psychology of mental lapses and everyday errors*. Englewood Cliffs, NJ: Prentice-Hall.

Reber, A. S., & Allen, R. (1978). Analogic and abstraction strategies in synthetic grammar learning: A functionalist interpretation. *Cognition, 6,* 189–221.

Reddy, R., & Newell, A. (1974). Knowledge and its representations in a speech understanding system. In L. W. Gregg (Ed.), *Knowledge and cognition.* Potomac, MD: Erlbaum.

Rescorla, R. A., & Wagner, A. R. (1972). A theory of Pavlovian conditioning: Variations in effectiveness of reinforcement and non-reinforcement. In A. H. Black and W. F. Prokasy (Eds.), *Classical conditioning II.* New York: Appleton-Century-Crofts.

Rock, I. (1983). *The logic of perception.* Cambridge, MA: Bradfort/MIT Press.

Rokeach, M. (1960). *The open and closed mind.* New York: Basic.

Rosch, E. H. (1975). Cognitive representations of semantic categories. *Journal of Experimental Psychology: General. 104,* 192–233.

Rosch, E. H., Mervis, C. B., Gray, W., Johnson, D., & Boyes-Bream, P. (1975). Basic objects in natural categories. *Cognitive Psychology, 7,* 573–605.

Rozin, P. (1976). The evolution of intelligence and access to the cognitive unconscious. In J. Sprague & A. Epstein (Eds.), *Progress in Psychobiology and Physiological Psychology.* New York: Academic Press.

Rumelhart, D. E., & McClelland, J. L. (1982). An interactive activation model of context effects in letter perception: Part 2. The contextual enhancement effect and some tests and extensions of the model, *Psychological Review, 189*(1), 60–94.

Rumelhart, D. E., & McClelland, J. E., & the PDP Research Group (1986). *Parallel distributed processing: Explorations in the microstructure of cognition, Vol. I: Foundations.* Cambridge, MA: Bradford/MIT Press.

Rumelhart, D., & Norman, D. A. (1975). The active structural network. In D. A. Norman & D. E. Rumelhart (Eds.), *Explorations in cognition* (pp. 35–64). San Francisco: Freeman.

Ryle, G. (1949). *The concept of mind.* London: Hutchinson.

Sagi, D., & Julesz, B. (1985). "Where" and "what" in vision. *Science, 7,* 1217–19.

Schachter, S., & Singer, J. E. (1962). Cognitive, social, and physiological determinants of emotional state. *Psychological Review, 69,* 379–99.

Scheibel, A. B. (1980). Anatomical and physiological substrates of arousal. In J. A. Hobson and M. A. Brazier (Eds.), *The reticular formation revisited* (pp. 55–66). New York: Raven.

Scheibel, M. C., & Scheibel, A. B. (1967). Anatomical basis of attentional mechanisms in vertebrate brains. In G. C. Quarton, T. Melnechuk, & F. O. Schmitt (Eds.), *The Neurosciences: A study program.* New York: Rockefeller University Press.

Schneider, W., & Shiffrin, R. M. (1977). Controlled and automatic human information processing: I. Detection, Search, and Attention. *Psychological Review, 84*(1), 1–57.

Shallice, T. (1972). Dual functions of consciousness. *Psychological Review, 79*(5), 383–93.

    (1978). The dominant action system: An information-processing approach to consciousness. In K. S. Pope & J. L. Singer (Eds.), *The stream of consciousness: Scientific investigation into the flow of experience.* New York: Plenum

Shannon, C. E., & Weaver, W. (1949). *The mathematical theory of communication.* Urbana: University of Illinois Press.

Shepard, R. N. (1967). Recognition memory for words, sentences, and pictures. *Journal of Verbal Learning and Verbal Behavior, 6*, 156–63.

Shevrin, H., & Dickman, J. (1980) The psychological unconscious: A necessary assumption for all psychological theory? *American Psychologist, 35*, 421–34.

Shiffrin, R. M., Dumais, S. T., & Schneider, W. (1981). Characteristics of automatism. In J. Long & A. Baddeley (Eds.), *Attention and performance IX* (pp. 223–38). Hillsdale, NJ: Erlbaum.

Shiffrin, R. M., & Schneider, W. (1977). Controlled and automatic human information processing: II. Perceptual learning, automatic attending, and a general theory. *Psychological Review, 84*, 127–90.

Simon, H. A. (1969). *The sciences of the artificial.* Cambridge, MA: MIT Press.

Singer, J. L. (1984). The private personality. *Personality & Social Psychology Bulletin, 10*(1), 1–29.

Skinner, B. F. (1974). *About behaviorism.* New York: Knopf.

Sokolov, E. N. (1963). *Perception and the conditioned reflex.* New York: MacMillan.

Spence, D. P., Scarborough, H. S., & Ginsberg, E. H. (1978). Lexical correlates of cervical cancer. *Social Science and Medicine, 12*, 141–45.

Sperling, G. (1960). The information available in brief visual presentations. *Psychological Monographs, 74*, No. 11.

Spiegel, D. (1984). Multiple personality as a post-traumatic stress disorder. *Psychiatric Clinics of North America, 7*(1), 101–08.

Spiegel, H., and Spiegel, D. (1978). *Trance and treatment: Clinical uses of hypnosis.* New York: Basic Books.

Spitzer, R. L. (Ed.), (1979) *Diagnostic and Statistical Manual of Mental Disorders (DSM III)*, Washington, DC: American Psychiatric Association.

Springer, S., and Deutsch, G. (1981). *Left brain, right brain.* San Francisco: Freeman.

Sternberg, S. (1966). High-speed scanning in human memory. *Science, 153*, 652–54.

Stevens, S. S. (1966). Operations or words? *Psychological Monographs: General and Applied, 80*, 33–38.

Straight, H. S. (1977). Consciousness as anti-habit. Unpublished paper, State University of New York at Binghamton.

Sutherland, N. S. (1967). Comments on the session. In W. Wathen-Dunn (Ed.), *Models for the perception of speech and visual form* (pp. 239–43). Cambridge, MA: MIT Press.

Sutton, R. S., & Barto, A. G. (1981). Toward a modern theory of adaptive networks: Expectation and prediction. *Psychological Review, 88*, 135–70.

Swinney, D. (1979). Lexical access during sentence comprehension. (Re)consideration of context effects. *Journal of Verbal Learning and Verbal Behavior, 18*, 645–60.

Szentagotai, J., & Arbib, M. A. (1975). Conceptual models of neural organization. *Neurosciences Research Bulletin, 12*, 307–510.

Szilard, L. (1964). On the decrease in entropy in thermodynamic systems by the intervention of intelligent beings (A. Rapaport and M. Knoller, Trans.). *Behavioral Science, 9*, 301–10. (Original German edition, 1929).

Tanenhaus, M. K., Carlson, G. N., & Seidenberg, M. S. (1985). Do listeners compute linguistic representations? In D. R. Dowty, L. Karttunen, & A. Zwicky (Eds.), *Natural language parsing: Psychological, computational, and theoretical perspectives* (pp. 359–408). London: Cambridge University Press.

Tellegen, A., & Atkinson, G. (1974). Openness to absorbing and self-altering experiences (''Absorption''), a trait related to hypnotic susceptibility. *Journal of Abnormal Psychology, 83,* 268–77.

Thatcher, R. W., & John, E. R. (1977). *Foundations of cognitive processes.* NJ: Erlbaum.

Thompson, R. F. (1967). *Foundations of physiological psychology.* New York: Harper & Row.

(1976). The search for the engram. *American Psychologist, 31,* 209–27.

Tighe, T. J., & Leaton, R. N. (1976). *Habituation: Perspectives from child development, animal behavior, and neurophysiology.* Hillsdale, NJ: Erlbaum.

Tomkins, S. S. (1962). *Affect, imagery, consciousness, Vol. 1: The positive affects.* New York: Springer Verlag.

Treisman, A. M. (1964). Selective attention in memory. *British Medical Bulletin, 20,* 12–16.

(1969). Strategies and models of selective attention. *Psychological Review, 76*(3), 282–99.

Treisman, A. M., & Gelade, G. (1980). A feature-integration theory of attention. *Cognitive Psychology, 12,* 97–136.

Treisman, A. M., & Schmidt, H. (1982). Illusory conjunction in the perception objects. *Cognitive Psychology, 14,* 167–41.

Tulving, E. (1972). Episodic and semantic memory. In E. Tulving & W. Donaldson (Eds.), *Organization of memory.* New York: Academic Press.

(1985). Memory and consciousness. *Canadian Psychology, 26*(1), 1–12.

Tversky, A., & Kahneman, A. (1973). Availability: A heuristic for judging frequency and probability. *Cognitive Psychology, 2,* 207–32.

Underwood, G. (1982). Attention and awareness in cognitive and motor skills. In G. Underwood (Ed.), *Aspects of consciousness* (Vol. 3, pp. 111–46). London: Academic Press.

Uznadze, D. N. (1966). *The psychology of set.* The International Sciences Series. New York: Consultants Bureau.

Valins, S. (1967). Cognitive effects of false heart-rate feedback. *Journal of Personality and Social Psychology, 4,* 400–8.

Wapner, M. A. (1986). Interview with Michael A. Wapner. In B. J. Baars (Ed.), *The cognitive revolution in psychology* (pp. 315–36). New York: Guilford Press.

Warm, J. (1984). *Sustained attention in performance.* New York: Wiley.

Warren, R. (1961). Illusory changes of distinct speech upon repetition – the Verbal Transformation Effect. *British Journal of Psychology, 52*(3), 249–56.

Warren, R. M. (1968). Verbal transformation effect and auditory perceptual mechanisms. *Psychology Bulletin, 70*(4), 261–70.

Watson, J. B. (1925). *Behaviorism.* New York: Harper Bros.

Weinberger, D. A., Schwartz, G. E., & Davidson, R. J. (1979). Low-anxious, high-anxious and repressive coping styles: Psychometric and behavioral and physiological responses to stress. *Journal of Abnormal Psychology, 88*(9), 369–80.

Weiner, B., (1986). *An attributional theory of motivation and emotion.* New York: Springer Verlag.

Weisskrantz, L. (1980). Varieties of residual experience. *Quarterly Journal of Experimental Psychology*, *32*, 365–86.

White, P. (1982). Beliefs about conscious experience. In G. Underwood (Ed.), *Aspects of consciousness* (Vol. 3, pp. 1–26). London: Academic Press.

Whyte, L. L. (1962). The unconscious before Freud. New York: Doubleday.

Wiener, N. (1961). *Cybernetics: On control and communication in the animal and the machine* (2nd ed.). Cambridge, MA: MIT Press.

Winograd, T. (1972). A program for understanding natural language. *Cognitive Psychology*, *3*, 1–191.

Winson, J. (1985). *Brain and Psyche: The biology of the unconscious*. New York: Doubleday.

Woodworth, R. S. (1915). A revision of imageless thought. *Psychological Review*, *22*, 1–27.

Woodworth, R. S., & Schlossberg, H. (1954). *Experimental Psychology*. New York: Holt, Rinehart, & Winston.

Wundt, W. (1912/1973). *An introduction to psychology*. London: G. Allen, Reprint, New York: Arno Press.

Yarbus, A. L. (1967). *Eye movements and vision*. New York: Plenum Press.

Name index

Subject index

Note: Most of the technical terms below are defined in the Glossary. Page numbers for Glossary entries are in italics; page numbers for figures are followed by "f"; for tables, by "t."

416